TOPICS ON CERVICAL CANCER WITH AN ADVOCACY FOR PREVENTION

Edited by **Rajamanickam Rajkumar**

Topics on Cervical Cancer with an Advocacy for Prevention
Edited by Rajamanickam Rajkumar

Published by InTech

Janeza Trdine 9, 51000 Rijeka, Croatia

Publishing Process Manager Masa Vidovic

Technical Editor Teodora Smiljanic

Cover Designer InTech Design Team

Additional hard copies can be obtained from orders@intechopen.com

Topics on Cervical Cancer with an Advocacy for Prevention,
Edited by Rajamanickam Rajkumar
p. cm.
ISBN 978-953-51-0183-3

For EU product safety concerns:
IN TECH d.o.o., Prolaz Marije Krucifikse Kozulić 3, 51000 Rijeka, Croatia,
info@intechopen.com or visit our website at intechopen.com.

Meet the editor

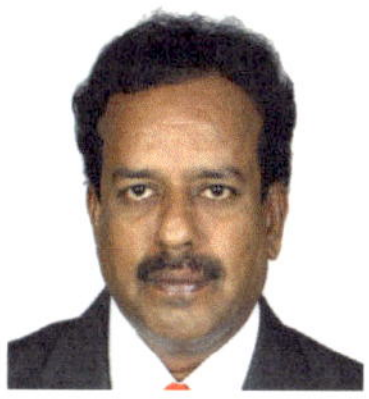

Dr Rajamanickam Rajkumar (BSC, MBBS, MD, PhD, Colposcopy (UK & Ireland), FUICC, Hon. Member SCCPS Singapore) was inspired to become a doctor at school age by Christine Matthews - an Irish Missionary who worked at the Christian Medical College, Vellore. He did his postgraduate in Community Medicine and worked at the Christian Fellowship Community Health Centre, Ambillikai, Tamil Nadu – under the mentorship of Padmabhushan Dr Jacob Cherian. Burdened by the large number of cervical cancer cases in this small rural hospital, Dr Rajkumar wrote to IARC/WHO for guidance to prevent and control cervical cancer. He initiated a rural population-based cancer registry with IARC in 1996, and following training in colposcopy and precancer management in UK and Ireland, he implemented a large scale screening program using the village workers in 2001. This IARC project was a great success. In 2011, in collaboration with the Society for Colposcopy and Cervical Pathology Singapore and The Ohio State University Medical Center, USA, Dr Rajkumar is forming the "Colposcopy and Cervical Pathology Society in South India – COLPI" for training doctors and nurses in cervical cancer prevention.

Contents

Preface

Cervical cancer is one of the leading cancers in women, especially among those living in the poor socioeconomic conditions in the developing world. Much research has been done into possible treatments and preventative measures to hep combat the disease, and while there is a wealth of information and statistical evidence in terms of incidence, survival and mortality rates the challenge is to communicate what this means to the average person on the street.

If we can ensure that cervical cancer can be screened for at an early stage, effective precancer treatment can be given and an evidence-based cure can be developed by meticulous follow up, then, we are justified. Women empowerment, education and screening/treatment of cervical cancer preceded by affordable, acceptable and accessible strategies, will play a critical role.

This book by InTech – Open Access Publisher is a commendable project. If the chapters could inspire a worldwide crusade to prevent cerrvical cancer, especially among the most underprivileged women in the developing countries, the mission is fulfilled.

Dr Rajamanickam Rajkumar
Professor, Community Medicine
Meenakshi Medical College Hospital & Research Institute,
Kanchipuram Tamil Nadu
India

1

Predictors of Cervical Cancer Screening: An Application of Health Belief Model

Sedigheh Sadat Tavafian
Tarbiat Modares University
Iran

1. Introduction

Worldwide, cervical carcinoma is one of the most common gynecologic malignant tumors and a leading cause of death from genital malignancies in women. Although, pap smear as a screening method has the potential to identify pre-cancerous lesions and could massively reduce the invasive disease in developed countries, developing countries could not significantly lower the rate of cervical cancer among general population through using this screening test. This chapter will review the factors influencing cervical cancer screening behavior. First, the state of pap smear up taking - as a method of screening - among women is described. Second, the structure of Health Belief Model and how the constructs of the model could predict health behavior of cervical cancer screening will be explained. Finally, the application of Health Belief Model intervention to improve the behavior of cervical cancer screening among women will be discussed.

2. Pap smear as a cervical cancer screening test

Cervical cancer is the second leading cause of death worldwide and the tenth leading cause of cancer-related deaths among women in the United States (Ben-Natan, & Adir, 2009). Despite, fully preventable, cervical cancer is a major health problem in developing countries (Sankaranarayanan et al., 2008 ; Tristen et al., 1996; Abdullahi, 2009; Akbari et al., 2010). Cervical cancer is also a common type of cancer among women, especially in women 20-39 years of age. In several developed countries, the incidence of invasive cervical cancer has declined, which is largely attributed to early detection efforts. However, several subpopulations remain under screened, Active young women, minority women with language difficulties, and women with specific cultural health beliefs are at risk for this disease (Harlan et al., 1996; Snider 1996). It has been argued that the majority of cervical cancer as well as the most related deaths occur in low and medium income countries (Akbari et al., 2010). The patients who have been early diagnosed had survival rate much more than who suffering from more advanced stage of the disease. Papanicolaou or Pap smear test is a powerful cervical cytology screening test that could detect cervical cancer in premalignant stage that could be fully curable (Gakidou et al., 2008). This method of cervical cancer screening detects abnormal precancerous cells before they advance to cancer. Routine cervical cancer screening - every one to three years - is recommended by American Society for Colposcopy and Cervical Pathology to be begun in women three years after becoming sexually active or no later than by age 21 and continue to age 65 depending on screening history . In developed countries, extensive screening program through pap smear test, has declined the incidence of cervical cancer. In contrast, in most developing countries, comprehensive cervical cancer screenings are rare. Low participation of cervical cancer screening and low follow up of screening were evidenced by studies done in low resource countries like Botswana (Ibekwe1 2010; McFarland, 2003). However, in spite of advances in screening and treatment of cervical cancer during the past several decades, this disease remain a major health problem for Hispanic women, as many women have never had a Papanicolaou smear, or were not tested regularly (Harlan et al., 1991; Matuk,1996, Salazar, 1996). It has been stated that current screening programs in developing countries or among minorities faced obstacles such as insufficient supplies, inadequate trained health care providers; limited available services and lake of patient follow up procedure. Additionally, lack of appropriate programs in these countries indicates that the population may be at relatively higher risk for cancer mortality and morbidity due to delayed diagnosis. Inappropriate allocation of funds and human resources could also be a barrier to an effective and organized screening program in developing countries. These deficiencies caused the majority of cervical cancer cases referred to health care providers with late stage disease (Were, 2011). There are many evidences from different countries to suggest that women of lower socio-economic status (SES) are less likely to participate in cancer screening than those who are more advantaged (Coughlin et al., 2006, Datta et al., 2006, Lofters et al., 2007, Ackerson 2010) . In addition, lack of enough knowledge regarding preventable cervical cancer and also socio-cultural barriers such as embarrassment for pelvic examination have been argued as leading factors of not using available screening services regularly (Sankaranarayanan, 2008). Fear of the result of the test is another socio cultural barrier among different countries. Studies with Hispanic women reported fear of cancer, embarrassment, and limited English ability as major perceived barriers. In Hispanic women, great fear of cancer was associated with extreme fatalism about the disease. Most believed that cancer cannot be cured, and a diagnosis is considered a death sentence. This fear leaded to the avoidance of the subject and discussion of cancer (Bakemeier et al., 1995, , Frank-Stromborg et al., 1998) As a result, educational programs were often avoided, contributing to lack of optimal knowledge of screening practices (Chavez , 1997, Mandelblatt , 1999). Embarrassment was a stronger predictor of screening than perceived susceptibility and perceived benefits of early detection in a study conducted by Richardson and colleagues (Richardson, 1987). A previous study examined the association between inadequate functional health literacy in Spanish among low-income Latinas and cervical cancer screening knowledge and behavior (Garbers & Chiasson, 2004). This study showed in compared to women with adequate and marginal health literacy, women with inadequate functional health literacy were significantly less likely to have ever had a Papanicolaou (Pap) test (odds ratio, 0.12; 95% confidence interval [CI], 0.04-0.37) or in the last three years (odds ratio, 0.35; 95% CI, 0.18-0.68) .This study verified even when controlling for other factors, women with inadequate health literacy were 16.7 times less likely to have ever had a Pap test. In 2006, American Cancer Society reported the American African women have a higher mortality rate due to cervical cancer when compared to all other groups of women. According to this report about 70 % of women diagnosed with cervical cancer had not received the Papanicolaou (Pap smear) test within the previous 5 years or had never obtained the screening test (American Cancer Society, 2006). One of the reasons for the deference in the mortality rate for American African women was that they tend to have less frequent screenings as compared to other racial groups of women. Subsequently, this group of women experienced discrepancies in mortality rates related to cervical cancer when compared to other groups It has been showed that individuals' beliefs about the causes and significance of a particular illness were interconnected with their healthcare seeking behaviors. Al-Neggar RA and co-workers concluded that despite adequate knowledge regarding risk factors of cervical cancer, some misconceptions and wrong beliefs among young women could be resulted in poor practice of pap smear test (Al- Neggar et al , 2010). One of theoretical models that could assess the beliefs of people regarding healthy behavior is Health Belief Model. In this section, the structure of Health Belief Model and its capability to predict the behaviors is explained. According to concepts of Health Belief Model, if individuals regard themselves as susceptible to a condition, believe that a course of action available to them would be beneficial in reducing either their susceptibility to or severity of the condition, and believe the anticipated benefit of taking action outweigh the barrier to action, they are more likely to take action so that their beliefs will reduce their risks.

3. Health belief model as a framework for predicting behaviors

The Health belief model was originally developed in the 1950s by a social psychologist in the U.S public Health Service to explain the widespread failure of people to participate in programs to prevent and detect disease. Later, the model was extended to study peoples' responses to symptoms and their behaviors in response to diagnosed illness, specially adherence to medical regimens (Glanz et al., 2008). This model aims to explain preventive health behaviors rather than behaviors in time of illness (Ben-Natan & Adir, 2009). Major health behaviors emphasized by the Health Belief Model focus on prevention exposure of diseases at their asymptomatic stage (Lee, 2000). The Health Belief Model contains several primary concepts that predict why people will take action to prevent, to screen for, or to control disease conditions. Thus, this model assumes that health behaviors are motivated by five elements of perceived susceptibility, perceived seriousness, perceived benefits and perceived barriers to behavior, cues to action and most recently factor of perceived self efficacy (Champion & Skinner, 2008).

3.1 Application of the Health Belief Model to cervical cancer screening behavior

The Health Belief Model has been used extensively to determine relationship between health beliefs and health behaviors as well as to inform interventions. In this section, the constructs of Health Belief Model is explained at the first and then the application of Health Belief Model constructs in the area of cervical cancer screening behavior is discussed.

3.1.1 Perceived susceptibility

The perceived susceptibility refers to beliefs about the likelihood of getting a disease or condition. Perceived risk of contracting a disease refers to individuals' subjective perception of their susceptibility to the disease. For example, women must believe there is a possibility of getting cervical cancer before they will be interested in uptaking Pap smear. The health belief model predicts that women will be more likely to adhere the cervical cancer screening recommendation if they feel that they are susceptible to cervical cancer (Glanz et al., 2008). Previous study has shown that individuals who believed they had risk factors for cervical cancer, were more likwely to take action to prevent an adverse outcome subsequent to getting the disease (Saslow et al., 2002). Perception of not being at risk for cervical cancer has been verified as a reason for not obtaining pap smear test in previous studies (Mutyaba et al, 2006; Basu et al, 2006, Winkler et al, 2008 , Ibekwe1, 2010). A common emerging belief to cervical cancer screening in Hispanic women is that it is unnecessary or not needed to prevent cervical cancer. Among this target group a substantial proportion of women perceived Papanicolaou smears as unnecessary diagnostic procedures, rather than preventive health measures. In a study (Stein & Fox , 1990) showed Hispanic women do not view preventive health, such as cancer prevention, as a priority; as a result, they have an increased risk for diseases because of their curative rather than preventive health practices. In this regard, Hispanic women do not perceive their own vulnerability to cervical cancer and do not see themselves at risk.

3.1.2 Perceived severity

The perceived severity of a disease refers to the severity of a health problem as assessed by the individual. This variable refers to feeling about the seriousness of contracting an illness or of leaving it untreated include evaluations of medical/ clinical consequences like death, disability and pain or social consequences such as effects of the conditions on work, family life and social relations. For example, if women think that cervical cancer is a sever disease and believe that getting cervical cancer would have serious medical, social and economical consequences for them, it is more likely to obtain cervical cancer screening test. Having personal knowledge regarding the importance of the Pap smear has been evidenced as an important factor to take action to prevent the adverse outcome of cervical cancer (Saslow et al., 2002). A survey on the severity of cervical cancer among adult females in Quebec, found that 57% of women were afraid of developing cervical cancer sometime in their life, and 93% thought cervical cancer has serious consequences. Cervical cancer related anxiety and perceived seriousness did not vary by age group or level of education (Sauvageau et al., 2007). Although most participants perceived cervical cancer as serious, the thought of believing that there was no treatment of cervical cancer, makes them uninterested to doing cervical cancer screening test (Ibekwe1, 2010) . However, Hoque and coworkers, compared two groups of ever screened and never screened for cervical cancer. In a cross sectional study. in this evaluation, it was observed that both groups equally believed that there is effective treatments for cervical cancer, and that cervical cancer makes a woman's life difficult. Both the screened and the never screened believed that cervical cancer is as serious as other cancers; that it causes infertility and that death from cervical cancer is not rare. This study showed no significant association between perceived severity and screening for cervical cancer that differs with the hypothesis of the Health belief model that predicts perceived seriousness of a disease necessitate people to engage in preventive actions. Further research should be done to explore the reasons why at risk women fail to participate in cervical cancer screening (Hoque, 2009).

3.1.3 Perceived benefits

Even if a person perceives personal susceptibility to a serious health condition (perceived treat) , whether this perception leads to behavior change will be influenced by the person 's belief regarding the perceived benefits of the various available actions for reducing the

Application	Definition	Concept
Define population(s)at risk, risk levels Personalize risk based on a person's characteristics or behavior	Belief about the Chances of experiencing a risk or getting a condition or disease	Perceived Susceptibility
Specify consequences of risks and conditions	Belief about how serious a condition and its sequel are	Perceived Severity
Define action to take; how where ,when; Clarify the positive effects to be expected	Beliefs in efficacy of the advised action to reduce risk or seriousness of impact	Perceived benefits
Identify and reduce perceived barriers through reassurance, correction of misinformation, incentives , assistance	Belief about the tangible and psychological costs of the advised action	Perceived barriers
Provide how-to information, promote awareness, Use appropriate reminder systems	Strategies to activate "readiness"	Cues to action
Provide training and guidance in performing recommended action. Use progressive goal setting Give verbal reinforcement .Demonstrate desired behaviors. Reduce anxiety	Confidence in one's ability to take action	Self efficacy

Table 1. Description of HEALTH BELIEF MODEL constructs.

disease treat (Glanz et al., 2008). For example, women must believe that a course of preventive behaviors available would be beneficial in reducing the risk of getting cervical cancer. Therefore, individuals exhibiting optimal beliefs in susceptibility and severity are not expected to accept any recommended health action unless they also perceive the action as potentially beneficial by reducing the treat. Ibekwel explored that either screened or never screened research participants overwhelmingly agree or strongly agree that it is important to do cervical cancer screening (Ibekwe1, 2010). This is consistent with studies in which the majority of subjects agreed that regular pap smear screening will give them peace of mind, find a problem before they become cancer and very necessary even if there is no family history of cancer (Leyva et al., 2006). The major reasons while both screeners and never screeners in Ibekwe1 study believed was that it is important to do cervical cancer screen because it could find changes in the cervix before they get cancer and the disease could easily be cured when found early. These reasons are consistent with findings of other studies (Agurto et al., 2004 ; Ibekwe1, 2010). As it was discussed before,Health belief model predicts that those with perceived benefits are more likely to take preventive actions, than those with no perceived benefits or low perceived benefits. Thus, it is most likely that the low uptake of cervical cancer screening among the participants took part in Ibekwel syudy could be attributed to other factors other than lack of perceived benefits (Ibekwe1, 2010). When in Ibekwe1 study participants and non-participants in cervical cancer screening were compared, it was found that there was no significant association between perceived benefits of doing cervical cancer screening and cervical cancer screening , and this was consistent with previous studies (Agurto et al., 2004; Leyva et al., 2006). The study did not find any significant association between socio-demographic characteristics and perceived benefits of doing cervical cancer screening as both the ever screened and the never screened irrespective of their socio-demographic characteristics overwhelming agree or strongly agree that it was important to do cervical cancer screening. (Ibekwe1, 2010). This finding is consistent with findings of other studies in which participants across all socio-demographic characteristics generally were aware of the benefits of cervical cancer screening (Leyva et al., 2006). However, continue education to clear misconceptions are still required to ensure increased uptake of cervical cancer screening among the eligible women especially among those that are high risk (Ibekwe1, 2010).

3.1.4 Perceived barriers

Perceived barriers to action refers to the negative aspects of health-oriented actions or which serve as barriers to action and/or that arouse conflicting incentives to avoid action. Perceived barrier refers to the potential negative aspects of particular health action may act as impediments to undertaking recommended behaviors. A kind of nonconscious, cost effective analysis occurs wherein individuals weight the action expected benefits with perceived barriers such as it could help me, but it may be expensive, have negative side effects, and be unpleasant, inconvenient or time consuming. Thus combined levels of susceptibility and severity provide the energy of force to act and the perception of benefits (minus barrier) provide a proffered path of action (Glanz et al., 2008). For example, if women believe that anticipated benefit of doing behaviors to prevent cervical cancer outweigh the barriers to or cost of the preventive behaviors, they are more probably to obtain cervical cancer screening test. Previous researchers also have reported that women who perceived the Pap smear testing process as painful and embarrassing due to visiting by male provider had lower rates of routine cervical cancer screening (Boyer etal.,2001 ; Hoyo et al., 2005; Jennings, 1997, Ackerson K , 2010, Abdullahi 2009). In this study, Some participants from the focus groups and interviews mentioned off-putting experiences that they had experienced themselves or heard from others acting as a barrier to attending screening. Such negative experiences included experiencing pain, bleeding and being faced with inexperienced sample takers who did not explain the process or enable them to ask questions (Abdullahi 2009). In this study, language difficulties were thought to not only detract from women's understanding of the test and thus the perceived need for screening, but also to prevent some women from attending, due to anxiety about not being able to understand the sample taker or not being able to ask questions and form a trusting relationship. Even if the participants took part in the study appreciated the need for screening, fear of the test was cited as a hindrance to some women, Furthermore, the metal speculum was perceived as a painful instrument and some did not trust the sterilization process. Fear of the test results was also thought to prevent some women from coming forward for screening. (Abdullahi 2009). Fear that abnormal test results mean existing cancer has been reported as a barrier to do Pap smear in previous researches (Mutyaba et al, 2006; Basu et al, 2006 ; Winkler et al., 2008, Were E1, 2011). The other factors that appeared to cause negative perceptions and act as barriers to cervical cancer screening was a previous history of trauma like childhood sexual abuse, intimate partner violence, and trauma related to medical procedures which was mentioned in previous study(Ackerson K , 2010). However, in previous research, a link between an interpersonal or medical trauma history and routine screening was not indicated (Bazargan et al., 2004; Hoyo et al., 2005). Chung HH conducted a cross sectional study to document currently cervical cancer screening practices of physicians in Korea These researchers verified that cost has been a major reason for selecting screening method of liquid-based cytology instead of Pap smear (Chung, 2006). Obesity was reported as a barrier for cervical cancer screening in previous study(Wee, 2002). In this study. it was shown that overweight and obese women were less likely to be screened for cervical cancer with Pap smears, even after adjustment for other known barriers. In a study was conducted in 1998, it was revealed that among women who sought outpatient care, screening rates decreased while co - morbidity/chronic disease increased (Kiefe, 1998). Embarrassment is known to be a barrier to cervical screening, regardless of ethnic background, but in the study conducted among some Somali women, there was additional embarrassment associated with the potential reaction of the sample taker when faced with a circumcised woman. The anxiety of potentially being faced with a male sample taker was a significant problem for these Muslim women (Abdullahi, 2009, Naish, 1994, Nichols, 1987). Time consuming was a barrier to cancer prevention in previous syudy. A study addressed the house staff adherence to cervical cancer screening recommendations by United States Preventive Services Task Force, reported lack of time during postgraduate training was frequently reported as a barrier to obtaining preventive care(Ross et al, 2006). Low socioeconomic status, poverty, low levels of education, lack of knowledge, and acculturation have been established as reasons for the low screening rates in Hispanic women. Cost of cytology have been cited as problems for Hispanic women in the United States (Austin et al, 2002). Many Hispanic women strongly believed that the fear of finding cancer would deter them from screening (Salazar MK. , 1996). Several studies reported that many Hispanic women would prefer not to know the diagnosis of cervical cancer (Hubbell et al., 1996; Mandelblatt , 1999). Suarez and associates (Suarez , 1993) noted that 48% of the Mexican-American women they surveyed thought that their chances of surviving cervical cancer were poor and those who preferred to speak in Spanish tended to have more fatalistic attitudes. They often believed that there was nothing one could do to prevent cervical cancer. This powerlessness may account for some of the anxiety associated with cancer. According previous evidences, a major barrier to cancer screening was culturally based embarrassment and similar emotions (Coyne , 1992, Bakemeier et al., 1995, Stein , 1990). The inability to speak English fluently interferes with Hispanic women's ability to obtain important health information and to communicate with health professionals. Women speaking only, or mostly, Spanish were consistently less likely to be screened for breast and cervical cancer. Language difficulties can deter referral and impede delivery of medical care (Harlan , et al1991).

3.1.5 Cues to action

Various early information of the Health Belief Model included the concept of cues that can trigger actions. Readiness to action (Perceived susceptibility and perceived benefits) could only be potentiated by other factors particularly by cues to instigate action such as bodily events or by environmental events such as media publicity (Glanz et al., 2008). For example, women would be more likely to have preventive behavior like uptaking Pap smear if they be reminded by their family members or heath care providers. The influence of cues on women to practice cervical cancer screening behavior has been reported by previous evidences. Ackerson has investigated the role of cues for obtaining pap smear test and resulted that health care providers were influential cues for studied participants by giving information regarding the importance of the test (Ackerson K , 2010). Furthermore, the Pap smear users in Ackerson study were more encouraged by health care providers and family members to do the test compared to other individuals who did not obtain the test. In the country of Australia, health care system is a good cues for women to obtain cervical cancer screening .In this country all people accessing high quality cancer control, whether it be prevention, screening, treatment or education. In addition, non-government organizations (NGOs) specializing in cancer control have been providing free or highly subsidized support services to patients and their families for over half a century in most states. These NGOs have also been very active in public education about cancer, especially cancer prevention and act as cues for women (Burton, 2002). In previous research recommendation by GPs and health care providers as well as written and oral information were considered as cues to action for cervical cancer screening (Abdullahi 2009). According to this study, many participants had first attended screening as a result of their GP's advice so that GPs were proactive in encouraging Somali women to take up screening. Regarding preferred formats of screening information, Somalian participants stated that it was necessary for information to be given in Somali language. They explained that, in view of the cultural significance of talking in this culture, they responded better to verbal than written information, such as being told by a friend or a Somali community worker through talks or workshops in community settings. Written information was considered unsuitable cues to action by some due to low levels of literacy among Somalis, although others felt that it was a useful adjunct (Abdullahi 2009). The integral role of nurses in educating women regarding health preventive care, especially the importance of routine cervical cancer screening was stressed in other study(Ackerson, 2010). This study confirmed nurses are in a position to influence positive health behavior, so they should inform women about the purpose of the Pap smear test, while assessing the woman's personal risk factors for cervical cancer, and her beliefs and perceptions regarding Pap smears. Many studies have identified positive cues to cancer screening in Hispanic women. These include physician recommendation, lay health workers, written materials, and media. Physician recommendation is one of the most important cues to cancer screening. Physicians play a key role in informing women of the benefits of screening (O'Malley , 2001) . Similar results were observed in previous evidence (Zambrana et al , 1999). The respect for authority is an important characteristic of Hispanic culture. Latinas consider doctors as powerful authority figures and have a tendency to listen to what doctors say, but rarely show self-initiated health care behaviors. The role of physician is especially important for older minority women (Rimer , 1994, Mandelblatt & Yabroff , 2000). Community outreach strategies are the most common health promotion, and probably most effective strategies employed by health care workers, researchers, and health promotion officers. Community outreach strategies include the use of appropriate language materials, involvement of lay health workers, and presentations at community and workplace settings. Lay health workers are trained personnel from the Hispanic community whose main job is to educate women on the benefits of Papanicolaou screening and mammography to reduce perceived barriers to screening. Several studies report that the involvement of the community is effective in the development, planning, and delivery of the screening programs (Eng et al., 1997, Zavertnik, 1993). Impressive results in cervical and breast screening behaviors were obtained in the Hispanic community living in California

(Perez-Stable , 1992). In Ontario, lay health workers have been found to be important positive cues to action for Hispanic women. Churches are also important vehicles to reach Hispanic women. Castro et al, reported positive church involvement in cancer screening practices of Latina women (Castro , 1995). Other researchers have found that churches provide a social influence to participation in cancer screening among Hispanic women (Frank-Stromborg , 1998, Zavertnik , 1993, Davis , 1994) The "Companeros en la Salud" program delivers educational programs at churches, and preliminary results are expected to show an increase in Papanicolaou smears and mammography among Latina women. Written materials are also used as cues to action. Specific educational materials (e.g., brochures, community newspapers), usually apart from community outreach programs, are effective in providing information to Hispanics if they are culturally sensitive, and written in Spanish at a grade (Snider et al., 1996) reading level to improve understanding among low-literacy individuals. One effective way to reach Hispanic women may be through media-based public health campaigns. However, such programs are effective only when delivered and implemented in a culturally meaningful and sensitive manner. Vellozzi et al. indicated that Hispanic women may be more receptive to media messages than are other ethnic groups (Vellozzi , 1996). In "A Su Salad" program, media messages (TV, radio, and newspaper) have been integrated successfully with community-based outreach(Suarez, 1993b, Anderson et al., 2009). Salazar indicated that the media increased Hispanic women's willingness to openly discuss breast cancer (Salazar , 1996).

3.1.6 Perceived self efficacy

Perceived self efficacy is defined as the conviction that one can successfully execute the behavior required to produce the outcomes. For behavior change to succeed, people must feel threatened by their current behavioral pattern (perceived susceptibility and severity) and believe that change of a specific kind will result in a valued outcome at an acceptable cost (perceived benefit). Then, they also must feel themselves competent (self - efficacious) to overcome perceived barriers to take actions. For example, women should be confident that they could uptake pop smear in a regular manner.

3.1.7 Other variables

Divers demographic, sociopsychological, knowledge, socio cultural, race , education and structural variables may influence perception and thus, indirectly affect on health related behavior (Glanze 2008). For example , socio demographic factors , particularly educational attainment, are believed to have an indirect effect on behavior of cervical cancer screening , through influencing the perception of susceptibility to getting the disease, severity of the disease and benefits of this screen behavior that overcome to the perceived barriers. Studies conducted among divers samples have found some differences in the specific types of beliefs about susceptibility, benefits and barriers among different racial and ethnic groups. Different groups have different beliefs about the causes of cervical cancer, which can affect perceived susceptibility. Hispanic women were afraid that they would not be able to cope with the disease. One research group noted that low-acculturated Mexican-American women expressed a stronger fear of cancer than did high-acculturated women (Balcazar , 1995). A study conducted in somali showed that knowledge about the purpose of cervical screening was limited among Somali women. There was also a lack of understanding of risk factors for cervical cancer, and many of the women held fatalistic attitudes, associated with the idea of 'God's will', about this cancer and other aspects of health. Somalis are almost all Muslim and their view of health is typically shaped by a combination of traditional Somali and Islamic beliefs, with most believing that illness and healing only occur by the will of God. It is important therefore to recognize that some Somalis may wrongly interpret Islam as not allowing disease prevention interventions (Abduullahi 2009). Researchers have found that Latinas hold more fatalistic attitudes about cervical cancer (Chavez , 1997). This attitude stemed from the belief that there was little an individual could do to alter fate or prevent cancer. Latinas often believed that cancer is God's punishment for improper or immoral behavior (Hubbell FA, 1996). Another culturally specific barrier was embarrassment associated with female circumcision, i.e. female genital mutilation. Embarrassment about discussion of private body parts and embarrassment at exposing private body parts during a physical examination may pose a barrier for some Hispanics, especially if examined by a male physician (Frank-Stromborg et al., 1998), Accordingly, gender of the physician may determine breast and cervical cancer screening uptake and compliance in this community. Hispanic women may also be embarrassed to disclose personal information related to their sexual activity to another person besides their partner. Limited proficiency in the language of the host country has also been identified as a barrier to cancer screening. This variable has been shown to provide a reliable prediction of the use of preventive health care among minority women (Stein & Fox , 1990). The other culturally barrier that was consistently mentioned by the participants who took part in the focus groups and interviewees from Somali was embarrassment as a hindrance to attending screening. Most of these women viewed the test as intrusive and uncomfortable, both physically and emotionally. For some, the embarrassment associated with having been circumcised was an additional barrier. Although they were not ashamed of this, they anticipated embarrassment associated with the shocked reaction of the sample taker to their circumcision. In all of the focus group discussions and six of the eight interviews, participants explained that for Muslim women, the possibility of having a man perform the test was a significant barrier. Many participants were unaware that they could request a woman to undertake the test (Abdullahi 2009) .Other variables suggested by the participants were: lack of knowledge about the need for cervical screening, practical problems such as appointment times and childcare needs, language difficulties, fear of the test and negative past experiences. Determinants of uptake of cervical cancer screening services include age, education, contraception use and being married (Objechina, 2009). Women with low educational achievement, low awareness of the risk factors for cervical cancer, and who do not have support from their husbands may also have poor uptake of screening services (Allahverdipour H, 2008; Abdullahi, 2009). In previous study which was conducted by Ackerson K, twenty-four participants were divided into two groups based on whether they did or did not get routine Pap smears . The results showed there were differences between the two groups in terms of demographic and social characteristics, having previous health care experience as well as cognitive appraisal related to beliefs and perceptions of vulnerability (Ackerson K , 2010). Monthly income and residential area were significantly associated with perceived severity (Houqe 2009). Certain types of barriers are more or less important for particular cultural or ethnic subgroups. Thus, women who had such belief might consider their susceptibility to cervical cancer was quite low. In a systematic review was conducted by Johnson CE in 2008, commonly held beliefs across several cultural groups emerged included fatalistic attitudes, a lack of knowledge about cervical cancer, fear of Pap smears threatening one's virginity, as well as beliefs that a

Pap smear is unnecessary unless one is ill (Johnson CE, 2008). This study revealed that some unique beliefs were common among specific cultural groups. For example, Hispanic women noted some body-focused notions and believed that childbirth, menses, sex, and stress play a role in one's susceptibility to cervical cancer. African Americans identified administrative processes in establishing health care as barriers to screening, whereas Asian immigrants held a variety of misconceptions concerning one's susceptibility to cancer as well as stigmatization imposed by their own community and providers. This study concluded health care providers and policy makers must be cognizant of the various sociocultural factors influencing health-related beliefs and health care utilization among immigrant and ethnic minorities in the United States. Culturally relevant screening strategies and programs that address these socio cultural factors must be developed to address the growing disparity in cervical cancer burden among underserved, resource-poor populations in the United States . Vietnamese American women are five times more likely to be diagnosed with cervical cancer than their White counterparts. Previous research has demonstrated low levels of Papanicolaou (Pap) testing among Vietnamese. Taylor VM and co-workers conducted a population-based, in-person survey of Vietnamese women aged 18 - 64 years to examine factors associated with interval Pap testing adherence. In this study the beliefs including Pap tests decrease the risk of cervical cancer , cervical cancer is curable if detected early, testing is necessary for women who are asymptomatic, sexually inactive, or postmenopausal , concern about pain/discomfort as a barrier to screening; family member(s) and friend(s) had suggested testing (social support); doctor(s) had recommended testing communication with health care providers were explored as predictor variables for obtaining pap smear (Taylor VM, 2004). In a multivariate analysis, this study showed being married, knowing Pap testing is necessary for asymptomatic women, doctor(s) had recommended testing, and had asked doctor(s) for testing were independently associated with screening participation (Taylor et al., 2004) . Fear, embarrassment, and cost were more likely to be barrier to adherence cervical cancer screening recommendation among Asian women compared to white women (Ross, 2008). Finally, in addition to differences in specific perceptions about susceptibility, benefits and barriers among different racial or ethnic groups, researchers have found differences by race in exploratory of Health Belief Model constructs. Racial and ethnic disparities in cervical cancer screening have been attributed to socioeconomic, insurance, and cultural differences. A previous study evaluated the relationship between U.S. citizenship status and the receipt of Pap smears among immigrant women in this study California Citizen immigrants were significantly more likely to report receiving a Pap smear ever (adjusted prevalence ratio [aPR], 1.05; 95% confidence interval [CI], 1.01 to 1.08), a recent Pap smear (aPR, 1.07; 95% CI, 1.03 to 1.11) as compared to immigrants who are not U.S. citizens (DE Alba, 2005).. Also variables like income, having a usual source care, and having health insurance were associated with receiving cancer screening. This study showed Hispanic women were more likely to receive Pap smears as compared to whites and Asians (DE Alba, 2005). Foreign birthplace may explain some disparities previously attributed to race or ethnicity, and is an important barrier to cancer screening, even after adjustment for other factors. Increasing access to health care may improve disparities among foreign-born persons to some degree. Results from previous research, showed black respondents were as or more likely to report cancer screening than white respondents; however, Hispanic and Asian-American and Pacific Islander (AAPI) respondents were significantly less likely to report screening for most cancers. When race/ethnicity and birthplace were considered together, U.S.-born Hispanic and AAPI respondents were as likely to report cancer screening as U.S.-born whites; however, foreign-born white (adjusted odds ratio [AOR], 0.58; 95% confidence interval [CI], 0.41 to 0.82), Hispanic (AOR, 0.65; 95% CI, 0.53 to 0.79), and AAPI respondents (AOR,0.28; 95% CI, 0.19 to 0.39) were less likely than U.S.-born whites to report Pap smears (Goel etal., 2003). A cross-sectional survey that was conducted among a convenience sample of 204 female post-graduate physicians examined adherence to United States Preventive Services Task Force cervical cancer screening recommendations, perception of adherence to recommendations, and barriers to obtaining care. This study showed just 83% of women were adherent to screening recommendations and 84% accurately perceived adherence or non-adherence. Women who self-identified as Asian were significantly less adherent when compared with women who self-identified as white (69% vs. 87%; Relative Risk [RR]=0.79, 95% Confidence Interval [CI], 0.64-0.97; P<0.01). Women who self-identified as East Indian were significantly less likely to accurately perceive adherence or non-adherence when compared to women who self-identified as white (64% vs. 88%; RR=0.73, 95% CI, 0.49-1.09, P=0.04). Women who self-identified as Asian were significantly more likely to report any barrier to obtaining care when compared with women who self-identified as white (60% vs. 35%; RR=1.75, 95% CI, 1.24-2.47; P=0.001). Women who self-identified as East Indian being more likely to report any barrier to obtaining care when compared with women who self-identified as white (60% vs. 34%; RR=1.74, 95% CI, 1.06-2.83; P=0.06) (Ross et al., 2008). A systematic review was conducted in 2008 showed most consistent associations between obesity and cervical cancer screening behavior. According to this review, most studies reported an inverse relation between decreased cervical cancer screening and increasing body size, and several studies reported that the association was more consistent among white women than among black women (Cohen et al., 2008). Participants from the focus groups and interviews in Abdullah study 2009 tended to discuss what they thought were other Somali women's reasons for not attending screening rather than the reason for their own non attendance. This study highlighted that 38% of participants had never been screened. Of these, when probed, four women said that they had never even heard of the screening test, eight said that they had never been sexual active and so thought that they did not need to attend for screening, and seven cited other reasons, including lack of understanding of the need to attend screening, hearing others' negative stories about the test, lack of knowledge and embarrassment. Participants within all focus groups and in the interviews identified that many Somali women had poor understanding of the need for cervical screening, and that this prevented them from attending screening. There is no cervical screening program in Somalia and the concept of preventative health was thought to be unfamiliar to many Somalis, especially to those new to the UK (Abdullahi 2009).

4. Cervical cancer screening behavior intervention based on Health Belief Model

A number of cervical cancer screening behavior promotion interventions have addressed at least one Health Belief Model construct - usually perceived barriers - and have had significant effects on cervical cancer screening behavior outcomes . This model, which emerged in the late 1950s, was used as an exploratory model to assess why people did not use preventive health services and eventually to understand why people use or fail to use health services. Many researchers now employ this model to guide the development of health interventions with the aim of changing behaviors. Here, the findings from several different types of interventions based on Health Belief Model are summarized. Perhaps because constructs in the Health Belief Model are fairly intuitive, they have been used in a number of community based interventions conducted among underserved groups with lower socio economic level. The development of efficacious theory-based, culturally relevant interventions to promote cervical cancer prevention among underserved populations is crucial to the elimination of cancer disparities. In a study by Scarinci and co-workers a theory-based, culturally relevant interventions used to promote cervical cancer prevention among underserved populations of Latina immigrants (Scarinci, 2011). The goal was to describe the development of a theory-based, culturally relevant intervention focusing on primary (sexual risk reduction) and secondary (Pap smear) prevention of cervical cancer among Latina immigrants using intervention mapping (IM). Health belief model provided theoretical guidance for the intervention development and implementation. IM provides a logical five-step framework in intervention development: delineating proximal program objectives, selecting theory-based intervention methods and strategies, developing a program plan, planning for adoption in implementation, and creating evaluation plans and instruments. We first conducted an extensive literature review and qualitatively examined the sociocultural factors associated with primary and secondary prevention of cervical cancer. We then proceeded to quantitatively validate the qualitative findings, which led to development matrices linking the theoretical constructs with intervention objectives and strategies as well as evaluation. IM was a helpful tool in the development of a theory-based, culturally relevant intervention addressing primary and secondary prevention among Latina immigrants (Scarinci,2011). To address the barrier of negative experience, in a qualitative study was performed in Somali, it was suggested that providing an explanation of the procedure prior to the test and allowing adequate time for questions could help to overcome negative past experiences. Some participants in focus group believed that attending as part of a group with a Somali-speaking community worker would make the experience less daunting, especially for first-time attendees. It was suggested by two participants in different groups and one interviewee that the fear of pain and poor hygiene could be helped by the provision of disposable plastic speculums, which were considered less aggressive and more hygienic (Abdullahi 2009). Beach and others in 2007 revealed in their study that the language could be as one potentially key factor in cancer screening disparities. They carried out secondary analyses of data from a randomized clinical trial that aimed to increase breast, cervical, and colorectal cancer screenings. The randomized clinical trial tested whether the intervention by Prevention Care Manager (PCM) which provided language-appropriate telephone support to help patients overcome barriers to cancer screening, was effective in helping women become up-to-date on these screening tests. Up-to-date status was based on recommendations of the U.S. Preventive Services Task Force .The intervention improved women's up-to-date status on all three screening tests, as reported elsewhere. This study included Spanish-speaking women seemed to benefit more than did English-speaking women from a bilingual telephone support intervention aimed at increasing cancer screening rates. (Beach et al, 2007). Some studies have compared the effectiveness of different media for delivering intervention addressing Health Belief Model constructs to women in clinic setting. Just as the Health Belief Model has guided community based interventions to deliver information or persuasive message to change perception and reduce barriers to cervical cancer screening behavior, it has guided interventions delivered through television campaign. To encourage the right women to attend for cervical cancer screening, a media complain program was developed and tested. In addition to drawing on findings from the published literature to assist campaign development, in-depth telephone interviews were conducted with 32 women aged from 30 to 69 who had previously had regular Pap tests, but had lapsed in their cervical screening for at least 3 years, to determine the barriers to returning for another test. There were three salient reasons for lapsing. A major factor was that women expressed a negative emotional disposition to Pap tests, indicating dislike, embarrassment, discomfort or anxiety about having the test. Second, for some women, Pap tests were not considered a high priority, in that they did not believe they were at risk of cervical cancer. Finally, a small group of women believed that they did not need a Pap test because they considered they would know if something was wrong with their own bodies. It was noted that lack of knowledge of the appropriate time interval between tests was not a barrier for these women, since they were aware that they were overdue for a Pap test. The findings from the interviews were used to develop a brief for an advertising agency to develop concepts for further testing with women. The brief Targeted cervical screening media campaign focused particularly on the importance of overcoming emotional barriers to having a Pap test. Ultimately, two rounds of focus groups were conducted (nine groups of women aged >40, some adequately screened and some lapsed screeners) to develop the final advertisement. A 30-s television advertisement was produced, with a 15-s cut-down version. A radio advertisement was also developed, but is not discussed in this paper, as very few women heard the radio advertisement without also being exposed to the television advertisement. The television advertisement aimed to acknowledge women's anxiety and discomfort about having the test, while reminding them there was a good reason for having one. However, it was also designed not to arouse concern for those women whose tests were up-to-date. The advertisement -Don't just sit there- featured a series of women's legs in a variety of situations and a voice-over acknowledging that although having a Pap test can be uncomfortable, being treated for cervical cancer can be far more uncomfortable. The voice-over concluded by saying If you haven't had a Pap test in the last two years, stop putting it off. Make an appointment today with your doctor or community health centre. The tag line of the advertisement on the screen indicated _Pap tests. Every two years. It could save your life._ The advertisement was broadcast for nearly 4 weeks from Sunday 18 July to Thursday 12 August 2004. The media-buying schedule indicated that during this time, the advertisement had the opportunity to be seen two or more times by 86% of women in the target age range and 73% would have had an opportunity to see it three or more times. Data were conducted at the last week of the media campaign. Numbers were randomly selected from the electronic telephone directory and trained female interviewers asked to speak to the woman in the household aged between 25 and 65 whose birthday was next. Contact was made with 3510 households and in 1600 of these someone was identified as being eligible to complete the survey. Overall, an interview was obtained in 63% of homes where someone had been identified as eligible. Among them, 1000 women completed the survey and 600 did not (433 refused, 114 terminated during the interview, 53 agreed to complete it later but did not). Women were told that the research was being conducted on behalf of a well known Victorian health organization, was for public health research purposes and had been approved by an ethics committee. Up to five attempts were made to reach each of the selected numbers. While collecting data, the advertisement was then described to the women who either did not recall a Pap screening advertisement at all or were unable to describe it accurately. A further 393 (51.8% of those asked, 42.0% of the total sample) remembered it when prompted. Thus, overall 61% of the women surveyed were aware of the television advertisement (19% unprompted recall and 42% prompted recall). Most of the 568 women who had seen the advertisement could describe its main message. About half (54.2%) reported a general message of everyone needing a Pap test, some saying that it should be regular but without specifying what regular meant, and some that it should be two-yearly. Some women (20.5%) indicated a more specific response that acknowledged that Pap tests are uncomfortable but still important to have and 9.7% reported a general message about prevention being important. Only 3.5% reported that the message was that Pap tests are unpleasant without adding the key point that they are worth having anyway. When asked what action they planned to take in response to seeing the advertising, 51.9% of women indicated that they would not do anything. However, women were most likely to respond in this way if their last Pap test had been more recent. Women who were overdue or lapsed screeners were less likely not to plan to take action. Overall, 15.9% of women indicated that as a result of seeing the advertisement, they planned to have a Pap test soon. Women overdue for a Pap test were significantly more likely to respond in this way than those who had a Pap test more recently. In total, 18.4% of women indicated they planned to have a Pap test when it was due, with no differences according to how long it had been since their last Pap test (Mullins, 2008). Mass media campaigns have been used with some success to improve participation in health screening. A meta-analysis of media health campaigns found that campaigns promoting mammography and cervical cancer screening caused 4% of women changed their behavior in response to a televised marketing campaign prompting these types of screening for women (Snyder, 2004). Several studies have used Health Belief Model variables to tailor cervical cancer screening behavior for particular recipients. In general, tailoring messages for cervical cancer screening behavior using Health Belief Model constructs have been found to increase cervical cancer screening behavior. In this study, Forsyth County Cancer Screening (FoCaS) was designed to improve beliefs, attitudes, and screening behaviors of women age 40 and older who resided in low-income housing communities. To develop effective interventions, results from the baseline women's survey, the health care provider survey, additional focus groups, and input from the Community Advisory Board were used. These sources provided information on barriers, attitudes, current breast and cervical cancer screening practices, and optimum strategies for delivering health education messages. The theoretical framework for the community-based interventions included the PRECEDE/PROCEED model for planning, the health belief model , for identifying and addressing barriers, social learning theory in terms of using lay health educators to deliver education messages and develop a sense of self-efficacy in the women, and the PENIII model, which incorporates cultural appropriateness and sensitivity in program development. Interventions implemented in the housing communities in Winston-Salem during the 2-year intervention period included: (*a*) "Women's Fest," a free party held in the community that included food, educational classes, cholesterol, blood pressure and diabetes screening, prizes, and information booths; (*b*) a church program that included a ministers' luncheon and a lay health educator program, "Taking Care of our Sisters," for female church members; (*c*) educational brochures especially designed to address identified barriers such as "Where to Get a Mammogram"; (*d*) mass media techniques (public bus ads, newspaper and radio ads on African-American media); (*e*) monthly classes in each housing community conducted by a lay health educator; (*f*) birthday cards with the FoCaS logo; (*g*) targeted mailings and door knob hangers with invitations to events; and (*h*) one-on-one educational sessions in women's homes. Clinic-focused interventions implemented at RHC were designed to address provider, system, and patient barriers to conducting breast and cervical cancer screening and included: (*a*) in-service and primary care conference training for providers on issues including clinical breast exam proficiency, cultural sensitivity, and techniques to integrate prevention in primary care; (*b*) visual prompts in the exam rooms, *e.g.*, "Have you screened today?"; (*c*) educational games, *e.g.*, "Find the Lump Game" to teach clinical breast exam techniques; (*d*) an abnormal test protocol that included alert stickers, a referral process for managing the care of women with abnormal test results, and a tracking system; (*e*) poster and literature distribution in the waiting rooms; and (*f*) one-on-one counseling sessions and personalized letters for follow-up testing for women who had abnormal test results. The delivery of the intervention components was monitored by the project manager through weekly reports, observations of classes, and process evaluation measures such as attendance rolls, number of classes taught, brochures distributed, and letters mailed. Results of this study showed the proportion of women who received a Pap smear within the last 3 years increased in the intervention city from 73 to 87%. The proportion of women reporting a Pap smear in the last 3 years in the comparison city decreased over time, from 67 to 60%. Thus, the Pap smear usage rate increased by 14 percentage points in the intervention city and decreased by 7 percentage points in the comparison city for an overall net change of 21 percentage points in favor of the intervention city (*P* 5 0.004, unadjusted Wald x2 test). Older women (65 and over) were less likely than younger women to have had a Pap smear within guidelines (70 *versus* 78%; *P* 5 0.013). Women who received regular examinations were more likely to have had a Pap smear within guidelines (79 *versus* 51%; *P* , 0.001). The more correct knowledge women had, the more likely they were to be within screening guidelines (*P* 5 0.001), and women who reported a higher number of barriers were less likely to be compliant with guidelines (*P* 5 0.005) than those reporting the least number of barriers. In the comparison city, married women were more likely than non married women (including divorced, separated, widowed, and never married) to be within guidelines (79 *versus* 60%). For Pap smears, significantly more women in the intervention city reported no barriers to screening at follow-up compared with women in the comparison city (55 *versus* 29%; *P*, 0.05). No significant differences were noted between the two cities in either time period in the proportion of women reporting positive beliefs (two or more) about cervical cancer and screening or the proportion of women with good knowledge (five or more correct answers) about cervical cancer and screening (Pasket al., 1999). Building on the tailored print cervical cancer screening behavior intervention finding, Dignan and co - workers examined the effects of health education on Increasing Screening for Cervical Cancer among Eastern-Band Cherokee Indian Women in North Carolina. The North Carolina Native American Cervical Cancer Prevention Project was a 5-year, National Cancer Institute-funded trial of health education designed to increase screening for cervical cancer among Native- American women in North Carolina.. This study was conducted to evaluate the effectiveness of this education program in the Eastern-Band Cherokee target population. Cherokee tribal lands were mapped and all households (N = 2223) were listed to ensure maximum coverage of the eligible population (women, aged 18 years and older, who were enrolled tribal members). Eligible women were identified by the use of a brief questionnaire administered to an adult member of the household. Of the 1279 households with eligible women, 1020 (79.8%) agreed to participate. The intervention was an individualized health education program delivered by female Cherokee lay health educators based on several theories and models including Health belief model. The participants were randomly assigned to receive or not to receive the intervention (i.e., to program and control groups, respectively) by use of the Solomon Four-Group design. Data were collected in face-to-face interviews conducted in the participant's home. Of the 996 women who were ultimately enrolled, 540 were randomly assigned to receive a pretest (pre intervention) interview that involved administration of a 96-item questionnaire designed to collect data on knowledge, intentions, and behaviors related to cervical cancer; of these 540 women, 263 were randomly assigned to receive the education program. The remaining 456 women did not receive the pretest, but 218 were randomly assigned to receive the education program. Six months after receiving the education program, the women in all four groups were administered a post-test that was identical to the pretest Logistic regression was used to assess the effects of the pretest and the educational program. All *P* values resulted from two-sided statistical tests. Results of this study showed eight hundred and fifteen (81.8%) of the 996 participants completed the post-test interview. The remaining 181 women who were lost to follow-up were evenly distributed among the four study groups. At the post-test, 282 (73.2%) of the 385 women who received the education program reported having had a Pap smear following the intervention, compared with 275 (64%) of the 430 control subjects. Women who received the education program were more likely to answer all knowledge items correctly on the post-test (odds ratio [OR] = 2.18, 95% confidence interval [CI] = 1.08- 439) and to report having obtained a Pap smear in the past year (OR = 2.06, 95% CI = 1.14-3.72) than women in the control groups. This study concluded women who received the education program exhibited a greater knowledge about cervical cancer prevention and were more likely to have reported having had a Pap smear within the past year than women who did not receive the program (DIgnan, 1996).

HEALTH BELIEF MODEL variables have also formed the basis for an interventional program to improve beliefs and behaviors of screening for cervical cancer among Iranian people. A quasi-experimental study was conducted in Hamadan , Iran, in 2010. In this study, 70 women aged 16 to 54 years - who had never done Pap test until the date of the study, participated voluntarily. The volunteers were divided into several small groups. For each group, 2-hour training session was held. The data collection tool was a self-administered multi-choice questionnaire that was developed based on HBM constructs. Health beliefs and practice of the target group were evaluated pre intervention and four months later. The findings indicated that education based on HBM was effective and could enhance the participants' knowledge significantly and improve the HBM constructs including perceived susceptibility, severity, benefits, and barriers. The training program enhanced the practice of screening test significantly. This study concluded that education program based on HBM can enhance women's knowledge of cervical cancer, change their health beliefs and improve their behaviors regarding screening programs like Pap test (Shojaeizadeh, 2011). In study that was conducted in Somali education about the purpose of the screening test and the programme was considered as key procedure in encouraging Somalis to take up screening. The participants felt that Somali health advocates or community workers should provide this information in a community setting. In their opinion, this would help women to understand the value of the test, and should aim to address some women's misinterpretation of the Islamic perspective regarding disease prevention and help to overcome fatalistic barriers to screening . Participants favored education from Somali speakers, and no participant suggested the need for increased opportunities to learn English. Overall, participants favored verbal modes of communication, reflecting Somali people having an oral culture. Participants suggested improving awareness of screening via the use of video, DVDs, CDs and audiotapes (Abdullahi , 2009) . In previous evidence, possible solutions suggested by the participants included the provision of education and information about cervical screening in the Somali language by Somali community workers. They also suggested that healthcare staff should be trained about Somali culture, particularly regarding female circumcision, and that general practitioners should more proactively encourage Somali women to attend screening (Abdullahi 2009).

5. Conclusion

This chapter highlighted the concepts of Health Belief Model that could be applied for cervical cancer screening test. In summary, Health Belief Model constructs generally have been found to predict participation in cervical cancer screening. In addition, a large number of interventions studied addressing Health Belief Model constructs have resulted in increased cervical cancer screening behavior. The interventions tailored to address recipient's specific Health Belief Model beliefs have been found to be particularly effective. It is entirely consistent with the Health Belief Model that intervention will be more effective if address the persons' specific perception about susceptibility, barrier and self efficacy. Women who already believe they are at risk for developing cervical cancer screening behavior do not need messages trying to conceive them to their susceptibility, those who know where to get a free pap smear but cannot find a way to get there need intervention addressing transportation not cost Just as it is important to be able to measure validity of Health Belief Model construct, tailoring technology has allowed interventions to address Health Belief Model constructs most relevant for particular intervention. Also in this chapter, the literature review summarized cervical cancer screening beliefs and attitudes of Hispanic women using the Health Belief Model. Perceived barriers (e.g., fear of cancer, embarrassment, fatalistic views of cancer, and language), as well as perceived susceptibility (e.g., belief that screening tests are not necessary/ needed impede screening. Physician recommendations and community outreach programs are effective strategies to increase breast and cervical cancer screening uptake among Hispanic women. The specific findings of this literature review indicate that cancer-screening programs should use multi sectorial approaches to address culture-specific issues and provide culturally sensitive and competent services.

6. References

Agurto, I., Bishop, A., Sanchez, G., et al (2004). Perceived barriers and benefits to cervical cancer screening in Latin America. *Prevtive Medicine*, Vol, 39. No,1.(Jul 2004), pp., 91-8.

Al-Naggar RA, Low WY, Isa ZM (2010). Knowledge and barriers towards cervical cancer screening among young women in Malaysia.. Asian Pacific Journal of Cancer Prevention., Vol,11. No,4. pp. 867-73.

Allahverdipour, H., Emami, A., Perceptions of cervical cancer threat, benefits, and barriers of Papanicolaou smear screening programs for women in Iran. *Women & Health,* Vol.47, No.3.pp.23-37.

Abdullahi, A., Copping, J., Kessel, A., Luck, M., Bonell, C.(2009). Cervical screening: Perceptions and barriers to uptake among Somali women in Camden. *Public Health,* Vol.123, No.10, (Oct 2009),.pp.680-5.

Ackerson, K. (2010). Personal Influences That Affect Motivation in Pap Smear Testing Among African American Women. Journal of Obstetrics, Gynecologic & Neonatal Nursing, Vol, 39.No,2, pp.136-146.

Akbari, F., Shakibazadeh, E., Pourreza, A., Tavafian, SS. (2010) . Barriers and Facilitating Factors for Cervical Cancer Screening: a Qualitative Study from Iran. *Iranian Journal of Cancer Prevention,* Vol,13. No,.4. pp. 178-84

Anderson1, Jo.,. Mullins, RM., Siahpush, M., Spittal, MJ, & Wakefield, M.(2009) .Mass media campaign improves cervical screening across all socio-economic groups. *HEALTH EDUCATION RESEARCH* , Vol,24.No, 5.(Apr 2009). pp. 867–875.

Balcazar, H., Castro, FG., Krull, JL (1995). Cancer risk reduction in Mexican American women: the role of acculturation, education, and health risk factors. Health Education Quarterly, Vol,21.No, 1.(Feb 1995). pp. 61–84.

Bakemeier, RF., Krebs, LU., Murphy, JR., Shen, Z., Ryals, T. (1995).Attitudes of Colorado health professionals toward breast and cervical cancer screening in Hispanic women. Journal of the Natlonal Cancer Institute, Monograph, Vol,18,. (1995), pp. 95-100.

Bazargan, M,. Bazargan, SH., Farooq, M., & Baker, RS. (2004). Correlates of cervical cancer screening among underserved Hispanic and African-American women. *Preventive Medicine,* Vol.39, No., 3. (Sep 2004), pp.465-473.

Beach, ML., Flood, AB., Robinson, CM. et al (2007). Can Language-Concordant Prevention Care Managers Improve Cancer Screening Rates? *Cancer Epidemioogy,l Biomarkers & Prevention* ,Vol.16, No.10, (Oct 2007),pp. 2058-2064.

Ben-Natan, M., & Adir , O. (2009) . Screening for cervical cancer among Israeli women. *International Nursing Review,* Vol. 56, No.4, (Dec 2009), pp.433–441.

Boyer, LE., Williams, M., Callister, LC., & Marshall, ES. (2001). Hispanic women's perceptions regarding cervical cancer screening. *Journal of Obstetrics, Gynecology, & Neonatal Nursing,* Vol. 30, No.2. pp (Mar 2001),. 240-245.

Burton, RC. Cancer control in Australia: into the 21(st) Century. Japanese Journal of Clinical Oncology, 32 Suppl:S3-9. (Mar 2002), pp.53-9.

Basu, P., Sarkar, S., Mukherjee, S., Ghoshal, M., Mittal, S. et al. Women's perceptions and social barriers determine compliance to cervical screening: results from a population based study in India. *Cancer Detection and Prevention* Vol.;30. No.4. (2006), pp.369-74.

Champion V.L., & Skinner C.S. (2008) . The Health belief model, In: *Health behavior and health education,* Glanz K, Rimer B.K, & Viswanath , K pp45- 66. Jossey-Bass, ISBN: 978-0-7879—614-7, U.S.A..

Chung, HH, Kim, JW, Kang, SB. (2006). Cost is a barrier to widespread use of liquid-based cytology for cervical cancer screening in Korea. Journal of Korean Medical Sciences, Vol .21,No.6.(Dec 2006), pp.1054-9.

Cohen, SS., Palmieri, RT., Nyante, SJ. Koralek, DO., Kim, S., et al. Obesity and screening for breast, cervical, and colorectal cancer in women: a Review. *Cancer*, Vol.112, No.9(may 2008), pp.1892-904.

Coughlin, SS., King, J., Richards, et al..(2006). Cervical cancer screening among women in metropolitan areas of the United States by individual-level and area-based measures of socioeconomic status, 2000 to 2002. *Cancer Epidemiology, Biomarkers & Prevention*, Vol. 15, No.11(Nov 2006), pp. 2154–9.

Castro, FG., Elder, JP., Tafoya-Barraza, HM., Moratto, S., Campbell, N., et al. (1995). Mobilizing churches for health promotion in Latino communities: Companeros en la Salud. *Journal of the National Cancer Institute, Monograph,* Vol.18 (1995) ,pp.127–135.

Chavez, LR., Hubbell, FA., Mishra, SI., Valdez, RB. (1997). The influence of fatalism on self-reported use of Papanicolaou smears. *American Journal of Preventive Medicine*, Vol.;13, No.6 (Nov-Dec 1997):418–424.

Coyne, CA., Hohman, K., Levinson, A. (1992). Reaching special populations with breast and cervical cancer public education. *Journal of Cancer Education*, Vol. 7, No.4,(1992) , pp. 293-303.

Datta, G., Colditz, G., Kawachi, I., et al.(2006). Individual-, neighborhood-, and state-level socioeconomic predictors of cervical carcinoma screening among U.S. black women. *Cancer*, Vol 106, No. 3 (Feb 2006), pp. 664–9.

Davis, DT., Bustamente, A., Brown, CP. (1994). The urban church and cancer control: a source of social influence in minority communities. *Public Health Reports* ,Vol.109, No.4 (Jul-Agu 1994), pp. :500-6.

Dignan, M., Michielutte, R., Blinson, K., Wells, HB., Douglas Case, LD., et al. (1996). Effectiveness of Health Education to Increase Screening for Cervical Cancer Among Eastern-Band Cherokee Indian Women in North Carolina. *Journal of the National Cancer Institute*, Vol, 88. No, 22 (Nov 1996) pp.1670-6.

De Alba, I., Hubbell, FA., McMullin, JM., Sweningson, JM., Saitz, R.(2005)..Impact of U.S. citizenship status on cancer screening among immigrant women. *Journal of General Internal Medicine* Vol. 20, .No. 3.(Mar 2005), pp.290-6.

Frank-Stromborg, M., Wassner, LJ., Nelson, M., Chilton, B., Wholeben, BE.(1998).A study of rural Latino women seeking cancer-detection examinations. *Journal of Cancer Education*, Vol. 13, No. 4 (winter 1998),pp. 231–241.

Gakidou, E., Nordhagen, S., Obermeyer, Z. (2008).Coverage of Cervical Cancer Screening in 57 Countries: Low Average Levels and Large Inequalities. *PLoS Medicine*, Vol.5, No.6, (June 2008), e132. doi:10.1371

Garbers, S., Chiasson, MA.(2004). Inadequate functional health literacy in Spanish as a barrier to cervical cancer screening among immigrant Latinas in New York City. *Preventive Chronic Disease*, Vol.1, No.4. (Oct 2004) , A07. Epub 2004 Sep 15.

Goel, MS., Wee, CC., McCarthy, EP., Davis, RB., Ngo-Metzger, Q., et al. (2003). Racial and ethnic disparities in cancer screening: the importance of foreign birth as a barrier to care. *Journal of General Internal Medicine*, Vol.18, No.12 (2003 Dec), pp 1028-35.

Hubbell, FA., Chavez, LR., Mishra, SI., Valdez, RB. (1996). Differing beliefs about breast cancer among Latinas and Anglo women. *Western Journal of Medicine* , vol. 164, No. 5 (May 1996), 405–409.

Harlan, LC., Bernstein, AB., Kessler, LG.(1991). Cervical cancer screening: who is not screened and why? *American Journal of Public Health*,Vol.81,No.7 (Jul 1991), pp.885-90.

Eng, E., Parker, E., Harlan, C. (1997) Lay health advisor intervention strategies: a continuum from natural helping to paraprofessional helping. *Health Education & Behavior*, Vol.24, No.4(Aug 1997),pp. 413- 417.

Hoque, M., Ibekwe, CM., Ntuli-Ngcobo, B. Screening and Perceived Severity of Cervical Cancer among Women Attending Mahalapye District Hospital, Botswana . *Asian Pacific Journal of Cancer Prevention, Vol 10 (2009*), 1095-1100.

Hoyo, C., Yarnall, KS H., Skinner, CS., Moorman, PG., Sellers, D. et al (2005). Pain predicts non-adherence to Pap smear screening among middle-aged African American women. *Preventive Medicine*, vol.41,No.2 (Aug 2005),pp. 439-445.

Ibekwe CM, Hoque ME, Ntuli-Ngcobo B (2010). Perceived Benefits of Cervical Cancer Screening among Women Attending Mahalapye District Hospital, Botswana. *Asian Pacific Journal of Cancer Prevention*, Vol. 11,No.4 (2010), pp., *1021*-1027.

Kiefe, CI., Funkhouser, E., Fouad, MN., May, DS. (1998). Chronic disease as a barrier to breast and cervical cancer screening. *Journal of General Internal Medicine*, Vol.13, No.6. (June 1998), pp.357-65.

Leyva, M., Byrd, T., Tarwater, P. (2006). Attitudes towards cervical cancer screening: A study of beliefs among women in Mexico. *Californian Journal of Health Promotion*, Vol. 4, No.2 (2006), pp.13-24.

Lee, M.C. (2000) Knowledge, barriers and motivators related to cervical cancer screening among Korean-American women: a focus group approach. *Cancer Nursing*, Vol. 23, No.3 (June 2000), pp.168–175.

Lofters, A., Glazier, R., Agha, M et al. (2007). Inadequacy of cervical cancer screening among urban recent immigrants: a population-based study of physician and laboratory claims in Toronto, Canada. *Preventive Medicine* Vol. 44, No.6 (2007), 536–42.

McFarland DM (2003). Cervical cancer and pap smear screening in Botswana: knowledge and perception. *International Nursing Review*, Vol, 50, No.3 (Sep 2003),pp.167-75.

Mandelblatt, JS., Gold, K., O'Malley, AS., Taylor, K., Cagney, K. et al.(1999). Breast and cervix cancer screening among multiethnic women: role of age, health, and source of care. *Preventive Medicine*, Vol.28, No.4 (Apr 1999), pp. 418–425

Mandelblatt, JS., Yabroff, KR. (2000). Breast and cervical cancer screening for older women: recommendations and challenges for the 21st century. *Journal of the American Medical Women's Association*, Vol.55,No.4 (Summer 2000) , pp.210–215.

Matuk, LC (1996). Pap smear screening practices in newcomer women. *Women's Health Issues*, Vol.6, No.2(Mar 1996), pp. 82–8.

Mutyaba, T., Mmiro, F., Weiderpass, E. (2006). Knowledge, attitudes and practices on cervical cancer screening among the medical workers of Mulago Hospital, Uganda. *BMC Medical Education*, Vol.6, No.13 (Mar 2006). doi: 10.1186/1472-6920-6-13

Naish, J., Brown, J., Denton, B. (1994). Intercultural consultations: investigation of factors that deter non-English speaking women from attending their general practitioners for cervical screening. *BMJ*, Vol. 309, No. 6962 (Oct 1994), pp.1126-1128.

Obiechina, NJ., Mbamara, SU. (2009). Knowledge, attitude and practice of cervical cancer screening, among sexually active women in Onitsha, southeast Nigeria. *Nigerian Journal of Medicine*, Vol.18, No.4 *(Oct*-Dec 2009), :384-7.

O'Malley, MS., Earp, JA., Hawley, ST., Schell, MJ., Mathews, HF. (2001). The association of race/ethnicity, socioeconomic status, and physician recommendation for mammography: who gets the message about breast cancer screening? *American Journal of Public Health* ,Vol.91, No.1(Jan 2009), pp. 49–54.

Paskett ED., Tatum CM., Ralph, D. Agostino, Jr. et al. (1999). Community-based Interventions to Improve Breast and Cervical Cancer Screening: Results of the Forsyth County (FoCaS) Project: *Cancer Epidemiology Biomarkers & Prevention*, Vol.8 (May 1999), pp. 453-459.

Perez-Stable EJ, Sabogal F, Otero-Sabogal R, Hiatt RA, McPhee SJ. Misconceptions about cancer among Latinos and Anglos. *The Journal of American Medical Association* ,Vol.268, No.62 (1992),pp.3219–3223.

Ross, JS., Nuñez-Smith, M., Forsyth, BA., Rosenbaum, JR.(2008). Racial and ethnic differences in personal cervical cancer screening amongst post-graduate physicians: results from a cross-sectional survey. *BMC Public Health*. 30, Vol.8,No,378 (Oct 2008). doi: 10.1186/1471-2458-8-378

Ross, JS. Forsyth, BA., Rosenbaum, JR(2006). Brief report: House staff adherence to cervical cancer screening recommendations. *Journal of General Internal Medicine.*, Vol. 21, N0.1(Jan 2006), pp.68-70.

Richardson, J., Marks, G., Solis, JM., Collins, LM., Birba, L.(1987). Frequency and adequacy of breast cancer screening among elderly Hispanic women. Preventive Medicine, Vol.16, No.6 (Nov1987), pp. 761–774.

Mullins,R., Wakefield1, M., Broun, K. (2008). Encouraging the right women to attend for cervical cancer screening: results from a targeted television campaign in Victoria. Australia. *Health Education Rresearch,* Vol, 23. No, 3 (Jan 2008), pp .477–486.

Rimer, BK. (1994). Interventions to increase breast screening: lifespan and ethnicity issues. *Cancer*, Vol. 74. No. 1 Suppl. (Jul 1994), pp. 323–328.

Salazar, MK.(1994). Hispanic women's beliefs about breast cancer and mammography. *Cancer Nursing*, Vol.19, No.6 (dec 1996), pp. 437–446.

Sankaranarayanan R, Thara S, Esmy PO, Basu P (2008). Cervical cancer: screening and therapeutic perspectives. *Medical Principal and Practice*, Vol. 17, No.5 (2008), pp.351-64.

Sauvageau, C., Duval, B., Gilca, V., Lavoie, F., Ouakki, M. (2007). Human papilloma virus vaccine and cervical cancer screening acceptability among adults in Quebec, Canada. *BMC Public Health*, Vol.7, No. 304. Published online Oct 2007 25. doi: 10.1186/1471-2458-7-304.

Scarinci, IC., Bandura, L., Hidalgo, B., Cherrington, A.(2011). Development of a Theory-Based (PEN-3 and Health belief model), Culturally Relevant Intervention on Cervical Cancer Prevention among Latina Immigrants Using Intervention Mapping. *Health Promotion Practice*,(Mar 2011). [Epub ahead of print]

Shojaeizadeh, D., Hashemi, Z., Moeini, B., Poorolajal, J. (2011). The Effect of Educational Program on Increasing Cervical Cancer Screening Behavior among Women in Hamadan, Iran: Applying Health belief model. *Journal of Research Health Sciences*, Vol, 11. No, 1 (2011), pp.20-25.

Snyder, L., Hamilton, M., Mitchell, E. et al. (2004).A meta-analysis of the effect of mediated health communication campaigns on behavior change in the United States. Journal of Health Commonunication;Vol. 9, No. Supp 1(2004), pp. 71–96.

Snider, J., Beauvaise, J., Levy, I., Villeneuve, P., Pennock, J. (1996). Trends in mammography and pap smear utilization in Canada. *Chronic Disease in Canada* , Vol.17, No.3-4 (1996). pp.108–117.

Stein, JA. & Fox, SA. Language preference as an indicator of mammography use among Hispanic women. Journal of the Natlonal Cancer Institute Vol 82, No. 21(Nov 1990), pp.1715–1716.

Suarez, L. Nichols, DC. Brady, CA. (1993a). Use of peer role models to increase Pap smear and mammogram screening in Mexican-American and Black women. *American Journal of Preventive Medicine* ;Vol 9, No.5 (Sep-Oct 1993), pp. 290–296.

Suarez, L., Nichols, DC., Pulley, L., Brady, CA., McAlister, A. (1993b). Local health departments implement a theory-based model to increase breast and cervical cancer screening. *Public Health Reports* 1993;Vol .108, No.4 (June 1993), 477–482.

Saslow, D., Runowicz, CD., Solomon, D., Moscicki, AB., Smith, RA. et al. (2002). American cancer society guideline for the early detection of cervical neoplasia and cancer. *A Cancer Journal for Clinicians*, vol.52, No, 6 (2002), pp. 342-362.

Tristen C, Bergstrom S (1996). Cervical cancer in developing countries. A threat to reproductive health. *Lakartidningen*, vol.93, No.39 (Sep 1996), pp.3374-6.

Taylor,VM., Yasui, Y., Burke, N., Nguyen, T., Acorda, E.(2004). Pap testing adherence among Vietnamese American women. *Cancer Epidemiology, Biomarkers & Prevention*, Vol.13,.No.4. (Apr 2004), pp.613-9.

Vellozzi, CJ., Romans, M., Rothenberg, RB. (1996).Delivering breast and cervical cancer screening services to underserved women: Part 1. Literature review and telephone survey. *Women's Health Issues* Vol 6, no.2: (Mar-Aug 1996), pp. 65–73.

Wee, CC., McCarthy, EP., Davis, RB. Phillips, RS. (2000). Screening for cervical and breast cancer: is obesity an unrecognized barrier to preventive care? Annals of Internal Medicine. Vol.132, No. 2 (May 2000), pp. 697-704.

Were, E., Nyaberi, Z., Buziba, N. (2011). Perceptions of risk and barriers to cervical cancer screening at Moi Teaching and Referral Hospital (MTRH), Eldoret, Kenya. *African Health Sciences*, Vol, 11, No,1 (Mar, 2011).pp. 58 - 64.

Winkler, J., Bingham, A., Coffey, P., Handwerker, WP. (2008). Women's participation in a cervical cancer screening program in northern Peru. *Health Education R*esearch, Vol. 23, No.1(Feb 2008) ,pp. 10-24.

Zambrana, RE., Breen, N., Fox, SA., Gutierrez-Mohamed, ML. Use of cancer screening practices by Hispanic women: analyses by subgroup. *Preventive Medicine;* Vol 29, No. 6, (Dec 1999), pp. 466–477.

Zavertnik, JJ. Strategies for reaching poor Blacks and Hispanics in Dade County, Florida. *Cancer*, Vol. 72, No. 3 Suppl(1993 Aug), pp. 1088–1092.

2

Community Based Cancer Screening – The 12 " I "s Strategy for Success*

Rajamanickam Rajkumar
Meenakshi Medical College Hospital and Research Institute, Enathur, Kanchipuram, Tamil Nadu India

1. Introduction

Background of the study, in which the Editor has served as the Investigator at source 1.

Cluster Randomized Controlled Trial of Visual Screening for Cervical Cancer in Dindigul District, Tamil Nadu, India

Supported by the Bill & Melinda Gates Foundation through the Alliance for Cervical Cancer Prevention (ACCP)

Collaborators:

1. Christian Fellowship Community Health Centre (CFCHC), Ambillikai, India
2. Cancer Institute (WIA), Chennai (Madras), India
3. PSG Institute of Medical Sciences and Research (PSGIMSR), Coimbatore, India
4. World Health Organization-International Agency for Research Cancer (WHO-IARC), Lyon, France

A communtiy based screening program was planned and the editor used the following strategies which ensured success.

The 12 " I"s Strategy

> "Our experience in a Community Based Cervical Cancer Screening Programme and the strategies which helped us to be successful"

The 12 " I " s

1. **INITIATION**
2. **INFERENCE**
3. **IMBIBE**
4. **INSTALL**
5. **INSPIRE**
6. **INVOLVEMENT**

---

* Experience and Evidence Based Recommendations for Health Care planners especially in developing countries who undertake Cervical Cancer Screening projects in limited resource settings

7. **INVITE**
8. **INSURE**
9. **INDIGENOUS**
10. **INSTITUTE**
11. **ILLUSTRATE**
12. **IMPROVE**

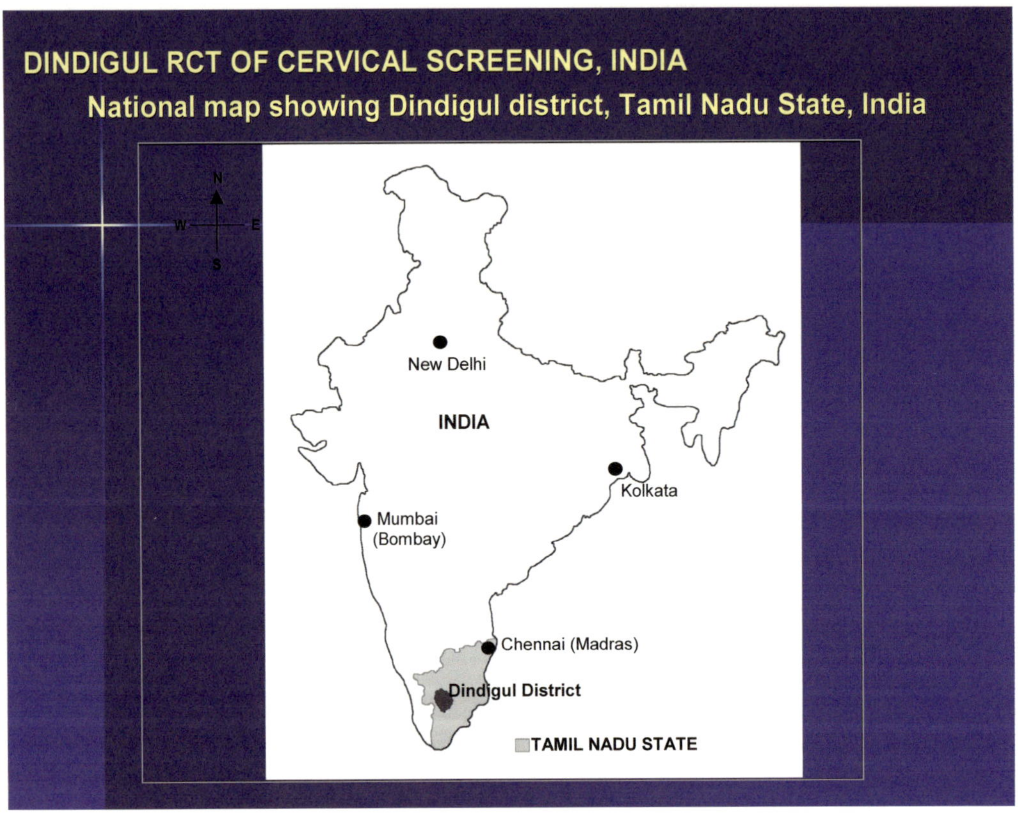

Fig. 1. Geographical location of the study area

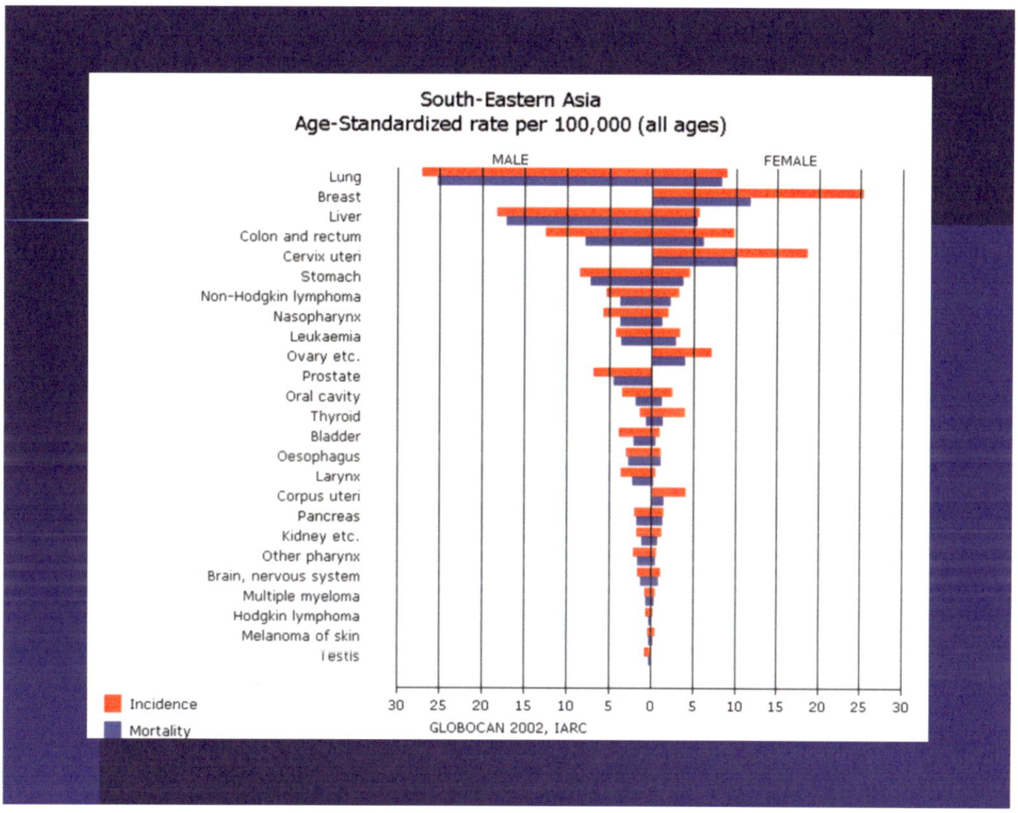

Table 1. Cancer Incidence in SE Asia: The need for screening is based on the following tables, showing high incidence of cervical cancer

World - Females

SITE	Incidence			Mortality			Prevalence		ICD-10
	Cases	Crude Rate	ASR(W)	Deaths	Crude Rate	ASR(W)	1-year	5-year	
Oral cavity	98373	3.2	3.2	46723	1.5	1.5	75769	273356	C00-C08
Nasopharynx	24247	0.8	0.8	15419	0.5	0.5	17786	63235	C11
Other pharynx	24077	0.8	0.8	16029	0.5	0.5	16630	52905	C09-C10,C12-C14
Oesophagus	146723	4.8	4.7	124730	4.1	3.9	54159	129394	C15
Stomach	330518	10.7	10.4	254297	8.3	7.9	166436	522156	C16
Colon and rectum	472687	15.4	14.6	250532	8.1	7.6	362911	1315195	C18-C21
Liver	184043	6.0	5.8	181439	5.9	5.7	46521	111446	C22
Pancreas	107465	3.5	3.3	107479	3.5	3.3	26002	66596	C25
Larynx	20011	0.7	0.6	11327	0.4	0.4	15463	57944	C32
Lung	386891	12.6	12.1	330786	10.7	10.3	162377	423467	C33-C34
Melanoma of skin	81134	2.6	2.6	18829	0.6	0.6	75940	332953	C43
Breast	1151298	37.4	37.4	410712	13.3	13.2	1060042	4406080	C50
Cervix uteri	493243	16.0	16.2	273505	8.9	9.0	381033	1409265	C53
Corpus uteri	198783	6.5	6.5	50327	1.6	1.6	183528	775542	C54
Ovary etc.	204499	6.6	6.6	124860	4.1	4.0	153761	538499	C56,C57.0-4
Kidney etc.	79257	2.6	2.5	39199	1.3	1.2	57234	223235	C64-C66,C68
Bladder	82699	2.7	2.5	36699	1.2	1.1	64673	249966	C67
Brain, nervous system	81264	2.6	2.6	61616	2.0	2.0	37721	118861	C70-C72
Thyroid	103589	3.4	3.3	24078	0.8	0.8	89315	394698	C73
Non-Hodgkin lymphoma	125448	4.1	4.0	72955	2.4	2.3	86221	324184	C82-C85,C96
Hodgkin lymphoma	24111	0.8	0.8	8352	0.3	0.3	20178	87449	C81
Multiple myeloma	39192	1.3	1.2	29839	1.0	0.9	27925	84521	C90
Leukaemia	129485	4.2	4.1	97364	3.2	3.1	68394	221134	C91-C95
All sites but non-melanoma skin	5060657	164.3	161.5	2927896	95.1	92.1	3490957	13022650	C00-C96/C44

Table 2. Cancer Incidence Rates- World – Females

India - Females

SITE	Incidence			Mortality			Prevalence		ICD-10
	Cases	Crude Rate	ASR(W)	Deaths	Crude Rate	ASR(W)	1-year	5-year	
Oral cavity	30906	6.1	7.5	17106	3.4	4.2	22600	77170	*C00-C08*
Nasopharynx	1150	0.2	0.3	841	0.2	0.2	854	2912	*C11*
Other pharynx	7793	1.6	1.8	5858	1.2	1.4	4979	14558	*C09-C10,C12-C14*
Oesophagus	20805	4.1	5.1	17938	3.6	4.4	7418	17442	*C15*
Stomach	11743	2.3	2.8	9962	2.0	2.4	5636	15996	*C16*
Colon and rectum	13555	2.7	3.2	9351	1.9	2.2	9534	33015	*C18-C21*
Liver	4477	0.9	1.1	4264	0.9	1.0	1031	2256	*C22*
Pancreas	3506	0.7	0.8	3073	0.6	0.7	757	2414	*C25*
Larynx	3157	0.6	0.8	2075	0.4	0.5	2246	8081	*C32*
Lung	8046	1.6	2.0	6934	1.4	1.7	2646	6394	*C33-C34*
Melanoma of skin	882	0.2	0.2	471	0.1	0.1	698	2557	*C43*
Breast	82951	16.5	19.1	44795	8.9	10.4	71493	269470	*C50*
Cervix uteri	132082	26.2	30.7	74118	14.7	17.8	101583	370243	*C53*
Corpus uteri	6937	1.4	1.7	2707	0.5	0.7	6046	23584	*C54*
Ovary etc.	21146	4.2	4.9	16319	3.2	3.8	15339	53627	*C56,C57.0-4*
Kidney etc.	2129	0.4	0.5	1459	0.3	0.3	1247	4685	*C64-C66,C68*
Bladder	3031	0.6	0.7	1907	0.4	0.5	2319	8452	*C67*
Brain, nervous system	7530	1.5	1.6	6149	1.2	1.4	3570	10525	*C70-C72*
Thyroid	8686	1.7	1.9	4538	0.9	1.0	7187	31918	*C73*
Non-Hodgkin lymphoma	7389	1.5	1.7	5227	1.0	1.2	4190	14718	*C82-C85,C96*
Hodgkin lymphoma	2155	0.4	0.5	1047	0.2	0.2	1674	6523	*C81*
Multiple myeloma	2525	0.5	0.6	2044	0.4	0.5	1549	4249	*C90*
Leukaemia	9778	1.9	2.1	7977	1.6	1.7	4164	10630	*C91-C95*
All sites but non-melanoma skin	447592	88.8	104.4	284636	56.5	67.6	306532	1089125	*C00-C96/C44*

Mortality: Incidence and survival
Prevalence: Incidence and survival

Crude and Age-Standardised (World) rates, per 100,000
GLOBOCAN 2002, IARC

Table 3. Cancer Incidence Rates – India – Females

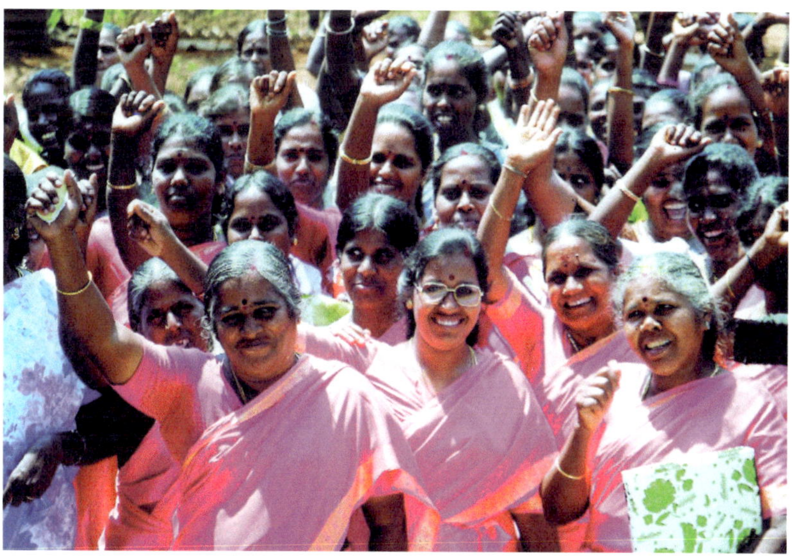

Fig. 2. The women need education and empowerment

2. INITIATION – of cancer registry

- POPULATION BASED CANCER REGISTRY IS A MUST FOR THE SUCCESSFUL IMPLEMENTAION OF A SCREENING PROGRAM
- There are Urban and Rural Population based Cancer registries
- Cancer registry is important to know the cancer pattern
- Priority for preventable cancers by screening, is an important use
- Our Ambillikai Cancer Registry, was population based rural cancer registry in India started in 1995, and its an Associate Member of the International Association of Cancer Registries

3. INFERENCE – of the cancer pattern

- Leads for the planning of control strategies
- Ambillikai cancer registry recorded one of the highest ASR for cancer cervix (65.4/ 100 000)
- This gave the lead for a community based cervical cancer screening programme

Supported by our publication:
"Leads to cancer control based on cancer patterns in a rural population in South India"
R.Rajkumar, R.Sankaranarayanan, A.Esmi, R.Jeyaraman, J.Cherian & D.M.Parkin,
Cancer Causes and Control 2000; 11:433-39

4. IMBIBE – the appropriate technology

- Developing countries can seek technical support from developed nations
- Low resource settings need appropriate, affordable and accessible technologies
- Technical & Financial constraints to be overcome by resource development
- In rural India - Cervical Cancer Screening was not a health care priority
- Hence we offered once a life time - VIA, Colposcopy
- High risk approach is needed for selected population
- 80% PARTICIPATION was targeted, and achieved

Supported by our publication:
"Effective screening programmes for cervical cancer in low-and middle - income developing countries"
Rengasamy Sankaranarayanan, Atul Madhukar Budukh, Rajamanickam Rajkumar,
Bulletein World Health Organisation, 2001, 79(10) 954-962

5. INSTALL – resources

- Political Will & Commitment
- Manpower - train local health staff
- Materials - locally available equipments and local maintenance expertise
- Money - internal and/or external funds

Supported by our publication:
"Early detection of cervical cancer with visual inspection methods, A summary of completed and on - going studies in India".

R.Sankaranarayanan , IARC/WHO, B.M. Nene , K.Dinshaw , R.Rajkumar , S.Shastri , R.Wesley ,P.Basu , R.Sharma , S.Thara , A.Budukh , D.M. Parkin , IARC/WHO
Public Health Journal of Mexico (Revista de Salud Publica de Mexico)

In commemoration with 80th Anniversary School of Public Health & 15th Anniversary National
Institute of Public Health, Mexico, July 2002

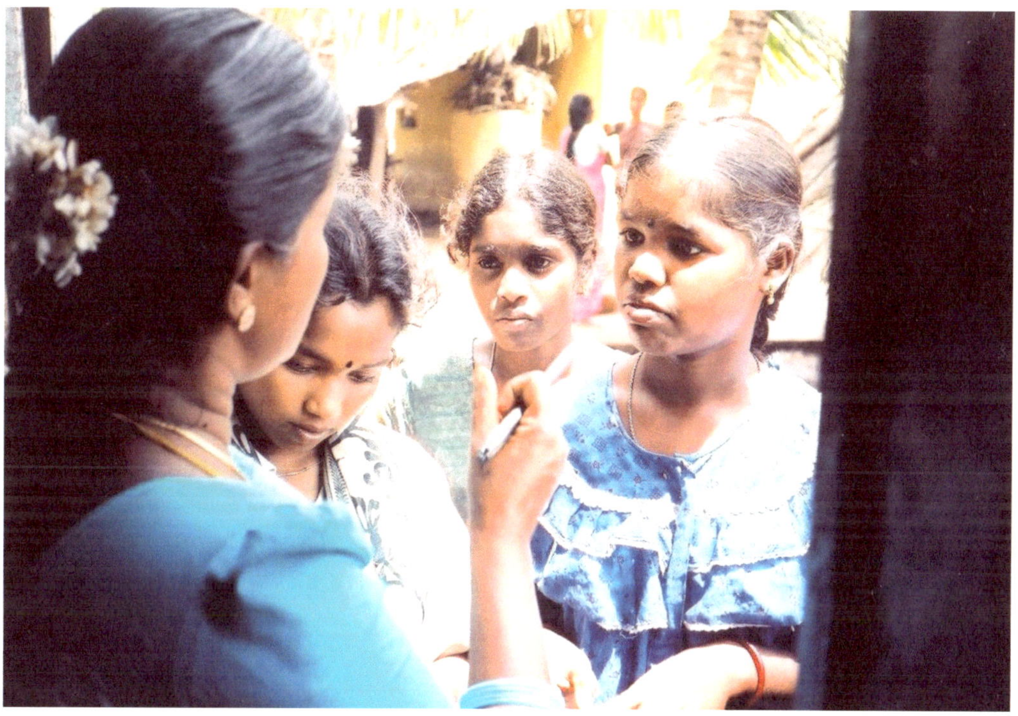

Fig. 3. Use local manpower

6. INSPIRE – personnel

- Lighted to lighten, the health care providers play key role
- Financial incentives, motivates them
- Social recognition is very important in team work
- Appreciation means a lot for the workers
- Awards, titles, honours, cost little but the gain is big

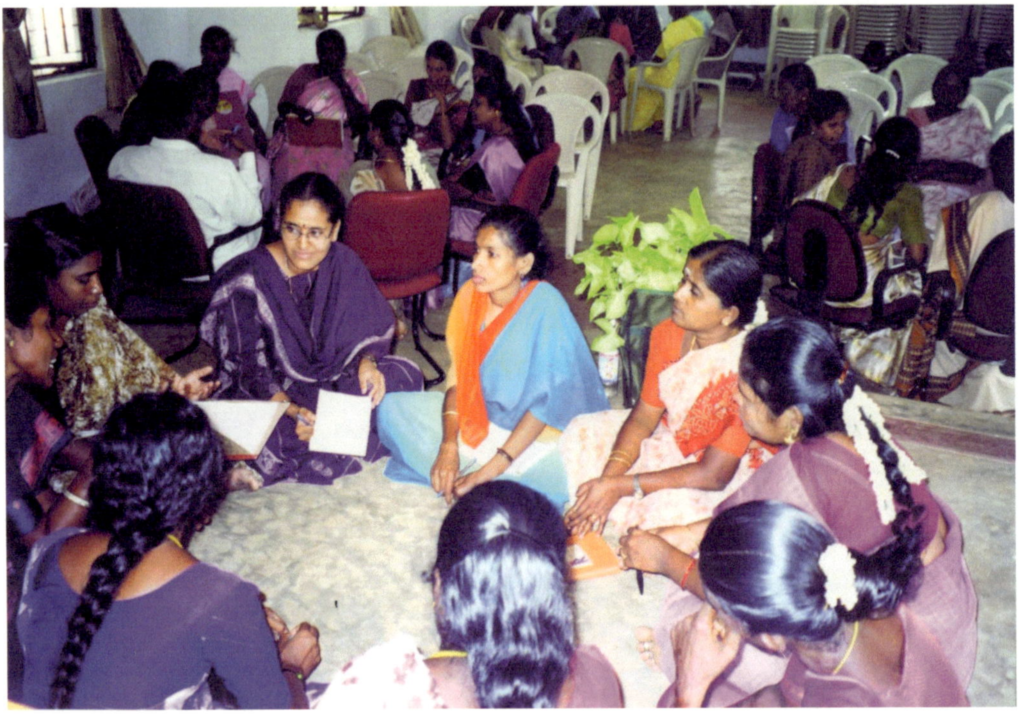

Fig. 4. Inspiration and motivation of the Health care providers ensure success

- Even in the Olympics it is a small "MEDAL" which matters

7. INVOLVEMENT

- Involve both " providers" & "recipients"
- All levels of micro & macro planning
- All levels of implementation
- When we hear we forget
- When we see we remember
- When we do we know

8. INVITE

- It is humans' innate desire to be invited for participation
- Advertisements, Propaganda, Bombardment with information - may not work
- Invitation with genuine Interest by Influencers works well

Methods of Invitation

- Mass - Appeal to "Emotions" - Use the words "Mothers", " Wives", "Sisters" instead of Women
- Families - Appeal to "Responsibilities" of the family towards the motherhood and their duty for " mother's" health
- Individuals - Appeal to their "self care and self esteem"

Who would invite ?

- The "Influencers"
- Medical personnel, village leaders, religious leaders, local healers, teachers
- Satisfied Customers
- Peer groups
- Family members
- Educating the school children have resulted in them bringing their mothers for screening - "tender roots split hard rock"

9. INSURE – holistic health

- Rural community does not appreciate "organ specific approach"
- Wholesome approach for holistic health is the demand
- Do whatever possible for total care - even counseling and advice are well received
- Health is a state of complete physical, mental and social well being and not merely an absence of disease or infirmity - Health for All

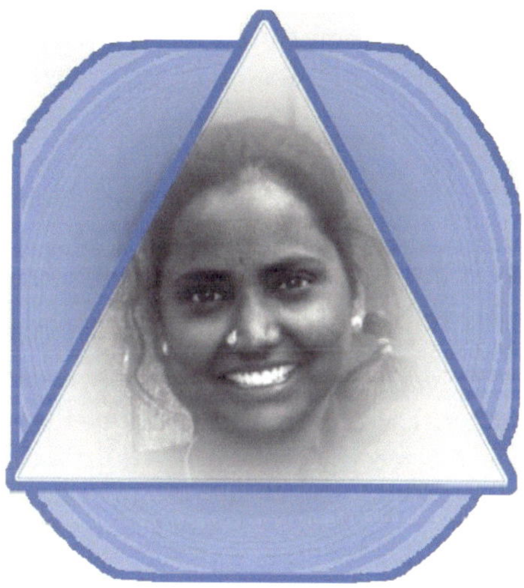

Fig. 5. A woman expects holistic health care from the provider

10. INDIGENOUS

- In thoughts, words and deeds
- "Cancer" is scaring, terrifying and people are afraid to get diagnosed as to have cancer
- Start from what they know and build from what they have
- Address their common complaints like "wdpv", "abnormal bleeding pv" and then explain about precancer and cancer.
- Perform VIA, colposcopy and cryotherapy/LEEP and the "women get rid of their complaints" and we have done our "screening for cervical cancer" . Thus we have made the very "problem" as "indigenous"

Indigenous - Screening Environment

- People in villages are reluctant to get in to the huge vans or buses for screening as these are unusual environments to them
- Hence, screening clinics could be arranged in places which are frequently visited by the people, like health centre buildings, schools, ration shops, public utility buildings

Indigenous – Health personnel

- Like begets like
- Birds of the same feather flock together
- Screening could be done by trained local nurses and health workers
- Examination - Female to female and male to male
- Identification with the people in all possible ways ensures good compliance

Indigenous in attitude

- Never say that the other is wrong, only that they may not be right
- Never call the local customs, beliefs, hopes, attitudes and practices as superstitions. It will hurt the feelings. Just guide them rightly.
- Screening clinics should ensure privacy, confidentiality in a pleasant atmosphere.
- All services under one roof and cordial relationship to be maintained
- No outside prescriptions, referrals
- Counsel the family as a whole, whenever possible

11. INSTITUTE – follow up

- In rural India, people greet each other by asking " How are you ? "
- People appreciate this gesture very much as it coveys one's concern and regard
- If this is done in a scientific way it is called the " follow up ", and it should be done meticulously and frequently. The possible outcomes of the screening should be well explained before hand and the need for passive follow up should be well understood by the beneficiaries and their families.

How we tackled some of the problems!

Post cryotherapy period

↓

Long term serous discharge

↓

Very distressing for women

↓

Good sign of healing "Ice" melting

↓

Convinced

Post Cryo - LEEP period

↓

Long period of sexual abstinence

↓

Husbands' uncooperative

↓

Abstinence for religious reasons , Abstinence during jaundice

↓

Convinced

Problem Solving

- Dialogues, Discussions would definitely Dissolve many of the Deterrent factors
- Communication gap closes the doors
- Careful and considerate listening are very important for community based programmes
- Counseling increases the community's compliance for the programme

Determinants of Participation

- Educational level
- Social status
- Economic status
- Type of family
- Severity of the disease
- Satisfactory services

Supported by our publication:
"Determinants of participation of women in a cervical cancer visual screening trial in rural south India"
Rengaswamy Sankaranarayanan, Rajamanickam Rajkumar, Silvina Arrossi, Rajapandian Theresa, Pulikattil Okkaru Esmy, Cerdric Mahe, Richard Muwonge, Donald Maxwell Parkin, Jacob Cherian
Cancer Detection and Prevention 27 (2003) 457 - 465

12. ILLUSTRATE – study findings

- The above strategies helped us to successfully complete one of the largest cervical cancer screening programmes done in rural areas.

Supported by our publication:
"Initial results from a randomized trial of Cervical Visual Screening in rural South India".
R. Sankaranarayanan. R. Rajkumar, et al.
International Journal of Cancer 2004; 109, 461 - 467

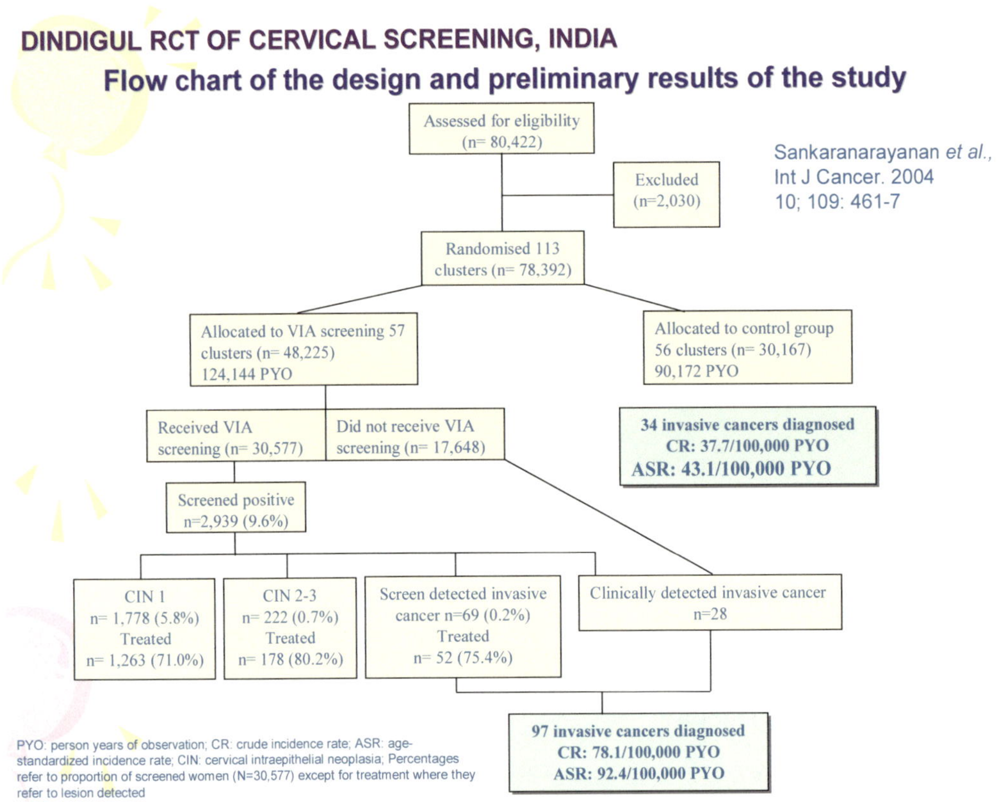

Fig. 6.

13. IMPROVE

Successful completion of a program improves capabilities of the health care providers and it leads to further research, like our other studies:

HPV Studies:

Study 1

Papillomavirus infection in rural women in southern India
Franceschi, R Rajkumar, PJF Snijders, A Arslan1, C Mahe, M Plummer, R Sankaranarayanan, J Cherian, CJLM Meijer and E Weiderpass, **British Journal of Cancer (2005) 92, 601 - 606**

Study 2

Worldwide distribution of HPV Types in Cytologically Normal Women: Pooled Analysis of the IARC HPV Prevalence Surveys
G. Clifford (PhD), S. Gallus (ScD), R. Herrero (MD), N. Muñoz (MD), P.J.F. Snijders (PhD), S. Vaccarella (ScD), P.T.H Anh (MD), C. Ferreccio (MD), N.T Hieu (MD), E. Matos (MD), M. Molano (PhD), R. Rajkumar (MD), G. Ronco (MD), S. de Sanjosé (MD), H.R. Shin (MD), S. Sukvirach (MD), J.O. Thomas (MD), S. Tunsakul (MS), C.J.L.M. Meijer (MD), S. Franceschi (MD) and the IARC HPV Prevalence Surveys (IHPS) Study Group, **Lancet 2005;366(9490):991-8.**

Study 3

HPV vaccine trial
"Preparation of a large, simple "phase IV" study of anti- HPV Vaccination in Asia"
Silvia Franceschi IARC/WHO, Richard Peto, T.Rajkumar, R.Rajkumar, Rengaswamy Sankaranarayanan, Soina Pagliusi, Teresa Aguado & Thomas Cherian, **Scientific Paper Submitted to the HPV International Conference - Floriano polis - June 2001.**

14. References

The editor is happy to enlist all his publications for further reference :

SCIENTIFIC PAPERS PUBLISHED IN PEER REVIEWED INTERNATIONAL JOURNALS

[1] Wright Thomas C; Blumenthal Paul; Bradley Janet; Denny Lynette; Esmy Pulikattil Okkaru; Jayant Kasturi; Nene Bhagwan M; Pollack Amy E; Rajkumar Rajamanickam; Sankaranarayanan Rengaswamy; Sellors John W; Shastri Surendra S; Sherris Jacqueline; Tsu Vivien Cervical cancer prevention for all the world's women: new approaches offer opportunities and promise. Diagnostic cytopathology 2007;35(12):845-8.

[2] Sankaranarayanan Rengaswamy; Esmy Pulikkottil Okkuru; Rajkumar Rajamanickam; Muwonge Richard; Swaminathan Rajaraman; Shanthakumari Sivanandam; Fayette Jean-Marie; Cherian Jacob Effect of visual screening on cervical cancer incidence and mortality in Tamil Nadu, India: a cluster-randomised trial. Lancet 2007; 370(9585):398-406.

[3] Sankaranarayanan R; Rajkumar R; Esmy P O; Fayette J M; Shanthakumary S; Frappart L; Thara S; Cherian J Effectiveness, safety and acceptability of 'see and treat' with cryotherapy by nurses in a cervical screening study in India. British journal of cancer 2007;96(5):738-43.

[4] Franceschi Silvia; Herrero Rolando; Clifford Gary M; Snijders Peter J F; Arslan Annie; Anh Pham Thi Hoang; Bosch F Xavier; Ferreccio Catterina; Hieu Nguyen Trong; Lazcano Ponce Eduardo; Matos Elena; Molano Monica; Qiao You-Lin; Rajkumar Raj; Ronco Guglielmo; de Sanjosé Silvia; Shin Hai-Rim; Sukvirach Sukhon; Thomas Jaiye O; Meijer Chris J L M; Muñoz Nubia Variations in the age-specific curves of human papillomavirus prevalence in women worldwide. International Journal of Cancer. Journal international du cancer 2006;119(11):2677-84.

[5] Vaccarella Salvatore; Herrero Rolando; Dai Min; Snijders Peter J F; Meijer Chris J L M; Thomas Jaiye O; Hoang Anh Pham Thi; Ferreccio Catterina; Matos Elena; Posso Hector; de Sanjosé Silvia; Shin Hai-Rim; Sukvirach Sukhon; Lazcano-Ponce Eduardo; Ronco Guglielmo; Rajkumar Raj; Qiao You-Lin; Muñoz Nubia; Franceschi Silvia Reproductive factors, oral contraceptive use, and human papillomavirus infection: pooled analysis of the IARC HPV prevalence surveys. Cancer epidemiology, biomarkers & prevention : a publication of the American Association for Cancer Research, cosponsored by the American Society of Preventive Oncology 2006;15(11):2148-53.. vaccarella@iarc.fr

[6] Clifford G M; Gallus S; Herrero R; Muñoz N; Snijders P J F; Vaccarella S; Anh P T H; Ferreccio C; Hieu N T; Matos E; Molano M; Rajkumar R; Ronco G; de Sanjosé S;

Shin H R; Sukvirach S; Thomas J O; Tunsakul S; Meijer C J L M; Franceschi S; Worldwide distribution of human papillomavirus types in cytologically normal women in the International Agency for Research on Cancer HPV prevalence surveys: a pooled analysis. Lancet 2005;366(9490):991-8.

[7] Franceschi S; Rajkumar R; Snijders P J F; Arslan A; Mahé C; Plummer M; Sankaranarayanan R; Cherian J; Meijer C J L M; Weiderpass E Papillomavirus infection in rural women in southern India. British journal of cancer 2005;92(3):601-6.

[8] Sankaranarayanan Rengaswamy; Rajkumar Rajamanickam; Theresa Rajapandian; Esmy Pulikattil Okkaru; Mahe Cedric; Bagyalakshmi Karur R; Thara Somanathan; Frappart Lucien; Lucas Eric; Muwonge Richard; Shanthakumari S; Jeevan D; Subbarao T M; Parkin Donald Maxwell; Cherian Jacob Initial results from a randomized trial of cervical visual screening in rural south India. International Journal of Cancer. Journal international du cancer 2004;109(3):461-7.

[9] Sankaranarayanan R; Nene B M; Dinshaw K; Rajkumar R; Shastri S; Wesley R; Basu P; Sharma R; Thara S; Budukh A; Parkin D M Early detection of cervical cancer with visual inspection methods: a summary of completed and on-going studies in India. Salud pública de México 2003;45 Suppl 3():S399-407.

[10] Sankaranarayanan Rengaswamy; Rajkumar Rajamanickam; Arrossi Silvina; Theresa Rajapandian; Esmy Pulikattil Okkaru; Mahé Cédric; Muwonge Richard; Parkin Donald Maxwell; Cherian Jacob Determinants of participation of women in a cervical cancer visual screening trial in rural south India. Cancer detection and prevention 2003;27(6):457-65.

[11] Sankaranarayanan R; Budukh A M; Rajkumar R Effective screening programmes for cervical cancer in low- and middle-income developing countries. Bulletin of the World Health Organization 2001;79(10):954-62.

[12] Rajkumar R; Sankaranarayanan R; Esmi A; Jayaraman R; Cherian J; Parkin D M Leads to cancer control based on cancer patterns in a rural population in South India. Cancer causes & control : CCC 2000;11(5):433-9.

3

Challenges to Cervical Cancer in the Developing Countries: South African Context

Nokuthula Sibiya
Durban University of Technology,
Head of Nursing Department, Durban
South Africa

1. Introduction

Despite the fact that cancer of the cervix is preventable, it is the commonest cancer cause of death in women in sub-Saharan Africa, Melanesia, South Central and South East Asia, the Caribbean and Latin America (Parkin et al., 2005). Southern Africa has one of the highest incident rates in the world, and in South Africa alone it caused the deaths of 3 700 women in 2002 (Denny, 2006). According to the International Agency for Research on Cancer (IARC), cervical cancer accounts for 23% of all cancers diagnosed in South Africa (International Agency for Research on Cancer, 2006 as cited in le Riche, 2006). Cervical cancer is the second most common cancer among South African women, with 1 in 41 women developing the disease in her lifetime (Sitas et al., 1998). Adar & Stevens (2000) noted that it was responsible for nearly 2% of deaths of women aged 15-44 years and 4% of women aged 45-59 years. In South Africa, the total age-adjusted incidence rate (ASIR) of cancer in Africans is far lower than that in the corresponding white population. According to the KwaZulu-Natal Department of Health (2004) in South Africa, cervical cancer accounts for 18.5% of female cancers, with approximately 5 000 new cases reported annually and black women being most at risk of getting cervical cancer compared to white and coloured women. African women seek help only when their particular disorder/disease is far advanced, thereby, as in the case of cervical cancer, rendering cure or control nearly impossible (Walker et al., 2002). A study done by De Jonge et al. (1999) found more aggressive tumours in black women compared to white women with cervical cancer in South Africa. In women of all race groups, the age specific cervical cancer rates for 1992 remained low up to 30 years of age, but thereafter increased rapidly until they peaked at 50 to 59 years (Denny, 2006). Similarly, Sitas et al. (1998) reported that the incidence of invasive cancer rises in the age group 35-39, with 87% of cases occurring in women over 35 years of age. It is a common cancer in poor women due to inadequate mass cervical cancer screening, and their cure rates are low as they present late (Denny, 2006).

The South African National Department of Health identified cervical cancer as a health priority and in 2000 introduced a national screening programme, based on models of the natural history of the disease (Department of Health, 2000). The cervical screening policy states that every woman attending public sector health services is entitled to three free smears from the age of 30 years at intervals of ten years provided no smears have been taken within the previous five years and a total of three smears will be taken in a woman's lifetime. The starting age was based on the fact that the disease affects women in early to late middle age. The goal is to screen 70% of women in the target age group within 10 years of initiating the programme. This model aims to decrease cancer incidence by 64% (Miller, 1992 as cited in Smith et al., 2003). According to Walraven (2003), cervical cancer develops slowly. Invasive cancer is usually preceded by long phases of pre-invasive disease (Sankaranarayanan & Wesley, 2003) and high-grade dysplasia can generally be detected 10 years before cancer develops (Population Reference Bureau & Alliance for Cervical Cancer Screening, 2004). It is widely believed that that invasive cervical cancer develops from dysplastic precursor lesions, progressing steadily from mild to moderate to severe dysplasia, then to carcinoma in situ, and finally to cancer. Based on resource considerations and best available evidence, the policy adopted a public health approach by targeting the age group most at risk of developing high-grade, precursor lesions of the cervix. The policy conformed to the recommendations of the World Health Organization [WHO] (1999 as cited in Smith et al., 2003) for the screening protocol for regions with limited resource.

There has been much debate as to the most suitable screening policy, particularly with age commencement and appropriate time intervals between smears. A number of studies revealed that nurses were opposed to and misunderstood the screening policy, probably limiting the performance of screening (Smith & Hoffman, 2000; Smith et al., 2003; Sibiya & Grainger, 2010). They were of the opinion that women should have their first smears at the age of 20 and thereafter at intervals of five years because women become sexually active at an early age. Screening programmes are effective provided that they are well organized (le Riche et al., 2006; Gaym et al., 2007). The aim of cervical cytology screening programme is to detect pre-malignant lesions on the transformation zone of the cervix. Those patients with abnormal cytologic results are then referred for further management, usually at dedicated colposcopy clinics. The current referral criteria are a single smear with a high-grade squamous intra-epithelial lesion (HSIL) or two low-grade squamous intra-epithelial lesion (LSIL) smears. The aim of colposcopy is to detect the most abnormal area on the cervix and to direct the clinician to the area of biopsy.

2. Cervical cytology screening programmes in developing countries

Cervical cytology screening programmes have been introduced in low- and middle-income developing countries, but generally have achieved very limited success (WHO, 2001). Although cytological screening is being carried out in some developing countries, there are no organized programmes. As a result, there has been a very limited impact on the incidence of cervical cancer, despite the large numbers of cytological smears taken in some countries such as Cuba and Mexico (Sankaranarayanan et al., 2001). Only 5% of women in developing countries undergo cervical screening compared with 40-50% in the developed world. Substantial costs are involved in providing the infrastructure, manpower, follow up and surveillance for cervical screening programmes. Owing to their limited health care resources, developing countries cannot afford the models of frequently repeated screening of women over a wide age range that is used in developed countries (Sankaranarayanan et al., 2001). Cervical cancer has been described as "a disease of the economically disadvantaged" because even in developed countries such as the United States, cervical cancer mostly affects women of low socio-economic status, rural and poor women (Dickson-

Tetteh, 1998). Lower socio-economic status has been associated with higher risk of developing cancer probably due to lack of access to good health care and screening programmes (Mqoqi, 2003). Barriers to screening uptake include a lack of knowledge about the disease, the geographical and economic inaccessibility of care, the poor quality of services and lack of support from families. Abrahams et al. (1996) state that in order for the cervical screening programme to be successful, among other things, strategies in low-resource settings should be socially and culturally appropriate.

3. Cervical screening in South Africa

South Africa, one of the better-resourced countries in sub-Saharan Africa provides opportunistic screening. Despite the existence of the guidelines, difficulties have occurred with the implementation of the South African cervical screening programme. A number of attempts were made in the past to introduce cervical screening programmes at national, provincial and local levels in South Africa. In the 1970s the Department of Health suggested that a Pap smear should be taken only if the cervix appears abnormal (Performance of the National Health System [NHS] Cervical Screening Programme in England, 1998 as cited by Hoffman et al., 2003). A number of cervical screening programmes that were introduced in the 1980s failed due to poor attendance of women at the health services. The findings of the study that was conducted by Abrahams et al. (1996) revealed that the poor attendance of women was due to lack of knowledge about cervical cancer and the significance of cancer screening. Fonn (2003) reported that implementation was slow, whilst Moodley et al., (2006) found that cervical screening in the public health service was conducted in an ad hoc manner and focused on younger women attending family planning and ante natal services. In South Africa, women have access to cervical screening at primary health care (PHC) clinics. The clinics serve a demarcated area and offer a variety of services. Due to the demand of services, it is not possible to concentrate on the prevention of cervical cancer, as cervical screening is one aspect of the total services rendered. This is a great concern given that the likelihood of reducing the incidence of cervical cancer is dependent upon a well-organized programme. A study was conducted in the eThekwini Region, previously named Ilembe in the province of KwaZulu Natal on the evaluation of the implementation of the cervical screening programme in PHC clinics (Sibiya & Grainger, 2007). This study consisted of a record review, a clinic audit and focus group discussions with the nurses. The findings confirmed that follow-up of clients was problematic, referral hospital feedback was poor, record keeping was inadequate, and rural clinics lacked resources. Despite the positive aspects, such as the good quality of smears and adequate drugs, the problems overall would have resulted in an ineffective programme. The following factors have been identified as the contributory factors to ineffective screening in South Africa:

3.1 Shortage of health care workers

According to the South African cervical screening policy, all service providers are expected to participate in the screening programme (Department of Health, 2000). The South African screening policy states that women should have Pap smears at least once every 10 years as from the age of 30 years. Therefore, the annual number of women requiring a Pap smear is the total number in the province divided by 10. It is worth noting that the finding of the study that was conducted by Fonn (2003) revealed that in order to achieve 100% coverage of women eligible for screening over a 10-year period, each nurse would have to perform on average less than one Pap smear per day. This author further argues that there is spare capacity and that any potential underestimate in the number of Pap smears required per year could be relatively easily accommodated. According to the Department of Health (2006) nurses constitute the largest professional group in South Africa's health care services and form the backbone of PHC in South Africa. Nurses provide the bulk of service provision in the public health sector. This emphasis is most striking at the primary care level. Given the emphasis the need for well-trained primary level staff is imperative. The South African yearbook (2004/05) states that patients visiting PHC clinics are treated mainly by PHC-trained nurses, or at some clinics, by doctors yet according to the Department of Health (2004) only about 40% of facilities have PHC qualified nurses. This means that the pace of training has been slower than planned. However, migration of nurses has also impacted on these figures. The gross shortage of health workers in developing countries may be a further limitation to effective screening.

A number of research studies have attempted to explore the 'push and pull' factors that lead to South African nurses working in other countries. Emigration is a commonly cited cause of PHC attrition rate in South Africa. Migration of health personnel, also dubbed the brain drain, partly from rural to urban areas, but more particularly out of the country, has become a debated issue in human resource circles not only in South Africa, but also on the continent of Africa itself. According to the Department of Health (2006) for many years before 1994 South Africa constituted a preferred destination for many health professionals, the majority being doctors from the African continent. This situation has however changed since the late 1990's when a policy of not recruiting from fellow developing African countries was adopted at the Southern African Development Community (SADC) Health Minister's level. The findings of the study that was done by Oosthuizen & Ehlers (2007) indicated that nurses' inadequate remuneration, poor working conditions, excessive workloads, lack of personal growth and career advancement possibilities were major factors that influenced nurses' decision to emigrate. Lucas (2005) argues that although African countries have a shortage of health workers, they continue to migrate from Africa to more developed countries. Tarimo (1991) argues that it is unrealistic to expect good performances under the difficult conditions from workers who are poorly rewarded. However, financial incentives alone are insufficient to improve health worker motivation. Investing in a functional health care system in which nurses feel motivated to work is an important part of human resource planning.

The capacity to read cervical smears at public sector laboratory level is limited in South Africa. The South African guidelines indicate that cyto-technologists reading population-based smears are expected to screen six smears per hour and to work for no longer than 8 hours per day, i.e. total of 48 smears per day. Thus if all technologists employed by the state only read cervical smears we would have just enough technologists employed in the public sector. However, they also have other smears to read (Fonn, 2003). It is important to note that if the first smear is done at the age of 20 years, it would mean that the annual number of smears would increase from 85 0740 to 127 5016. This would mean that cyto-technicians would have to read 69 smears per day. The capacity to read the cervical smears at public sector laboratory is limited (Fonn, 2003). In developing countries, because of lack of the trained cyto-technicians, there is often a long interval of 1-3 months between the Pap screening and when the test result is available (Jeronimo et al., 2005). This is further supported by the findings of the study that was conducted by Moodley et al. (2006) which revealed that long cytology turnaround time is attributed to poorly functioning administrative and transportation systems. The study that was conducted by Denny et al, (2006) revealed that a large number of women did not return for the cervical screening results. Cytology-based screening programmes can only be successful if infrastructure is in place and laboratory quality assurance is consistent (Alliance for Cervical Cancer Prevention, 2004).

3.2 Poor system of follow up and referral process

The South African policy on cervical screening maintains that a working follow-up system needs to be in place for effective implementation of the cervical screening programme (Department of Health, 2000). The policy further states that the time lapse between screening and follow-up should be 1–4 weeks depending on the circumstances and every attempt possible should be made to find those patients who do not return voluntarily. The results of the study that was done in the KwaZulu-Natal province of South Africa revealed that there was poor follow up of patients with abnormal smears and that if patients were referred to the hospital from the PHC settings there was no feedback that was provided to the clinic (Sibiya & Grainger, 2007). Lack of capacity in terms of infrastructure and human resources were cited as factors for poor follow up and referral process. However, the findings of the study that was conducted by Nene et al., (2007) showed that the lowest compliance rate with follow-up care was found among unmarried women, those with low level of education and those with a high number of pregnancies. Some studies have reported that women with abnormal screening results were confused and did not understand the information provided by the nurse (Kavanagh et al., 1997; Yabroff et al., 2000 as cited in by Nene et al., 2007).

There are also challenges regarding the referral process of women with abnormal smears for further investigation and management.When the protocol for cervical screening was evaluated in the province of KwaZulu-Natal, the results reveled that none of the 88 reviewed documents showed evidence of feedback from the referral hospital (Sibiya & Grainger, 2007). Interview data with nurses revealed that none of the referral hospital provided feedback to the referral hospital. This means that there was lack of effective liaison with referral centres for diagnosis and treatment to ensure follow-up and monitoring. According to Smith and Hoffman (2000) nurses work diligently to achieve good rates of follow-up but there is one group of women that they cannot monitor, namely those with high-grade lesions. Once a woman is referred for colposcopy, the nurses do not receive feedback regarding whether she kept her appointment, or what the outcome was. This is further supported by the findings of a study that was done by Abraham et al. (1996) where the health workers expressed disappointment that they continued to not receive feedback from hospital specialists to whom they referred women found to have abnormal smears, which merited further clinical investigations. The only way that feedback of a referral to a hospital was gained was that all patients were encouraged to report back to the clinic to give information as to the outcome of their hospital visit. Improving communication would allow the nurses to remain involved with their clients, and help to ensure that follow-up takes place. The referring doctor has a responsibility to the woman to ensure that she has fully understood the significance of her abnormal smear, the options for evaluation and management of that smear, and has been involved in the decision-making.

3.3 The impact of HIV and AIDS

The growing number of women in resource-poor areas, such as sub-Saharan Africa, who have immunodeficiency virus (HIV), appears to compound the problem because they have an increased risk of human papillomavirus (HPV) infection, the causal agent of cervical cancer (Goldie et al., 2001). South Africa remains one of the countries with a high HIV and AIDS prevalence rate - there are currently about 5.27 million people who are infected with HIV and AIDS in South Africa (UNAIDS, 2008). About 70% of the HIV positive pregnant women attending antenatal clinics are below the age of 30 years (Department of Health, 2007). The prevalence rate among young people aged 20-24 years was estimated to be 30%, with the highest prevalence rate of about 40% being among women aged 25-29 years. Cervical cancer is regarded as an important AIDS-related disease and since 1993 has been considered as an AIDS-defining illness in women with HIV virus (KwaZulu-Natal Department of Health, 2004). HIV positive women have a high rate of persistent HPV infections, and a higher rate than HIV negative women with the types of HPV that are associated with the development of high grade dysplasia and cervical cancer (Hoytt, 1998). HIV-positive women are almost five times more likely to present with dysplasia than HIV-negative women (KwaZulu-Natal Department of Health, 2004). One case-controlled case study reported that 60% of HPV positive women had initiated sex prior to reaching 16 years old. The report further stated that this may expose women to STIs, which may lower a woman's immune response and contribute to malignant transformation of HPV infections (Kenney, 1994).

Of particular concern was the lack of acceptance of the age at first screening criterion. According to the findings of the study that was conducted by Smith et al (2003), of the interviewed nurses, 90% were that some screening policy exists, and 57% could correctly state the policy. However, all the participants were of the opinion that women should have their first smear at the start of the sexual activity, which is at the age of 20 years, and the interval period should be five years due to high rate of HIV/AIDS in this province. They argued that there was an association between cervical cancer and HIV/AIDS and STIs hence younger women were at risk. This is in contrast with what the policy states as discussed above (Sibiya & Grainger, 2010). Many health professionals feel that as a result of the increased incidence of HIV/AIDS and sexually transmitted infections (STIs), younger women are at risk of getting cervical cancer (Kenney, 1994; KwaZulu-Natal Department of Health, 1999). Smith & Hoffman (2000) reported that approximately half of the nurses they sampled in Mitchell's Plain, Cape Town were of the opinion that women should have their smears done at the start of sexual activity, whilst a quarter thought that this should occur when the woman is under the age of 30 years. The participants in our study also believed that the age for first smear should be lowered to 20 years and that they should be repeated at five year intervals thereafter. They recommended this because of the high rate of HIV/AIDS in this province. Such sentiments have been criticized on the grounds that the nurses do not understand the natural course of the disease or the rationale behind the screening programme (Fonn, 2003; Smith et al., 2003). Worth noting are the results of the study that was conducted in the province of KwaZulu-Natal in South Africa by Gaym et al. (2007), which revealed that all the high-grade squamous intra-epithelial lesions occurred in women younger than 30 years of age, which is much lower than the usual age distribution for high grade lesions (around 35-40 years of age).

4. Recommended measures to improve screening programmes in developing countries

Many low-income developing countries currently have neither the financial and manpower resources nor the capacity in their health services to organize and sustain a screening programme of any sort (Sankaranarayanan et al., 2001). Efforts to organize effective screening programmes in developing countries will have to find adequate financial resources, develop the infrastructure, train the needed manpower, and elaborate surveillance mechanisms for screening, investigating, treating and follow-up of the targeted women. The following measures need to be put in place in order to improve cervical screening in developing countries:

4.1 Effective screening tests

The developing countries should consider cost effective screening test to use. Newer alternative methods for cervical screening have being developed and tested (Denny, et al., 2000; Goldie et al., 2006; Sankaranarayanan et al., 1998). These include DNA testing for HPVand visual inspection with acetic acid (VIA). The most promising of these being DNA testing for HPV as cervical cancer is caused mainly by HPV. The key barriers to HPV testing in developing countries are the costs and technical requirements associated with the test (Sankaranarayanan et al., 2005). VIA also called cervicoscopy, consists of naked eye visualization of the uterine cervix after the application of diluted acetic acid, to screen for cervical abnormalities. A solution of 3% to 5% acetic acid is used, and the cervix is illuminated with a light source and the purpose is to identify aceto-white areas which may indicate tissue undergoing precancerous changes (Sankaranarayanan et al., 1998). A study of the cost effectiveness of several cervical cancer screening strategies, based on the South African experience, indicated that strategies using VIA or HPV DNA testing may offer attractive alternatives to cytology-based screening programmes in low-resource settings (Goldie et al., 2001). In developing countries, because of the lack of trained cytotechnologists and cytology laboratories, there is often a long interval (1-3 months) between the Pap screenings and when the test result is available. VIA has the advantage of requiring only low-technology equipment and the result is available immediately (Jeronimo et al., 2005). Therefore, the treatment of abnormal lesions can be done during the same consultation. This is further supported by the findings of the study that was conducted by Goldie et al., (2005) which revealed that VIA or HPV DNA testing offer cost-effective alternatives to conventional cytology-based screening in low resource settings as these require only one or two clinical visits. The results of the study that was conducted by Maree et al. (2009) revealed that VIA screening is acceptable to women due to the fact that the results are available immediately. The use of VIA as a screening tool should be considered as it is a realistic alternative for low-resource settings. VIA training should be instituted and registered nurses trained to perform it effectively. Part time registered nurses, possibly including the retired registered nurses, could perform VIAs at primary health care clinics, together with breast examinations. The major drawback of this approach that was identified by Sankaranarayanan et al. (1998) is that lesions are not detected early enough to prevent invasion because of a large proportion of the cancers detected are relatively advanced, requiring complex medical therapy that is difficult to provide in many settings. Cytology remains the best method available in screening for cervical cancer. However, in countries with limited resources, an inexpensive and easy alternative is needed. Choosing a suitable screening test is only one aspect of a screening programme. A more fundamental and challenging issue is the organization of the programme in its totality. Whichever screening test is to be used, the challenges in organizing a screening programme are more or less the same. However, screening tests that require additional recalls and revisits for diagnostic evaluation and treatment may pose added logistic difficulties and these may emerge as another barrier for participation in low-resource settings (Sankaranarayanan et al., 2001).

4.2 Improving health human resources

Due to task shifting, cervical screening previously the exclusive domain of doctors and family planning nurses was extended to all registered nurses in the public sector (Department of Health, 2000). This led to the greater availability of screening services as well as increasing the demand for additional competent nurses to do Pap smears. Making the registered nurses the primary cervical screening providers is logical, given the need to increase the services. However, Kawonga & Fonn (2008) argues that this solution fails to recognize that a screening programme entails more than just taking Pap smears. These authors further argue that there are several components that should be well-co-ordinated including the facilities for follow-up and referral of women with abnormal smears. South Africa has not invested sufficiently in health systems strengthening nor in building the management capacity to co-ordinate and monitor the screening programme (Moodley et al., 2006). In South Africa, registered nurses have an important responsibility for the implementation of the programme. Health workers in South Africa are poorly distributed, being concentrated in urban areas, private sectors and hospitals (Wadee & Khan, 2007). In order to ensure efficient utilization of registered nurses, appropriate skills mix at the PHC clinics must be ensured.

According to the South African cervical screening policy, all nurses at the clinics are expected to conduct screening but this is not happening, mainly because nurses have not been equipped with knowledge and skills (Moodley et al., 2006; Sibiya & Grainger, 2007; Smith et al., 2003). In order for the nurses to be knowledgeable about the disease and understand, accept and comply with the programme, they must be trained through continuing professional development system. Education concerning the rationale of the policy, and the natural history of the disease, may encourage nurses to perform more screening tests. Zweigenthal (1998) found a correlation between a high level of screening and nurses' knowledge or a personal interest in the level of nurses' education. This researcher reported that the screening rates increased with an increase in the level of nurses' education. If nurses have a positive attitude towards the cervical screening programme, they are likely to motivate women to have a smear done. According to the cervical screening policy, all service providers must have access to information and be technically competent to perform adequate smears with effective management of abnormal results. The policy further states that the adequacy rate of a screening facility must reach at least 70% and if the facility consistently achieves below 70%, the programme stipulates that the staff will have to be re-trained (Department of Health, 2000). Smith et al. (2003) suggested that low coverage may be due to nurses' opposition to and poor understanding of the programme. Given that the participants disagreed with the starting age and intervals for smears, and mentioned inappropriate criteria, there is a clear need for further training.

In order to address the limited capacity to read cervical smears, the alternative methods for cervical screening, for example the DNA testing for HPV and VIA will relieve pressure on the cyto-techicians. Additional posts will have to be established or, in addition, methods of contracting private sector resources could be investigated (Fonn, 2003).

4.3 Good follow up and referral systems

It is unethical to offer screening without ensuring that follow-up and treatment services are available for women with abnormal smears (Sackett, 1975 as cited in Kawonga & Fonn, 2008). The WHO (2002) states that for success, the cervical screening programme must have the ability to "ensure high levels of coverage of the target population, to offer high quality, caring services, to develop and monitor good referral systems that ensure good patient follow-up and to ensure that the patients receive appropriate, acceptable and caring treatment in the context of informed consent." The manner in which the health professionals perform can have a profound effect on the achievement of these. The relationship between primary and referral sites and good monitoring systems is essential in order for a screening programme to be effective. The fact that screening services offered at PHC settings are not available outside office hours can also be seen as an obstacle. A system must be put in place to ensure that working women have access to the clinics even after office hours. A booking system can also be used to increase access of the screening services.

5. Conclusion

The South African government has produced a commendable screening programme and made a commitment to reduce cervical cancer. However, there are still challenges with the implementation of the cervical screening policy. South Africa is better placed than most sub-Saharan countries, but will not attain a successful screening programme without increased effort. An important consideration that needs to be taken into account is the cost. Frequent screening of women has considerable cost and resource implications. The limited health care budgets in most developing countries preclude initiating and sustaining such programmes. Despite calls for screening, implementation difficulties include shortages both of health funds and of number of skilled personnel. Strategies to reduce the burden on registered nurses may include training of less skilled cadres of nurses, like enrolled nurses and enrolled nursing auxiliaries for cervical screening. In order for a cervical cancer screening programme to succeed in South Africa, there must be greater political commitment so as to improve resources that are required for implementing the policy. The political will to see a national screening programme implemented is required from government, the health sector, the various medical, nursing and allied health and professional boards. Communication methods and delivery strategies aimed at encouraging women from developing countries are needed in order to increase screening uptake.

6. References

Abrahams, N., Wood, K. & Jewkes, R. (1996). *Cervical screening in Montagu District: Women's experiences, coverage and barriers to uptake. Research Report.* CERSA-Women's Health: Medical Research Council. ISBN: 1-874-826 48-X

Adar, J. & Stevens, M. (2000). *Women's health.* (In: Ntuli, A (ed). *South African Health Review.* Durban: Health Systems Trust)

Alliance for Cervical Cancer Prevention. (2004). Planning *and implementing cervical cancer prevention and control programmes:a manual for managers.* Alliance for Cervical Cancer Prevention: Seattle

De Jonge, E.T.M., Makin, J.D. & Lindeque, B.G. (1999). Is cancer of the cervix a more aggressive disease in black women? *The South African Journal of Epidemiology and Infection,* 14(2), pp.40-45

Denny, L., Kuhn, L., Pollack, A., Wainwright, H. & Wright, T. (2000). Evaluation of alternative methods of cervical cancer screening for resource-poo settings. *Cancer,* 89, pp. 826-833

Denny, L. (2006). Cervical cancer: The South African perspective. *International Journal of Gynaecology and Obstetrics,* 95(supplement 1), pp. S211-214

Department of Health. (2000). National *guidelines for cervical cancer screening programme.* Government Printers: Pretoria

Department of Health. (2004). Strategic *priorities for the national health system 2004-2009.* Department of Health: Pretoria

Department of Health. (2006). A *national human resources plan for health.* Department of Health: Pretoria

Department of Health. (2007). Report: *National HIV and syphilis prevalence survey South Africa* 2006. Government Printers: Pretoria

Dickson-Tetteh, K. (1998). Cervical cancer: A global health problem. *Health and Hygiene,* January: 18-20

Fonn, S. (2003). Human resource requirements for introducing cervical screening-who do we need where? *South African Medical Journal,* 93(12), pp. 901-903

Gaym, A., Mashego, M., Kharsany, B.M., Walldorf, J., Frohlich, J. & Abdoll Karim, Q. (2007). High prevalence of abnormal Smear smears among young women co-infected with HIV in rural South Africa - implications for cervical cancer screening policies in high HIV prevalence population. *South African Medical Journal,* 97(2), pp. 120-123

Goldie, S.J., Kuhn, L., Denny, L., Pollack, A. & Wright, T.C. (2001). Policy analysis of cervical cancer screening strategies in low-resource settings. Clinical benefits and cost-effectiveness. *The Journal of American Medical Association,* 285(24), pp. 3107-3115

Goldie, S.J., Gaffikin, L., Goldhaber-Fiebert, J.D., Gordillo-Tobar, A., Levin, C., Mahe, C. & Wright, T.C. (2005). Cost-effectiveness of cervical cancer screening in five developing countries. *The New England Journal of Medicine,* 353(20), pp. 2158-2168

Hoffman, M., Cooper, D., Carrara, H., Rosenberg, L., Kelly, J., Stander, I., Williamson, A-L., Denny, L., du Toit, G. & Shapiro, S. (2003). Limited pap screening associated with reduced risk of cervical cancer in South Africa. *International Journal of Epidemiology,* August, 32, pp. 573-577

Hoytt, M.J. (1998). Cervical dysplasia and cancer. *Community research initiative on AIDS (CRIA) Update,* 7(2) http://www.thebody.com/cria/spring98/dysplasia (accessed on 19/04/2005)

Jeronimo, J., Morales, O., Horna, J., Pariona, J., Manrique, J., Rubinos, J. & Takahashi, R. (2005). Visual inspection with acetic acid for cervical cancer screening outside of low-resource settings. *Review Panam Salud Publica,* 17(1), pp. 1-5

Kawonga, M & Fonn, S. (2008). Achieving effective cervical screening coverage in South Africa through human resources and health systems development. *Reproductive Health Matters*, 16(32), pp. 32-40

Kenney, J.W. (1994). Comparison of risk factors, severity and treatment of women with and without AIDS. *Cancer Nursing*, 17(4), pp. 308-316

KwaZulu-Natal Department of Health. (1999). *Cervical and breast cancer screening programme*. Department of Health: KwaZulu-Natal

KwaZulu-Natal Department of Health. (2004). *Sexual, reproductive and youth health: Student training modules: Professional Nurses*. Department of Health: KwaZulu-Natal

le Riche, H.R. & Botha, M.H. (2006). Cervical conisation and reproductive outcome. *South African Journal of Obstetrics and Gynecology*, 12(3), pp. 150-154

Lucas, A. (2005). Human resources for health in Africa. *British Medical Journal*, Volume 331, pp. 1037-1038

Maree, J.E., Lu, X., Mosalo, A. & Wright, S.C.D. (2009). Cervical screening in Tshwane, South Africa: Women's knowledge of cervical cancer, acceptance of visual inspection with acetic acid (VIA) and practical lessons learnt. *Africa Journal of Nursing & Midwifery*, 11(1), pp. 76-90

Moodley, J., Kawonga, M., Bradley, J. & Hoffman M. (2006). Challenges in implementing a cervical screening programme in South Africa. *Cancer Detection and Prevention* 30, pp. 361-368

Mqoqi, N. (2003). National Department of Health Systems Research, Research Co-ordination and Epidemiology. Research Update, 5(4). Available from http://www.doh.gov.za/docs/research

Nene, B., Jayant, K., Arossi, S., Shastri, S., Budukh, A., Hingmire, S., Muwonge, R., Malvi, S., Dinshaw, K. & Sankaranarayanan, R. (2007). Determinants of women's participation in cervical screening trial, Maharashtra, India. *Bulletin of the World Health Organization*. 85(4), pp. 264-272

Oosthuizen, M. & Ehlers V.J. (2007). Factors that may influence South African nurses' decisions to emigrate. *Health SA Gesondheid*, 12(2), pp. 14-26

Parkin, D.M., Whelan, S., Ferlay, J. & Storm, H. (2005). Cancer incidence in five continents. *IARC Database No. 7. Vols I-VIII*. Lyon: IARC

Sankaranarayanan, R., Wesley, R., Somanathan, N., Dhakad, N., Shymalakumary, B., Amma, N.S., Parkin, D.M. & Nair, M.K. (1998). Visual inspection of the uterine cervix after the application of acetic acid in the detection of cervical carcinoma and its precursors. *Cancer*, 83, pp. 2150-2156

Population Reference Bureau & Alliance for Cervical Cancer Screening. (2004). *Preventing cervical cancer worldwide. Population Reference Bureau: Washington*

Sankaranarayanan, R. Budukh, A.M. & Rajkumar, R. (2001). Effective screening programmes for cervical cancer in low- and middle-income developing countries. *Bulletin of the World Health Organization*, 79(10), pp. 954-962

Sankaranarayanan R. & Wesley, R. (2003). *A practical manual on visual screening for cervical neoplasia*. International Agency for Research on Cancer (IARC) Press: Lyon

Sankaranarayanan, R. Gaffikin, L., Jacob, M., Sellors, J. & Robles, S. (2005). A critical assessment of screening methods for cervical neoplasia. *International Journal of Gynecology and Obstetrics*, *89* pp. S4-S12

Sibiya, M.N. & Grainger, L.D. (2007). An assessment of the implementation of the provincial cervical screening programme in selected Primary Health Care Clinics in the Ilembe region, KwaZulu-Natal. *Curationis*, 30(1), pp. 48-55

Sibiya, M.N. & Grainger, L.D. (2010). Registered nurses' perceptions of the cervical screening programme in primary health care clinics in the KwaZulu-Natal Province of South Africa. *Africa Journal of Nursing & Midwifery*, 12(1), pp. 15-26

Sitas, F., Madhoo, J. & Wessie, J. (1998). Cancer in South Africa, 1993-1995. National Cancer Registry of South Africa: Johannesburg

Smith, N., & Hoffman, M. (2000). *A situation analysis of cervical cancer screening in Mitchell's Plain Health District.* Unpublished Masters in Public Health. University of Cape Town.

Smith, N., Moodley, M & Hoffman, M. (2003). Challenges to cervical cancer screening in the Western Cape Province. *South African Medical Journal*, 93(1), pp. 32-35

South African Yearbook 2004/05. [Accessed on 14 December 2007: http://www.gcis.gov.za/docs/publications/yearbook.htm]

Tarimo, E. (1991). *Towards a healthy district: Organizing and managing district health systems based on Primary Health Care.* WHO: Geneva

UNAIDS. (2008). Report *on the global AIDS epidemic.* UNAIDS: Geneva

Wadee, H & Khan, F. (2007). Human resources in health. In: Harrison, S., Bhana, R. & Ntuli, A., editors. *South African Health Review, 2007.* Health Systems Trust: Durban

Walker, A.R.P., Michelow, P.M. & Walker, B.F. (2002). Cervix cancer in African women in Durban, South Africa. *International Journal of Gynaecology and Obstetrics*, 79, pp. 45-46

Walraven, G. (2003). Prevention of cervical cancer in Africa: a daunting task? *African Journal of Reproductive Health*, 7 pp. 7-12

World Health Organization. (2001). Effective screening programmes for cervical cancer in low- and middle-income developing countries. *Bulletin of the World Health Organization* 79(10), pp. 954-962

World Health Organization. (2002). Cervical *cancer screening for developing countries. Report of a WHO consultation.* Geneva. ISBN: 9241545720.

Zweigenthal, V. (1998). *An assessment of the effectiveness of the implementation of the cervical screening following policy guidelines into the routine services of the Eastern Metropolitan Local Council.* The South African Institute for Medical Research. University of Witwatersrand: Johannesburg

4

Cervical Cancer in Sub Sahara Africa

Atara Ntekim
Department of Radiation Oncology,
College of Medicine, University of Ibadan
Nigeria

1. Introduction

"Cervical cancer is fully preventable and curable, at low cost and at low risk, when screening to facilitate the timely detection of early precursor lesions in asymptomatic women is available together with appropriate diagnosis, treatment and follow-up" (Lewis, M. Pan American Health Organization, 2004).

The burden of cervical cancer is quite low in the developed countries of the world. The situation is quite the reverse in developing countries where it constitutes a major health problem. While the incidence is decreasing in the former, it is on the increase in the later. This is a source of great concern considering the fact that cervical cancer is preventable and curable at low cost with currently available methods. Sub Sahara Africa is the region with the highest incidence of cervical cancer in the world with concomitant high mortality affecting women at their prime. There are no screening programs for early detection of precancerous lesions within the countries of Sub Sahara Africa. Most screening activities are done as pilot or research projects which are discontinued on completion. South Africa is the only country in the region with a national cytology based screening program since 2001 but then coverage remains poor and the impact on invasive cervical cancer is unknown (Louie et al.2009). The onset of HIV/AIDS epidemic that is highest in the sub region has elevated the problem of cervical cancer to a serious level. To compound the problem is the widespread lack of resources associated with the region. The countries of Sub Sahara Africa are shown in figure 1.

2. Aim

The aim of this work is to appraise the incidence, mortality, state of prevention and treatment of cervical cancer in sub-Sahara Africa. This highlight is necessary so that health professionals, philanthropists, policy makers, advocates and other stake holders can appreciate and understand the state of the disease and respond through the development of treatment, preventive and control programs that will lessen the burden and mortality from this disease in the sub region. It is also aimed at highlighting the need to see that cervical cancer should be considered a public health problem in the region.

3. Methods

The method used was through the synthesis of data and information derived from available current published scientific works from peer reviewed journals, workshop proceedings,

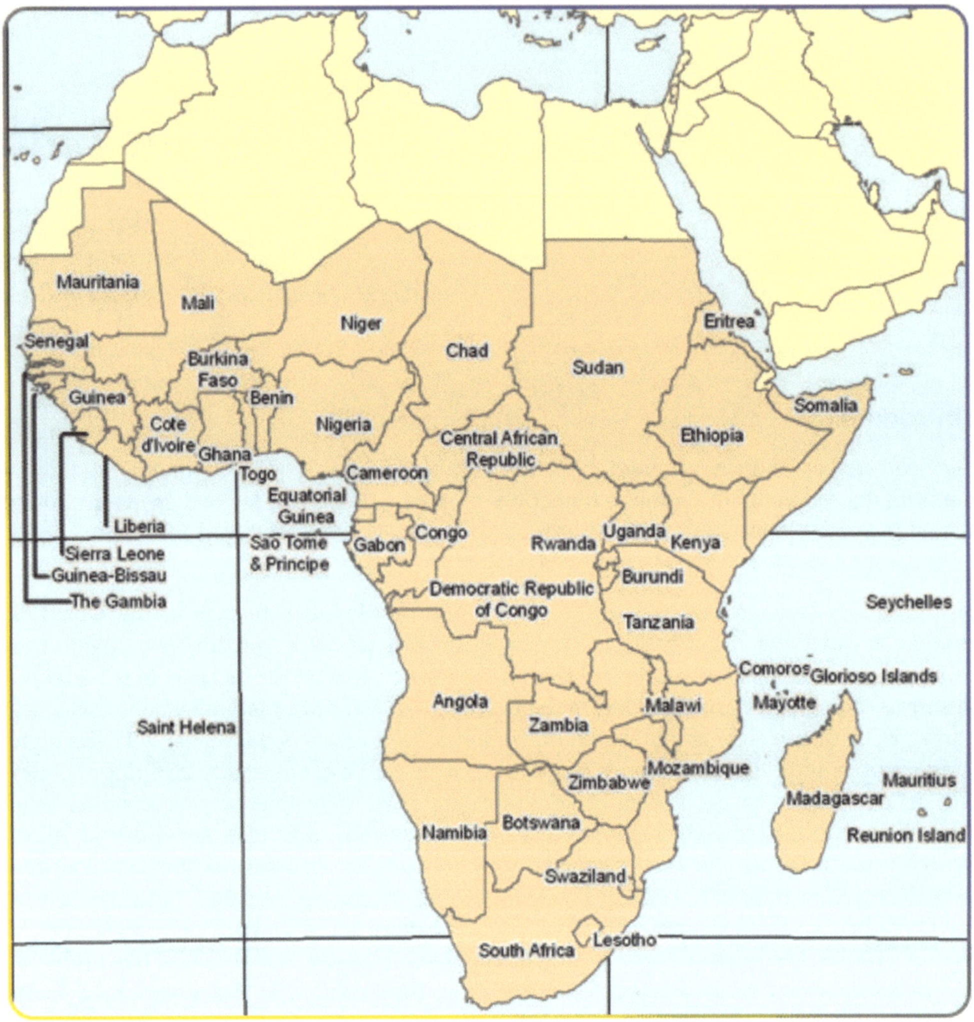

Fig. 1. Map showing the countries of Sub Sahara Africa (Map Source: www.world map .org) (NB Southern Sudan became independent July 2011)

hospital and regional based cancer registry figures , reports from specific centres, conference proceedings and a review of work done on cervical cancer in the authors institution The University College Hospital Ibadan Nigeria.

4. Findings and discussions

Cervical cancer occurs worldwide but the highest incidence and mortality rates of cervical cancer are in Eastern, Western, and Southern Africa, as well as South-Central Asia and South America. Rates are lowest in Western Asia, Australia/New Zealand as shown in table 1.

In sub-Saharan Africa cervical cancer accounts for 22.2% of all cancers in women and it is also the most common cause of cancer death among women (Parkin et al.,2003). Cervical

World Area	Incidence per 100,000	Mortality per 100,000
Eastern Africa	**34.5**	**25.3**
Western Africa	**33.7**	**24.0**
Southern Africa	**26.8**	**14.8**
South - Central Asia	24.6	14.1
South America	24.1	10.8
Melanesia	23.7	16.6
Middle Africa	**23.0**	**17.0**
Central America	22.2	11.1
Caribbean	20.8	9.4
South - Eastern Asia	15.8	8.3
Central and Eastern Europe	14.5	6.3
Micronesia/ Polynesia	13.4	4.9
Eastern Asia	9.6	3.9
Northern Europe	8.3	2.4
Southern Europe	8.0	2.6
Western Europe	6.9	2.0
Northern Africa	6.6	4.0
Northern America	5.7	1.7
Australia/ New Zealand	5.0	1.0
Western Asia	4.5	2.1

Table 1. Age Standardized Cervical Cancer Incidence and Mortality Rates by World Area (Extracted from GLOBOCAN 2008 by Jemal et al., 2011).

cancer is however the second common cancer among women after cancer of the breast in some areas like Ibadan in Nigeria (Adebamowo et al. 1999). About 60-75% of women in sub-Saharan Africa who develop cervical cancer live in rural areas. Many of these women go untreated, mostly due to lack of access (financial and geographical) to health care. Women in sub-Saharan Africa lose more years to cervical cancer than to any other type of cancer. Unfortunately, it affects them at a time of life when they are critical to the social and economic stability of their families (Parkin et al., 2002).

The true incidence of cervical cancer in many African countries is unknown as there is gross under-reporting. Only very few countries have functional cancer registries and record-keeping is minimal or non-existent in many countries. Some of the figures quoted in the literature are hospital-based, which represents a small fraction of women dying from cervical cancer, as most women cannot access hospital care and die at home. A mortality rate of 35 per 100,000 is reported in Eastern Africa. The reported mortality rates in developed countries with successful screening programs seldom exceed 5 per 100,000 women (Chokunonga et al., 2002).

4.1 Factors responsible for the high prevalence

4.1.1 Socio-cultural factors

Human papillioma virus (HPV) has been isolated in most cases of cervical cancer in all parts of the world. Epidemiologic studies have shown that the association of genital human papilloma virus (HPV) with cervical cancer is strong, independent of other risk factors, and consistent in several countries .The International Biological Study on Cervical Cancer (IBSCC) Study Group led by Bosch, F. in 1995 reported that HPV DNA was detected in 93% of the tumors, with no significant variation in HPV positivity among countries. HPV 16 was present in 50% of the specimens, HPV 18 in 14%, HPV 45 in 8%, and HPV 31 in 5%. HPV 16 was the predominant type in all countries except Indonesia, where HPV 18 was more common. There was significant geographic variation in the prevalence of some less common virus types. A clustering of HPV 45 was apparent in western Africa, while HPV 39 and HPV 59 were almost entirely confined to Central and South America. In squamous cell tumors, HPV 16 predominated (51% of such specimens), but HPV 18 predominated in adenocarcinomas (56% of such tumors) and adenosquamous tumors (39% of such tumors). The report concluded that the results confirm the role of genital HPVs, which are transmitted sexually, as the central etiologic factor in cervical cancer worldwide (Bosch F et al., 1995). Epidemiological studies employing a variety of HPV typing protocols have been collated in meta-analyses. HPV-16/18 is estimated to account for 70% of all cervical cancers worldwide, although the estimated HPV-16/18 fraction is slightly higher in more developed (72–77%) than in less developed (65–72%) regions. About 41–67% of high-grade squamous intraepithelial lesion (HSIL), 16–32% of low-grade squamous intraepithelial lesion (LSIL) and 6–27% of atypical squamous cells of undetermined significance (ASCUS) are also estimated to be HPV-16/18-positive, thus highlighting the increasing relative frequency of HPV-16/18 with increasing lesion severity. After HPV-16/18, the six most common HPV types are the same in all world regions, namely 31, 33, 35, 45, 52 and 58; these account for an additional 20% of cervical cancers worldwide.(Clifford et al., 2006)

Human papillomavirus (HPV), the necessary cause of cervical cancer, is endemic in Africa. In a study to investigate the prevalence of and the risk factors for cervical infection with human papillomavirus (HPV) in an inner-city area of Ibadan, Nigeria, Thomas et al., (2004) interviewed and obtained a sample of cervical cells from 932 sexually active women aged 15 years or older. A total of 32 different HPV types were identified with an HPV prevalence of 26.3% overall and 24.8% among women without cervical lesions; or age-standardised to the world standard population of 28.3 and 27.3%, respectively. High-risk HPV types predominated, most notably HPV 16, 31, 35 and 58. In all, 33.5% of infections involved more than one HPV type. Unlike most populations studied so far,

HPV prevalence was high not only among young women, but also in middle and old age. Single women (odds ratio, OR=2.1; 95% confidence interval, CI=1.1-3.9) and illiterate women (OR=1.7; 95% CI=1.1-2.5) showed increased HPV positivity.. High prevalence of HPV in all age groups may be a distinctive feature of populations where HPV transmission continues into middle age and cervical cancer incidence is very high. Many of the factors that increase both HPV acquisition and promote the oncogenic effect of the virus are also very widespread in Africa (Schmauz et al 1989). These include: early marriage, polygamous marriages and high parity. Polygamy is reported to increase the risk of cervical cancer two-fold and the risk increases with increasing number of wives (Bayo et al., 2002). This is part of the male factor in addition to prostitution that lead to the high prevalence of HPV in Sub Sahara Africa.

High parity, which is the norm in some cultures in Africa, is also a recognised, HPV-related co-factor for the development of cervical cancer (Brinton et al 1989).

The prevalence of HPV has been shown to be higher in uncircumcised men than in circumcised men. In a study to investigate the association between male circumcision (MC) and high risk human papilloma virus (HR-HPV) prevalence, Auvert and colleagues (2009) using urethral swabs collected during a period of 262 consecutive days among participants from the intervention (circumcised) and control (uncircumcised) groups who were reporting for a scheduled follow-up visit reported that HR-HPV prevalences among intervention and control groups were 14.8% (94/637) and 22.3% (140/627). Confounder factors (ethnic group, age, education, sexual behaviour including condom use, marital status, and HIV status) had no effect on the results. Multiple HR-HPV prevalence was 7.0% (89/1267) It was significantly lower among men of the intervention group compared with men of the control group (4.2% vs. 9.9%) .The prevalence of HR-HPV infections in their study was even thought to be underestimated since detection in the urethra is significantly lower than detection in the glans, corona sulcus or the penis shaft. As a corollary, some randomized controlled trials have shown a partial protective effect of male circumcision (MC) on the acquisition of HIV by males in Africa. The effect of MC on HR-HPV reinforces the WHO-UNAIDS recommendation for the implementation of MC programs in countries with a high HIV prevalence, a low MC prevalence and a high MC acceptability (Auvert et al., 2009). In Sub Sahara Africa these countries are mainly in Southern and Eastern Africa. Drain et al., in 2006, published an analysis of classification of developing countries according to prevalence of male circumcision. The categories were low, 20%, intermediate 20-80% and high > 80%. The classification for developing countries in Africa is presented in table 2.

This report noted that male circumcision, which is routinely practiced in the Middle East, Northern and Western Africa, and Western Asia, was associated with lower rates of certain STIs, HIV and cervical cancer (a proxy for HPV), but not with infections transmitted by non-sexual routes. In general, more male circumcision was strongly associated with lower cervical cancer rates and fewer HIV cases, independent of religion. Furthermore, male circumcision was independently associated with HIV among countries with primarily heterosexual HIV transmission, and not among countries with primarily homosexual or injection drug use HIV transmission. These findings all suggest that male circumcision is a true protective factor that reduces the sexual transmission of HIV and possibly HPV, independent of Muslim and Christian religions.

Male circumcision prevalence			
Low (<20%)	Intermediate (20-80%)	High (>80%)	
Botswana	Central African Republic	Algeria	Guinea-Bissau
Burundi	Cote d'ivoire	Angola	Kenya
Cape Verde	Ethiopia	Benin	Liberia
Malawi	Lesotho	Burkina Faso	Libya
Namibia	Mozambique	Cameroon	Madagascar
Rwanda	South Africa	Chad	Mali
Swaziland	Sudan	Congo (Brazzaville)	Mauritania
Zambia	Tanzania	Dem Rep of Congo	Mauritius
Zimbabwe	Uganda	Djibouti	Morocco
		Egypt	Niger
		Equatorial Guinea	Nigeria
		Eritrea	Senegal
		Gabon	Sierra Leone
		Gambia	Somalia
		Ghana	Togo
		Guinea	Tunisia

Table 2. Category of male circumcision prevalence for developing countries in Africa (Adapted from Drain et al., 2006)

4.1.2 Socio-economic factors

Worldwide women of low socio-economic status have a greater risk of having cervical cancer. Cervical cancer is often referred to as a disease of poverty and of poor women. A recent study in Mali in West Africa showed that within a population widely infected with HPV, poor social conditions, high parity and poor hygienic conditions were the main co-factors for cervical cancer (Palacio-Mejia et al., 2003). Sub Sahara Africa also has widespread conditions that encourage sub standard living conditions. These include wars, political chaos, internal conflicts, natural disasters, famine and drought. These often lead to large populations being displaced externally and internally for long periods of time. Under this refugee- like conditions, social vices like rapes, prostitution and multiple marriages and cohabitation prevail encouraging the transmission of HPV. War is associated with male sexual promiscuity, which in turn contributes to the development of cervical cancer among sexually monogamous women. In 1996, a case–control study sponsored by Stanford University documented that the Vietnam War had contributed substantially to the problem of cervical cancer in contemporary Vietnam, and the Vietnam/American Cervical Cancer Prevention Project was established as an all-volunteer non profit organization. Publication of data linking war to disease was delayed for 8 years in an attempt to ease the process of reconciliation by offering what most would acknowledge to be a remedy in advance of what some will perceive to be an accusation. (Suba et al., 2006)

High rates of invasive cervical cancer was noted in coastal areas of Coasta Rica and this was attributed to difficulties in having access to treatment. Most countries of Sub Sahara Africa are located within the Tropical Rain Forest with difficult terrain as there are lots of swampy areas and thick and mountainous forests. This makes access to screening, health education and treatment difficult.

4.1.3 Biological factors

Poor nutritional status and infections, e.g. malaria, HIV and TB, are ravaging sub-Saharan Africa and have made many people immuno-compromised. Several studies have demonstrated the association of HIV with HPV. The prevalence of CIN has been estimated to be as high as 20–40% in HIV-positive women (Wright et al 1994). HIV-positive women are more likely to have persistent HPV infections than HIV-negative women. In a study of 2,198 women who attended gynaecological clinics in Abidjan, Côte d'Ivoire, HIV-positive women had a significantly higher prevalence of squamous intraepithelial lesion (SIL) (La Ruche et al., 1998). Temmerman et al (1999) reported a five-fold increased risk of high-grade SIL among 513 HIV-positive women in a family planning clinic in Kenya. Other reports from the region show that women with HIV develop cervical cancer at an earlier age than women who are HIV-negative(Moodley 2001). Gichangi et al(2003) in Kenya found that young women under the age of 35 who had invasive cervical cancer were 2.6 times more likely to be HIV positive than controls of similar age (35% vs. 17%, OR 2.6, p=0.043). A recently published study from Tanzania showed that the prevalence of HIV-1 was much higher among the cervical cancer patients (21.0%) than among the controls (11.6%). HIV-1 was a significant risk factor for cancer of the cervix (OR=2.9, 95% CI=1.4–5.9).(Moodley et al., 2006) Sub-Saharan Africa harbours 67% of the world's population of people living with HIV and AIDS (Buga G 1998).

4.1.4 Lack of awareness and knowledge of cervical cancer in Africa

Cervical cancer is yet to be recognised as an important public health problem in sub-Saharan Africa. In Sub Sahara Africa, priority is given to infectious diseases such as malaria, tuberculosis, leprosy, diarrheal diseases, acute respiratory infections and HIV/AIDS all of which have preventive and management strategies. Several studies have shown poor knowledge of cervical cancer in Africa, which cuts across different literacy levels. Among 500 attendees of a maternal and child health clinic in Lagos-Nigeria only 4.3% were found to be aware of cervical cancer. (Anorlu et al., 2004) In 2004, also in Lagos-Nigeria, 81.7% of 139 patients with advanced cervical cancer had never heard of cervical cancer before, and 20%, 30% and 10% respectively thought the symptoms they had were due to resumption of menses, lower genital infection and irregular menses. Almost all the women (98%) believed that their advanced disease was curable, 12% thought it was not a serious disease and only 9% understood that it was cancer and therefore serious (Ajayi et al., 1998). Similar studies in Kenya and Tanzania also reported very poor knowledge of the disease in patients. (Gichangi et al., 2003 & Kidanto et al., 2002). Poor knowledge is not limited to patients alone, however; health care workers who are supposed to be better informed do not have good knowledge of the disease either. In Lagos Nigeria, delay by primary health care providers in referring cases of cervical cancer was found to be an important cause of women presenting with late-stage disease. It took a mean of 9.35 ± 12.9 months for primary health care providers to diagnose and refer women with cervical cancer to a tertiary hospital for management. (Anorlu et al., 2004).

Education improves knowledge and acceptability of preventive measures against cervical cancer. In a study on cervical cancer awareness and HPV vaccine acceptance among 375 female university students in Northern Nigeria, a total of 133 participants knew of HPV (35.5%), 202 (53.9%) had heard of cervical carcinoma and 277 (74.0%) were willing to accept HPV vaccination. (Ilyasu et al., 2010). Apochie and colleague (2009) conducted a cross sectional survey among college students aged 18 years and above, attending a large university in Accra, Ghana. A sample of 157 students was selected to study knowledge and beliefs about cervical cancer screening. In general, respondents seemed to understand that cervical cancer screening had benefits. Over 64 percent believed that the test could find cervical changes before they became cancerous while 78.5% thought those changes could be easily cured. Among the perceived barriers to screening, the most prevalent perceived barrier was that only half of respondents believed that the purpose of cervical cancer was to diagnose cancer, the second commonest reported barrier (40.6%) was the belief that their partner would not allow them to obtain cervical cancer screening. The following barriers were also important; cost (23.2%), not knowing where to go (24.3%), and belief that everyone would think they were sexually active (24.6%). Encouragingly, few believed that a pap test would be painful (9.4%). While more than 68% perceived that young women were susceptible to cervical cancer, a lower percentage (52.5%) believed that they themselves were at risk for cervical cancer. About three quarters of respondents (73%) believed that cervical cancer was a serious disease that would make a woman's life difficult and about 62% of students also believed that there were effective cures for cervical cancer. In general, a low percentage received screening cues from their social environment by way of knowing peers who had screened or from a healthcare worker's recommendation. Six of the fifteen respondents who had received at least one recommendation from a healthcare worker to get cervical screening, scheduled and obtained one. The subset reporting having received a health care worker recommendation but that reported not having the test, indicated the following reasons; they could not afford it, they did not know where to get screening, they had no time to schedule and obtain screening and they felt it was embarrassing to expose themselves for screening. About a third reported ever having heard a mass media discussion on cervical cancer while a fifth have at least once listened to a discussion on cervical cancer at a church or other social gathering. About half also stated that they would be willing to obtain the cheaper alternative cervical cancer screening using visual inspection and mild acetic acid, if a doctor recommended it. Overall there was good awareness of the issues related to screening, although there were specific gaps in knowledge about risk factors and screening intervals. For instance, it was found that although the relationship between sex and cervical cancer was known, less was known about other risk factors like their partner's prior sexual experiences and very little was known about the link between HPV and cervical cancer.

4.1.5 Poor cervical cancer screening

Very few women in sub-Saharan Africa are ever screened for cervical cancer. None of the 500 women attending a maternal and child health clinic in a poor area of Lagos in 1999 had ever had a Pap smear .Only 9% of health care workers in two health institutions in Nigeria had ever had a Pap smear. In a study among medical workers in a Ugandan hospital (doctors , nurses and medical students) Only 19% of the female medical workers had ever had a cervical cancer screening test done. The reasons for not having been screened included: not feeling at risk, lack of symptoms, carelessness, fear of vaginal examination, lack of interest, test being unpleasant and not yet being of risky age. Moreover, 25% of the female respondents said that they would only accept a vaginal examination by a female health worker.(Mutyaba et al., 2006) In a similar study among nurses in a Tanzanian hospital concerning nurses' own cervical cancer screening practices most (116/137) of the respondents had never had a Pap smear the most common reason (54.7%) was not knowing where to go for the test, followed by seeing no reason for the test (13.1%), being afraid of the procedure (9.5%) and being afraid of bad results (7.3%).(Urasa & Darj 2009)

Some of the few women who do have access to screening do not get themselves screened because they have wrong beliefs about cervical cancer. (Anorlu et al., 2007). Less than 1% of women in four West African countries had ever been screened (Gichangi et al., 2003). Moreover, there are very few cervical screening services in Africa and many of them are based in secondary and tertiary health care facilities located in urban areas. Only 5% of 504 general practitioners in Lagos Nigeria in 2004 screened their patients (Denny et al 2006). Women who use these services are generally young, and smears are thus being taken from a relatively low-risk group.

Screening in most developing countries like the countries within the sub region is mainly opportunistic, characterized by an estimated low coverage, coexisting with over-screening of women with access to health services, and an absence of quality control procedures. Policies for cervical cancer screening in most countries vary and, most often nonexistent . Formulation and ensuring compliance with national program guidelines is an essential step toward significantly reducing the burden of cervical cancer (Arrosi et al. 2010). This type of service does not reach women most at risk, i.e. older women aged 35–60 years, especially those who live in rural areas. Cytology-based screening, which is used in developed countries, is resource intensive, and difficult to realise in very many countries in sub-Saharan Africa because of poor health care infrastructure and lack of resources. There are very few cytopathologists, cytoscreeners and cytotechnicians; some have inadequate training. Quality control is inadequate. Histopathological services are extremely limited in many countries. Malawi, a country with a cervical cancer incidence rate of 47 per 100,000 women, had one pathologist, one colposcope, no cyto-technicians and no facilities for cervical cancer screening or treatment as at 2001. The situation is not much different presently. The default rate among those with cytological abnormalities reaches 60–80% due to the absence of effective mechanisms for recall of women with abnormal smears.

The effectiveness of direct visual inspection [visual inspection with acetic acid (VIA) and visual inspection with Lugol's iodine (VILI)) as a form of population-based screening has been studied across the continent, mainly sponsored by international agencies (Chirenje et al., 2001) VIA is similar to colposcopy in that 4% acetic acid is applied to the cervix and any acetowhite lesion is visualized, although with VIA there is no magnification. It is a simple procedure and in most centres has been carried out by trained nurses. Candidates with suspicious lesions are selected for treatment. Studies have shown the sensitivity of VIA to be the same as that of Pap smear while its specificity is lower than 85% (Urasa & Darj 2011). The specificity is also noted to be even lower among HIV positive patients possibly due to high rates of coinfections in the lower genital tract (Denny et al., 2002). Visual inspection method is however a subjective method and prone to different interpretations by different observers depending on experience and competence. Other screening methods include HPV DNA assay (which has been shown to be even superior to PAP smear test) and colposcopy.

4.1.6 Treatment of cervical cancer in sub-Saharan Africa

Treatment of cervical cancer is dependent on the stage of the disease, age and medical state of the patient, tumor characteristics, patients' preferences and resources within the health sector of each country. Options can be monotherapy or combined; they range from conisation of the cervix, simple hysterectomy with or without lymphadenectomy, radical hysterectomy with pelvic lymphadenectomy, pelvic exenteration, chemotherapy, radiotherapy, to palliative chemotherapy. Treatment at an early stage has the best prognosis with the highest cure rates (Urasa & Darj 2011)

4.1.6.1 Treatment of pre-invasive cervical cancer

It may not be too wrong to say that there are apparently more cases of invasive cancer than pre-invasive cancer; this is mainly because there are very few facilities for screening and very poor access to the screening services. Because so few women are ever screened, not many cases of pre-cancerous lesions are diagnosed or detected. Colposcopy is available only in very few centres. Hysterectomy and cone biopsy are the usual treatment modalities for pre-cancerous lesions, as the equipment and expertise for large loop excision of the transformation zone (LLETZ), also known as loop electrosurgical excision (LEEP), are scarce.

4.1.6.2 Treatment of invasive cervical cancer

The treatment of invasive cervical cancer continues to be a major challenge in many sub-Saharan African countries, due to the lack of surgical facilities, skilled providers and radiotherapy services. Management of women with invasive cervical cancer requires a multidisciplinary approach, including: gynaecologists, radiation oncologists, medical oncologists, pathologists, medical physicists, technicians, nurses and counsellors. These specialists are lacking in many places across the continent, and where they exist they tend to work in isolation rather than in teams.

There are few cases that present in the operable stage of the disease. In Lagos Nigeria, less than 10% of cases are operable at the time of presentation. Some of the few who do present early may not have surgery as there are very few certified gynaecologists who perform radical gynaecological cancer surgery. Follow-up after surgery is often very poor as some patients who believe they have been cured never come back. Others just cannot afford the cost of transportation back to urban centres for follow-up (Ashraf, H. 2003). For patients who present late, radiotherapy becomes the preferred treatment. Unfortunately, only a few receive this treatment due to the paucity of resources and very advanced disease at presentation. Chirenje et al. (2001) found in Harare, Zimbabwe that in 70% of patients, radiotherapy was the most commonly used treatment modality, as many of the cases presented with stage 2B and above.

Radiotherapy is not available in many places in Sub Sahara Africa. In 1997, radiotherapy was not available in 32 African countries. (Levin et al.,1997). In 2003, 15 countries in Africa did not have a single radiotherapy machine. Nigeria, the most populous country in Africa, had only five radiotherapy centres as at 2009: four government-owned and one privately owned. WHO recommends 0.4 radiotherapy machines per million of population. Nigeria's five machines to 140 million people translates to ~0.04 per million, well below WHO's recommendation. In contrast, in the United States, there are 12 machines per million people. (Sepulveda et al., 2003). Besides few machines, those that exist frequently do not function most of the time because the resources for their proper maintenance and repair do not exist. In addition, there is a shortage of trained staff such as radiotherapists and medical physicists, as well as essential materials.

4.1.7 Supportive care

Pain is the most common presenting symptom in many cancer patients in Africa because of late presentation. In a survey of terminally ill patients in five countries in Africa - Uganda, Ethiopia, Tanzania, Zimbabwe and Botswana - the greatest need expressed by the patients was pain relief. (Harding et al., 2005) In another study comparing the concerns of terminally ill patients in a developed country (Scotland) and an African country (Kenya), it was found that the main concern of the Scottish patients was the emotional pain of facing death, while for their counterparts in Kenya it was physical pain and financial worries. Unfortunately, there is inadequate availability of pain-relieving medications, especially opioids. Only 11 out of 47 African countries use morphine for chronic pain and of these 11, the amount consumed is small. (Murray et al 2003) .

Oral morphine is not available to very many cancer patients in sub-Saharan Africa. Insufficient funds due to low priority accorded to palliative care by governments, regulatory and pricing obstacles, ignorance, and false beliefs are responsible. In some instances, where drugs are available to patients, sustainability of pain relief is hampered by poverty, as many cannot afford the cost of the drugs. Poverty, poor infrastructure, lack of health care workers adequately trained in palliative care and poor priority accorded to palliative care by African governments are all obstacles to effective palliative care in sub-Saharan Africa. There are very few hospices to take care of terminally ill patients. However, countries like South Africa, Uganda, Kenya, Tanzania, Nigeria and Zimbabwe have made some progress in palliative care. Uganda is the first African country to follow the WHO guidelines on palliative care. It has made oral morphine freely available to districts that have specialist palliative care nurses or clinical officers, and has promoted morphine use down to the villages. Laws have also been passed to allow trained nurses, especially those in the rural areas, where there are very few or no doctors, to prescribe morphine. Cancer is believed in certain cultures to be a punishment from the gods, and terminally ill patients often seek help from traditional healers and spiritual leaders. A good model for palliative care in Africa should therefore integrate the culture, beliefs and traditions of the people. Some countries are making efforts in this direction by incorporating traditional healers into mainstream medicine. However, a feasible, accessible, and effective palliative care is yet to be developed in sub-Saharan Africa. (Merriman & Kaur 2005).

4.2 Improvements in outlook

There is need to improve the outlook of this condition in Sub Sahara Africa. There should be improvement in attitude towards education needs of the populace so as to create and improve awareness and knowledge about the disease. Disease prevention requires social change, which in turn requires the participation of those for whom the change is intended, including demographic groups at high risk for disease, appropriate governmental authorities, and essential medical personnel. Both locally and globally, socio-political problems associated with sustaining working coalitions from groups with shared interests but competing incentives constitute critically important real-world obstacles to successful cervical cancer prevention and will remain so irrespective of the screening method(s) eventually used. In settings where health systems cannot afford to ignore such incentives, laboratory data constitute an essential yet sometimes overlooked fulcrum against which to leverage the social change required to preserve life (Suba et al., 2006)

There is need for sensitisation of health workers about cervical cancer and importance of screening. Based on studies carried out in countries where organized screening is available, it is known that screening uptake can be influenced by cultural beliefs, the social position of women, characteristics of the health care system, the physician's attitudes towards screening and women's comprehension of the screening process. Embarrassments about undergoing a gynecological examination, fear of the procedure or belief that little can be done to prevent cancer are other factors that might decrease screening participation. Lower socio-economic background, lack of health insurance and low literacy also compromise participation in screening. Attending cervical cancer screening may have a negative connotation or stigma when it is combined with a gynecological examination and treatment for reproductive tract infections. The gender of health care professionals and limited time that they allocate to patient education may negatively influence screening participation as well. Other influences that may influence participation in screening in particular in low resource countries are gender imbalances and whether illness is perceived as traditional or modern. Adequate knowledge about cervical cancer influences early detection and treatment seeking pattern (Mutyaba et al., 2007). In Botswana a national cervical cytology screening committee was formed in 1996 with a role in planning and advising the government. Just six years later a national guidance document for the national cervical cytology programme was drawn up and implemented. In this short space of time public awareness has been successfully raised resulting in an increased uptake of Pap smears from 5000 per year before the start of the programme to an impressive 32,000 per year in 2009. Despite considerable success, progress is hampered by inadequate resources, the high prevalence of HIV in the country and the long waiting list for treatment.

There is now a need to build upon the scope of cervical cancer prevention. This problem is not limited to Botswana as many African countries have similarly inadequate resources to treat patients even when abnormal cervical cytology is detected (sSACCWG 2010). Training curricula of nurses and medical students need to be revised to include more practical cervical cancer screening skills. There is need to change attitudes that screening is only for gynaecologists. For opportunistic screening to work, health workers in other departments need to be sensitised on the gravity of cervical cancer and to remember to refer all eligible women who come into their care for screening (Mutyaba 2006). Nurses in high income countries play a role in cancer prevention and participate in cervical cancer screening by carrying out Pap smear tests . Due to the lack of logistics and scarcity of gynecologists and pathologists in Sub Sahara Africa ,nurses could be used effectively in the prevention of cervical cancer, by being enabled to collect Pap smear tests specimen and using the visual inspection by acetic acid technique which is less costly and does not require high expertise (Urasa & Darj 2011).

Facilitation of screening activities through the provision of more PAP smear facilities while the evaluation and adoption of non cytological based screening methods such as use of VIA and Lugols iodine and HPV DNA testing and ensuring wider coverage of screening activities is desirable. In developed area with low mortality rates from cervical cancer , it has long been established that organized screening programs has great impact on the reduction of cervical cancer mortality. Time trends in mortality from cervical cancer in Denmark, Finland, Iceland, Norway, and Sweden since the early 1950s were investigated in relation to the extent and intensity of organised screening programmes in these countries. In all five countries the cumulative mortality rates (0-74 years) fell between 1965 and 1982. In Iceland, where the nationwide programme has the widest target age range, the fall in mortality was greatest (80%). Finland and Sweden have nationwide programmes also; the mortality fell by 50% and 34%, respectively. In Denmark, where about 40% of the population are covered by organised programmes, the overall mortality fell by 25%, but in Norway, with only 5% of the population covered by organised screening, the mortality fell by only 10%. The results support the conclusion that organised screening programmes have had a major impact on the reduction in mortality from cervical cancer in the Nordic countries.(Laara E et al., 1987)

It has been established that cytologic screening programs that detect and treat precancerous lesions decrease mortality from cervical cancer in countries that have been able to achieve broad screening coverage at frequent intervals. However, in the majority of low-income countries like Sub Sahara Africa, cytologic screening has proven difficult to sustain, in large part because of its reliance on highly trained cytotechnologists, high-quality laboratories, and an infrastructure to support up to 3 visits for screening, colposcopic evaluation of abnormalities, and treatment.

Several factors have led to an expansion of the options for cervical cancer control. First, the availability of reliable HPV DNA assays has led to numerous studies documenting its higher sensitivity for detecting precancerous lesions compared with a single cytology test. Second, recent studies suggest that alternate screening strategies that use HPV DNA testing or simple visual screening methods may be more practical in some areas of the world like Sub Sahara Africa. Third, regardless of initial screening test (e.g., cervical cytology, HPV DNA testing, simple visual screening), strategies that enhance the linkage between screening and treatment, and seek to minimize loss to follow-up, have the best chance of measurable success. Additionally, economic evaluations of these alternatives have concluded that they are promising (Goldhaber-Fierbat & Goldie 2006). It has been suggested that the most efficient and cost-effective screening techniques in low-resource countries include visual inspection using either acetic acid or Lugol's iodine and DNA testing for human papillomavirus (HPV) DNA in cervical cell samples (Sankaranarayanan et al., 2009 cited in Jemal A. et al., 2011) A recent clinical trial in rural India, a low-resource area, found that a single round of HPV DNA testing was associated with about a 50% reduction in the risk of developing advanced cervical cancer and associated deaths. The limitations of HPV DNA testing include the cost (i.e. US$20–30 per test), infrastructure, and time needed to obtain a result . However CareHPV (Qiagen Gaithersburg Inc., MD, USA) has been developed as a simple, rapid and operational HPV test for low-resource settings that can produce results within 3 h. The compact, portable and battery-operated technology has stable conditions, and the test can be conducted by workers with minimal training. Data from China showed that, compared to VIA, CareHPV has a higher sensitivity (90% vs. 41%) and a reasonably comparable specificity (84% vs. 94%) to detect high-grade lesions. Moreover, a modelling analysis found that CareHPV has the potential to reduce the incidence of cervical cancer by 56% in China if given just three times over a woman's lifetime and effective treatment is available, suggesting its potential impact in reducing the burden of invasive cervical cancer in comparable settings. Regulatory approval is anticipated in developing countries in the near future, and CareHPV test if provided at a low cost, represents a promising alternative screening test, however, its performance and diagnostic value to detect pre-cancerous lesions need to be evaluated in African settings (Louie et al., 2009).

Widespread adoption of HPV vaccination to the recommended target population will reduce the disease incidence in the future. The vaccine is however seen to demobilize efforts towards setting up and improving screening services in places with poor screening coverage. The high cost of the vaccines is a constraint on low resource countries that have high incidence of the disease. It has been submitted that the vaccines if given to girls before onset of sexual activity, have the potential to dramatically reduce the incidence of HPV infection and therefore cervical cancer. Mclntyre, P. (2011) however also reported that one problem is that it is unlikely that the benefits will start to be felt in 15-20 years, and the full population impact will take 50 years or more to be felt. He is of the view that implementing an HPV Vaccination program is no substitute for organizing an effective screening system. The vaccine is of little value to the population of women who have already become sexually active as it cannot eradicate the virus if already present or retard the growth of incipient cancer. The report also noted that despite impressive results in clinical trials, they have not yet proven themselves in country programs. An example was the program in Romania where free vaccine was provided to girls 11 years old and a school - based campaign program of vaccination was started. It was reported that the take up rate was as low as 4%. Some parents prevented their daughters from getting vaccinated raising public health aspect issues towards high coverage and acceptance. The vaccine is therefore seen by some as a possible distraction from the main challenge as "the vaccine is not an alternative to cytology. We cannot fight cancer without regular cytology examination and that must be clearly stated" (Chil, A., quoted in Mclntyre 2011) . The expectations that vaccines which primarily protect against the most common strains of HPV infections (HPV types 16 and 18), which cause about 70% of cervical cancers, may prevent cervical cancer worldwide are at present high. The vaccines have shown high safety, efficacy and immunogenicity for both the quadrivalent HPV 16/18/6/11 vaccine (Gardasil_, Merck & Co., Inc.) and the bivalent HPV 16/18 vaccine (Cervarix_, GlaxoSmithKline Biologicals) (Schiller et al. 2008 cited in Louie Et al., 2009). A number of countries in sub-SaharanAfrica have licensed the HPV vaccines

(Table 3). However, implementation plans are lagging and will depend largely on the affordability of the vaccines, and a clear cost benefit ratio. However, affordable pricing is the most critical factor to facilitate the introduction of HPV vaccines in low- and medium-resource countries like Sub Sahara Africa in the short term. It is also extremely important that women continue to receive screening services because the current vaccines are being given to adolescent girls only, and even vaccinated girls should begin screening when they

Quadrivalent HPV 6/11/16/18 Vaccine (Gardasil ® Merck, SA)	Bivalent HPV 16/18 Vaccine (Cervarix ®, GSK)
Botswana	Congo
Burkina Faso	Cote d'Voire
Cameroon	Gabon
Central African Republic	Ghana
Chad	Kenya
Congo	Namibia
Cote d'Ivoire	Nigeria
Democratic Republic of Congo	Senegal
Equatorial Guinea	South Africa
Ethiopia	Uganda
Gabon	
Kenya	
Malawi	
Mauritania	
Mauritius	
South Africa	
Togo	
Uganda	

Table 3. HPV Vaccines licensure in Sub Sahara Africa as of March 2009 (Source: HPV Information centre, 2009 cited in Louie et al., 2009)

HPV Prevalence				
HPV type	Any histology	squamous cell carcinoma	Adenocarcinoma	unspecified
6	0.4	0.2	0.0	1.4
11	0.5	0.3	0.0	1.1
16	51.6	53.4	36.5	49.4
18	18.1	15.1	29.4	24.8
31	2.5	2.8	0.0	2.3
33	6.2	6.4	5.3	5.9
35	4.1	2.5	1.5	8.4
39	1.1	1.5	0.0	0.3
45	9.1	8.3	8.2	11.3
51	3.1	1.4	1.5	8.5
52	3.4	1.9	0.0	8.7
56	0.7	0.8	0.0	0.5
58	1.3	1.1	0.0	2.4
59	0.7	0.6	1.5	0.7
66	0.6	0.6	0.0	0.8
68	1.1	1.1	0.0	1.4
70	0.1	0.0	0.0	0.0
73	0.7	0.8	0.0	0.0
82	0.0	0.0	0.0	0.0

Table 4. Type - specific HPV prevalence among invasive cervical cancer cases in Africa by histology.(Source: WHO/IDC HPV information centre).

reach the recommended screening age since the vaccines do not provide protection for the 30% of chronic infections by HPV types other than HPV 16, 18, 6 and 11 that cause cervical cancer as shown in table 4 and that even in the recommended strains, protection is not 100% (Sankaranarayanan , 2009a, 2009b).

Prevention and early diagnosis through vaccination and screening requires effective mobilization of the target groups and this has been a problem in developing countries like the countries of Sub Sahara Africa. An approach to improve this has been formulated by Alliance for Cervical Cancer Prevention (ACCP) as follows. Since cultural and emotional barriers and practical needs are among the main reasons why women choose not to be screened, addressing these barriers and needs will help increase women's awareness and willingness to seek services. Screening, treatment, and follow-up services need to address women's cultural, emotional, and practical needs and concerns.

Community involvement is essential for: Using a community-based education approach as a way of building a discourse with women and promoting women's participation will help reduce fear and misunderstanding about cervical cancer screening and treatment and strengthen prevention knowledge and practices. Making women's experiences with services more positive ensures greater follow-up rates and increases the likelihood that women will share information about their good experience with peers. Reducing their fear of screening and treatment Strengthening women's understanding of prevention. Efforts in creating effective messages to improve women's awareness is needed. Messages should be targeted to reach women at highest risk of cervical cancer (generally aged 30 -50 years). Women should be involved in creating prevention messages and programs. Recognized barriers to women's participation in screening include: little understanding of cervical cancer, limited understanding of female reproductive organs and associated diseases , lack of access to services, shame and fear of a vaginal exam, fear of death from cancer, lack of trust in health care system, lack of community and family support. Common misconceptions about cervical cancer include the fact that people often do not know that it is preventable and the belief that screening involves Sexually Transmitted Infections (STI)/HIV screening including the belief that a positive/abnormal Pap smear result means a woman will die. In South Africa and Kenya, women often think a positive screening test means they have HIV infection While in Mexico, women fear that treatment will leave them sexually disabled.

Direct personal contact can facilitate screening exercises. This can be done through community meetings, posters, pamphlet newspaper advertisements or articles and radio or television messages. Key sources of information include peers who have received messages or been screened, leaders or members of women's groups, midwives and traditional healers ,community health promoters, community leaders ,nurses, nurse practitioners, or doctors. The target groups have to be located. Places to reach women are local women's groups community centres, women's workplaces, places of worship ,health facilities, women's homes, schools (parent's groups) and markets and key cervical cancer prevention messages should include the facts that good health practices can help prevent cancer, cervical cancer develops slowly and is preventable, screening can detect treatable, precancerous lesions before they progress to cancer, women aged 30 and older are more likely to develop cervical cancer than younger women, women in their 30s and 40s should be screened and that the screening procedure is relatively simple, quick, and is not painful. A small number of women who need treatment after screening can receive a simple procedure to remove the lesion. Screening test that is positive is not a death sentence but it provides the opportunity to eliminate abnormal cells before they become cancerous

Helping women discuss cervical cancer can bring the message home. This can be done through community health or outreach workers who can facilitate communication at the community level. Counselling by health care providers can both inform women and help them talk to their families. Women who receive treatment for precancerous lesions and who must abstain from sexual intercourse for several weeks especially need good counselling

To ensure women's positive experiences with screening, there is need to build and maintain positive provider-client relationships. This is needed because women are more likely to participate when they are treated well, health care providers are sensitive, responsive and respectful. Health care providers should develop a respectful rapport with clients. Women with positive experiences will become advocates when talking to other women.

Important counselling tips include listening and encouraging women to express their concerns being sensitive to cultural and religious considerations expressing support through non-verbal communication, such as nodding, keeping messages simple and answering questions directly, calmly, and in a reassuring manner and providing adequate information to remind them of the instructions. Services should be made accessible and appropriate through review of internal policies and procedures to ensure that programs are accessible and friendly to women. Having female health care providers in settings where women are uncomfortable with male health care providers, if possible can help. Ensuring affordability of the services and having settings that will ensure confidentiality and privacy including easy access to the women are essential. Local languages should be incorporated into the counselling medium. This can be done through involving women helps who can also assist in developing, implementing and evaluating programs and messages. Advisory team of women and other key community leaders can be consulted in order to deliver a package that will meet women's cultural, emotional and practical needs. This is aimed at increasing women's awareness of and willingness to seek services and improve women's experience with cervical cancer prevention services in addition to increasing program participation among women at risk.

High parity is associated with increased incidence of HPV infection leading to increased cases of cervical cancer. Most women in the region have high number of children resulting in worsening poverty and predisposition to the disease. Education on the need for reduced family size through the adoption of effective family planning methods can help in improving the general living condition of the people. This will eventually lead to sizeable population that can be easily reached with cervical cancer control programs.

Onset of sexual activities among teenage girls in the sub region from the age of 15years is high . This predisposes such girls to high risk of cervical cancer. The promotion of use of condom early through sex education programs in early school days can also help in reducing the transmission of HPV in the sub region. Closely linked to this is the issue of circumcision which should be encouraged among those with low level of practice.

Adoption of radiotherapy facilities based on less sophisticated technology like the Cobalt 60 based teletherapy and brachytherapy equipments that give acceptable good treatment outcome can help in the treatment of those already diagnosed with the disease. At The University College Hospital, Ibadan Nigeria, cobalt 60 brachytherapy source is used for high dose brachytherapy services with satisfactory outcome. This has served the purpose and is quite economical as the source is changed every 5 years instead of every 4 months as the case with the more popular iridium 190 source.

The HIV epidemic in the sub region has further increased the problem of cervical cancer as those so infected have rapid progression of the disease and usually have poorer outcome. Efforts to improve the control of the infection will also lead to the reduction in the mortality of cervical cancer.

4.2.1 Pre-requisites for cervical screening: Infrastructure, funding, training

The following were the submissions of Oxford University's Africa - Oxford Cancer Consortium (AFROX) meeting towards prevention of cervical cancer in Africa at St Catherin's College Oxford in March 2009. The meeting was chaired by Professor David Kerr of Oxford University and Professor Fiander Alison of The University of Cardiff. The following were the suggested prerequisite towards setting up effective screening programs in the sub region.

To set up a cervical screening programme, it is vital to address the associated infrastructure, funding and training needs. The delegates at this workshop recommended that it would be important for:

- Screening to be free at point of service and ideally as close to the people as possible.
- The health systems for African countries differ, and so a unique approach would be required for each country. However, each African Government should be lobbied to set aside a certain amount of money per year to carry out cervical screening. It would be important to have this recognised by a separate sub-section of the national budget. Finding sustainable funding for screening programmes is important - one way to achieve this could be for donors to insist that they would only fund a cervical cancer screening programme if the government agreed to provide funding support for the programme to continue after set-up funding ended.
- Building up political will and support for national funding support towards cervical cancer screening would be required. The First Ladies of Africa could have an important role in leading this. In Nigeria, the Governors' wives have been keen supporters of cervical cancer screening. Community advocates and the media would also need to be mobilised. These groups would also have a key role in raising public awareness about the causes of cervical cancer and why treatment would be important.
- Records and documentation of those being screened should be kept so we can tell how often or if they go for screening. This would also help to monitor whether it was simply the same people getting screened, or if the programme was succeeding in reaching new women.
- If possible, screening should be integrated into existing programmes, such as programmes for breast cancer screening, sexual health programmes, etc
- Training of health professionals to take smear tests and/or HPV tests would be necessary. Training of pathologists to read smear tests would also be critical.

4.2.2 Evaluation & cost effectiveness of cervical screening

The participants of this workshop discussed how to evaluate and measure the cost effectiveness and success of cervical screening programmes. They identified the following areas as being critical for consideration:

1. Training
   - Are programs easy to staff?
   - Should pap smears be abandoned for developing countries due to lack of people to read them?
   - Work must be done by another health care level other than doctor - but problems arise when empowerment of lower personnel is met by resistance from doctors
   - Brain drain an issue - we must address the retention of health care personnel
2. Cost
   - Need more interaction with health economists
   - Sustainability?
   - We must look into different financial flows, the idea of marketing campaigns and alternate financing schemes to raise substantial sums
3. Coverage
   - Feasibility of "mother-daughter" screening and vaccination project?
   - Feasibility of self-screening?
4. Political will
   - Need to sell a product to the policy makers? It is problematic to make a set of recommendations for African countries. The right screening depends on where you are. This is a highly heterogeneous environment and we can't settle on a one-size-fits-all approach
   - Dogmatic decisions to be replaced by research-based decisions…lobbying is good if it is on the basis of data.
   - Screening must be made part of a country's health policy
   - Demonstration projects are a good way to show political leaders the efficacy of screening programs
   - Millennium Development Goals (MDG) goals 4 and 5 (reduction in child mortality and improvement in maternal health) are a useful platform to use - argue that HPV is part of maternal health.

4.2.3 Creating a climate for informed decision-making in screening and vaccination

The delegates at this workshop suggested the following steps should be taken, to create a climate of informed decision-making about screening and vaccination programmes:

- Informed consent has to be tailored appropriately to population. Informed consent means different things in different situations and with different people, so it has to be appropriate to population.
- Screening should become part of routine care.
- Policy makers are not yet aware of the cost/toll of cervical cancer in their countries. Consequently, the development of cancer registries is important.
- Scientific evidence is important but a consensus statement can also be useful, for example from the world health organisation.
- Need to show politicians that the impact of screening would be seen now.

- Survivors' stories and the family stories of the women who have died of cervical cancer need to be told. Doctors and nurses should also tell stories about cervical cancer. We should not be afraid to tell individual stories; these are the ones that touch people.

5. Conclusion

Cervical cancer is still a problem in sub Sahara Africa. Concerted and focussed effort towards the reduction in the burden of the disease is urgently needed. The intensification of preventive, screening and therapeutic measures including education of the populace on these aspects can bring the disease under control as it is in the developed countries. Each country of Sub Sahara Africa should develop and implement sustainable preventive and screening programs using any of the available methods suitable and appropriate for their own setting instead of the present opportunistic screening activities prevalent in the region. Functional cancer registries are needed to analyze the pattern of the disease so as to help in planning control programs. There is also the need to address some of the conditions that predispose to practices that favor the development and spread of the disease. These conditions include poverty, illiteracy, political instability and widespread underdevelopment.

6. References

Abotchie, P. & Shokar, N (2009). Cervical Cancer Screening Among College Students in Ghana: Knowledge and Health BeliefsInt J Gynecol ; Vol 19 No.3 (April 2009):pp. 412–416.

Adebamowo CA and Adekunle O O(1999). Case control study of epidemiologic risk factors for breast cancer in Nigeria. Br J Surg. No. 86: (1999) pp. 771-775

AFROX Towards Prevention of Cervical Cancer in Africa 2009 www.afrox.org accessed on 2oth July 2011

Ajayi IO, Adewole IF (1998). Knowledge and attitude of out patients' attendants in Nigeria to cervical cancer. Central African Journal of Medicine ;44(2):41–44.

Anorlu RI, Banjo AAF, Odoemhum C, et al. (2000) Cervical cancer and cervical cancer screening: level of awareness in women attending a primary health care facility in Lagos. Nigeria Postgraduate Medical Journal 2000;70:25–28.

Anorlu RI, Orakwue CO, Oyeneyin L, et al. Late presentation of cervical cancer in Lagos: what is responsible? European Journal of Gynaecological Oncology 2004; 25(6):729–32.

Anorlu RI, Rabiu KA, Abudu OO, et al. Cervical cancer screening practices among general practitioners in Lagos, Nigeria. Journal of Obstetrics and Gynaecology 2007;27(2):181–84

Arrossi S, Paolino M, Sankaranarayanan R (2010)Challenges faced by cervical cancer prevention programs in developing countries: a situational analysis of program organization in Argentina. Pan American Journal of Public Health. 2010 Oct;28(4):249-57

Ashraf H. Poor nations need more help to slow growing cancer burden. Lancet 2003; 361:2209.

Auvert B., Sobngwi-Tambekou,J. Cutler, E., Nieuwoudt, M Lissouba, P, Puren, A & Taljaard D. Effect of male circumcision on the prevalence of high-risk human papillomavirus in young men: results of a randomized controlled trial conducted in Orange Farm, South Africa. Jounal of Infectious diseases Jan Vol.199 No.1(2009) pp. 14-19

Bayo S, Bosch FX, de Sanjose S, et al. Risk factors of invasive cervical cancer in Mali. International Journal of Epidemiology 2002;31:202–09.

Bosch F, Manos M, Munoz N., Sherman M, Jansen A et al. Prevalence of Human Papillomavirus in Cervical Cancer: a Worldwide Perspective. Journal of The national cancer Institute Vol. 87 No 11(1995) pp 796- 8Brinton LA, Reeves WC, Brenes MM, et al. Parity as a risk factor for cervical cancer. American Journal of Epidemiology 1989; 130:486–96.

Buga GA. Cervical cancer awareness and risk factors among female university students. East African Medical Journal 1998;75(7):411–16.

Chirenje ZM, Rusakaniko S, Kirumbi L, et al. Situation analysis for cervical cancer diagnosis and treatment in east, central and southern African countries. Bulletin of WHO 2001;79:127–32.

Chokunonga E, Levy LM, Bassett MT, et al. Zimbabwe cancer registry. In: Parkin DM, Whelan SL, Ferlay J, et al, editors. Cancer Incidence in Five Continents. Vol. VIII. Lyon: IARC Press, 2002. pp.104–05.

Clifford G, Franceschi S., Diaz M et.al HPV type- distribution in women with or without cervical neoplastic disease Vaccine Volume 24, Supplement 3, 21 August 2006, Pages S26-S34

Denny l., Kuhn L, Pollack A & Wright T. (2002) Direct visual inspection for cervical cancer for cervical cancer screening: an analysis of factors influencing test performance. Cancer No. 94 2002 pp 1699-1707.

Denny L, Quinn M, Sankaranarayanan R. Screening for cervical cancer in developing countries. Vaccine 2006; 24(Suppl 3):S3/71–S3/77 Male circumcision, religion, and infectious diseases: an ecologic analysis of 118 developing countries

Drain, P. Halperin, D Hughes, J Klausner, J & Bailey R Infect Dis. 2006; 6: 172

Gichangi P, Estamble B, Bwayo J, et al. Knowledge and practice about cervical cancer and Pap smear testing among patients at Kenyatta National Hospital, Nairobi, Kenya. International Journal of Gynecological Cancer 2003;13:827–33.

Goldhaber-Fiebert J & Goldie S. Estimating the cost of cervical cancer screening in five developing countries Cost Eff Resour Alloc. 2006; 4: 13.s 1186

Harding R, Profrene J, Higginson PJ. Palliative care in sub-Saharan Africa. Lancet 2005;365:1971–77.

Jemal,A.; Freddie Bray, Melissa M. Center, Jacques Ferlay,; Elizabeth Ward, David Forman. Global Cancer Statiatics A Cancer J Clin 2011;61:69–90 volume 61 No 2 March/April 2011 pp 79

Iliyasu Z, Abubakar IS, Aliyu MH, Galadanci HS Cervical cancer risk perception and predictors of human papilloma virus vaccine acceptance among female university students in northern Nigeria J Obstet Gynaecol. 2010;30(8):857-62

Kidanto HL, Kilewo CD, Moshiro C. Cancer of the cervix: knowledge and attitudes of female patients admitted at Muhimbili National Hospital, Dar es Salaam. East African Medical Journal 2002;79:467–69.

Laara, E. Day, N. & Hakama M.(1987) Trends in mortality from cervical cancer in the Nordic countries: association with organized screening programs. The Lancet Vol.329 No. 8544 (May 1987) pp 1247-1249

La Ruche G, You B, Mensah-Ado I, et al. Human papillomavirus and human immunodeficiency virus infections: relation with cervical dysplasia-neoplasia in African women. International Journal of Cancer 1998;76: 482–86.

Levin V, el Gueddari B, Meghzifene A. Radiation therapy in Africa: distribution and equipment. Radiotherapy and Oncology 1997;52:79–83.

Louie K, Sanjose S & Mayaud P (2009)., Epidemiology and prevention of human papilloma virus and cervical cancer in sub- Saharan Africa: a comprehensive review. Tropical Medicine and International Health Vol. 14 NO. 10 (October 2009) pp 1287-1302

Mclntyre, P. (2011) Cutting unnecessary deaths from cervical cancer. Cancer World No 42 June 2011 pp 58-62

Merriman A, Kaur M. Palliative care in Africa: an appraisal. Lancet 2005;365:1909–11

Moodley M, Moodley J, Kleinschmidt I. Invasive cervical cancer and human immunodeficiency virus (HIV) infection: a South African perspective. International Journal of Gynecological Cancer 2001;11(3):194–97.

Moodley JR, Hoffman M, Carrara H, et al. HIV and pre-neoplastic and neoplastic lesions of the cervix in South Africa: a case-control study. BMC Cancer 2006;6135.

Murray SA, Grant E, Grant A, et al. Dying from cancer in developed and developing countries: lessons from two qualitative interview studies of patients and their caretakers. British Medical Journal 2003; 326:368–72

Mutyaba Twaha Mutyaba, Elisabeth Faxelid, Florence Mirembe, & Elisabete Weiderpass 1 . Influences on uptake of reproductive health services in Nsangi community of Uganda and their implications for cervical cancer screening Reprod Health. 2007; 4: 4. 1186

Mutyaba T, Mmiro F & Weiderpass. Knowledge, attitudes and practices on cervical cancer screening among the medical workers of Mulago Hospital, Uganda BMC Med Educ. 2006; 6: 13. Pp.1186

Palacio-Mejía LS, Range-Gomez G, Hernandez Avila M, et al. Cervical cancer, a disease of poverty: mortality difference between urban and rural areas in Mexico. Salud Pública de México 2003;45(Suppl 3): S315–25

Parkin DM, Ferlay J, Hamdi-Cherif M, et al. Cancer in Africa: Epidemiology and Prevention. IARC Scientific Publications. No.153. Lyon: IARC Press, 2003.

Parkin DM, Whelan SL, Ferlay J, et al, editors. Cancer Incidence in Five Continents, Vol VIII. IARC Scientific Publication No.155. Lyon: IARC, 2002.

Sankaranarayanan R, Nene BM, Shastri SS, et al. HPV screening for cervical cancer in rural India. N Engl J Med. 2009;360: 1385-1394.

Sankaranarayanan R. HPV vaccination: the promise & problems. Indian J Med Res. 2009;130:322-326.

Schmauz R, Okong P, de Villiers EM, et al. Multiple infections in cases of cervical cancer from a high incidence area in tropical Africa. International Journal of Cancer 1989;43:805–09

Sepulveda C, Habiyambere V, Amandua J, et al. Quality care at end of life in Africa. British Medical Journal 2003;327:209–13.

Suba, E, Murphy, S, Donnelly, A. Furia,L Huynh, M &. Raab, S. Systems Analysis of Real-World Obstacles to Successful Cervical Cancer Prevention in Developing Countries American Journal of Public Health Vol. 96, No. 3(March 2006) pp 480-487

sSACCWG (sub Sahara Africa Cervical Cancer Working Group)Scientific Communiqué number 3. November 2010

Temmerman M, Tyndall MW, Kidula N, et al. Risk factors for human papillomavirus and cervical precancerous lesions: the role of concurrent HIV-1 infection. International Journal Gynecology and Obstetrics 1999;65:171–78.

Thomas J, Herrero R, Omigbodun A, Ojemakinde K, Ajayi ! , Fawole A, Oladepo O, Smith J et al. Prevalence of papillomavirus infection in women in Ibadan, Nigeria: a population-based study. British Journal of Cancer No 90 (Feb 2004) pp.638-645

The Alliance for Cervical Cancer Prevention (ACCP) Developing Cervical cancer screening programs that meet women's needs. www.alliance-cxca.org Accessed 19th July 2011

Urasa M & Dar E. Knowledge of cervical cancer and screening practices of nurses at a regional hospital in Tanzania African Health Sci Vol 11 No. 1 March2011 pp 48-57

Wright TC Jr, Ellerbrock TV, Chiasson MA, et al. Cervical intraepithelial neoplasia in women infected with human immunodeficiency virus: prevalence, risk factors, and validity of Papanicolaou smears. Obstetrics and Gynecology 1994;84(4):591–97.

5

The Indicators of Predicting Disease Outcome in HPV Carcinogenesis

Coralia Bleotu[1,2] and Gabriela Anton[1]
[1]*Stefan S. Nicolau Institute of Virology, Romanian Academy, Bucharest*
[2]*Faculty of Biology, University of Bucharest, Bucharest*
Romania

1. Introduction

Cervical cancer is one of the most common cancers among women worldwide, currently ranked as the third cancer causing death for females (Ferlay et al., 2010). Since the screening programs have been implemented the incidence and mortality associated with cervical cancer have declined (Gustafsson et al., 1997) but in developing countries it still remains a cause of death in women.

Although essential for the transformation of cervical epithelial cells, HPV is not sufficient, a number of other cofactors and molecular events being also incriminated (Woodman et al., 2007). Cervical HPV infection is a sexually transmitted disease which occurs in women short time after beginning the sexual life. In young women, the disease is usually transient, its prevalence decreasing around 30 years (de Sanjosé et al., 2007). A second peak of infection is found in older women and is superposed to the peak of cervical cancer incidence (Anton et al., 2011). Near 40 of the more than 140 HPV types identified so far can infect the cervix (Bernard et al., 2010). Differences in carcinogenicity of cervix specific HPV types are partially related to the expression of the E6 and E7 oncogenes which, among other functions, interfere with tumour suppressor proteins p53 and pRb, respectively (Sinal et al., 2005). By these interactions viral oncogenes abrogate the mechanisms of cell-cycle control and apoptosis.

As many studies sustain, in the absence of persistent infection the risk of cervical cancer is low (Schiffman et al., 2011). Persistent infection with high risk genotypes and the inability of the immune system to clear viral infection are the main factors contributing to tumors genesis. Thus, according to new concepts (Snijders et al, 2006), both the immune mechanisms of the host and the nature of infected cells are decisive for cervix lesions development. It takes 12-15 years before a hrHPV persistent infection may lead to cervical carcinoma, thus underlying the multistep process of cervical oncogenesis. Aberrant functions of tumour-suppressor genes as a result of their interaction with hrHPV viral genes, determine the genomic instability. These alterations cumulated with the action of various cofactors lead to progressive lesions and finally to cancer. The epithelial cells transformation is a 4 steps process, as proven by *in vitro* analysis: extended life span, immortalization, loss of anchorage and tumorigenic growth (Snijders et al, 2006). Each step is characterized by accumulation of (epi) genetic cell changes.

There is a continuing interest in the molecular mechanism of HPV oncogenic induction program, especially for clinicians who need new markers. Together with HPV DNA and PAP tests, these new markers may have additional value for risk assessment of cervical cancer and may reduce the number of biopsies. A major challenge for gynaecologists is to implement more markers in the routine practice, in order to have a better estimation of the risk a cervical lesion has to progress to cancer. Taking into account the contribution of oncogenic HPVs to malignant phenotype development by several interrelated mechanisms we evaluated the molecular markers (used in a variety of techniques) which might characterize different stages of HPV-associated epithelial lesions. The next step is to determine their suitability as "surrogate markers". In order to point host genes involvement, viral cell cycle has to be known.

2. HPV life cycle

All the HPV types infecting cervix are non-enveloped small sized viruses and have about 8000-base pairs in their double-stranded circular DNA. Their genome has overlapped open reading frames, coding for eight proteins, divided into an early (genes E1-E7) and a late region (genes L1-L2). The early genes are expressed in the infected basal cells while the late proteins are synthesized only in well differentiated cells. The early proteins have regulatory functions, being involved in HPV genome replication and transcription, cell cycle, cell signalling and apoptosis control, immune modulation and structural modification of the infected cell (Molijn et al., 2005; Sinal & Woods, 2005).

The replication cycle of HPV is tightly linked to differentiation of the epithelium it infects. For the initial infection to occur microlesions in the stratified epithelium are requested. Although some cell surface receptors have been mentioned, as heparin sulphate (Giroglou et al., 2001) and alpha-6 integrin, the controversy persists. It has been suggested that for a lesion to be maintained, the virus must infect an epithelial stem cell (Egawa, 2003). Following infection, in the basal cells of the epithelium, where low levels of viral early proteins (E1, E2, E5, E6 and E7) are observed, a low number of viral genome copies are maintained as episome. For viral DNA synthesis, beside E1 and E2 proteins that are necessary for viral replication, papilomaviruses use the host cell machinery. Viral transcription increases in differentiated cells while assembly of new virions occurs only in the squamous epithelia undergoing terminal differentiation. E4 is the first protein expressed late in infection and it may be accompanied by E5. The late proteins L1 and L2, are expressed in the granular layer of the epithelium and the assembled viruses are released from the fully differentiated cells. This pattern of gene expression is characteristic to productive infection and its pathological effect is specific for CIN 1 and some CIN 2 lesions. A deregulated E6 and E7 expression in proliferating cells and the interference of these viral oncogenes with tumour supressor genes p53 and pRB respectively, determine the cells to overcome senescence barrier and to develop a transformed phenotype (Fehrmann & Laimins, 2003). Recent studies have provided data on how different types of stimuli activate signalling pathways leading to senescence. It seems that these stimuli are funnelled through p53 and pRB (Narita et al., 2003) whose combined levels of activity determine the cells to enter senescence or to remain in a competent state for proliferation (Dirac & Bernards, 2003). Usually, the up-regulation of viral oncogenes expression is associated with viral genome integration into the host cell chromosome and with viral E2 gene disruption. Loss of the E2 leads to the uncontrolled expression of viral oncoproteins, which in turn leads to disruption of the normal cell cycle regulation and progres of HPV-associated cervical cancer (Hung et al., 2010). E6 and E7 oncoproteins are also required for the maintenance of the transformed status of infected cells (Longworth & Laimins, 2004). This pattern is characteristic for high grade CIN and carcinoma.

In terms of HPV pathogenesis, depending on the HPV genotyope involved in the infections, there are three types of clinical manifestations: (a) productive infection, characterized by virions production and a strictly regulated expression of the viral genes at well defined sites. CIN 1 represents the histological manifestation of productive infections. (b) latent/inactive infection, rarely visible, without clinical signs (asymptomatic), characterized by maintenance of the viral genome in basal layers and early viral proteins expression at levels below those necessary to produce an effective immune response. Viral persistence may be the consequence of infection in case of immune system depletion and may result from silencing expression of viral gene through methylation (Kalantari et al., 2004). (c) abortive infection, as a precursor to cancer, is associated in particular with hrHPV genotypes which induce changes in virus-infected cells causing cancer. HPV-induced cancers often arise in sites which are non-optimal for productive infection. Low risk HPV types are only occasionally associated with mucosal cancers.

3. Biomarkers – Indicators of the disease state

According to Wentzensen and von Knebel Doeberitz (2007), there are several applications for the cancer biomarkers including: (1) early detection of cancers (identification of individuals prone to develop cancer at a time point that still allows for a successful curative intervention); (2) improved reproducibility of the histopathological diagnoses (allowing for risk assessment of detected lesions and stratify intermediate lesions); (3) surveillance of persons at risk (allowing for non-invasive monitoring or reduce invasive procedures); (4) post therapy monitoring (predicting the progression and monitoring recurrences after treatment).

Approximately 80% of CIN1 lesions regress spontaneously (Follen and Richards-Kortum, 2000) and usually are managed conservatively. On the other hand, CIN2 and CIN3 have a considerable risk of progression toward invasive cancer and are therefore usually treated by conization or other less invasive procedures. Anyway, despite its rather low rate of progression, CIN2 is frequently treated, fact that leads to contradictory discussions (Spitzer et al, 2006; Wright et al, 2003). In order to restrict treatment to CIN1/2 groups, there is a need for biomarkers that could discriminate between CIN1/2 with high risk of progression and those with high chance to regress spontaneously (Ozaki et al., 2011). Additional markers are also necessary to overcome diagnostic inaccuracies due to the existence of several CIN mimics, such as immature squamous metaplasia (Duggan et al, 2006; Geng et al, 1999), or to heterogeneous distribution of dysplastic lesions that can result in over- and under-diagnosis.

A hrHPV positive test without associated important cytological changes would always require monitoring. The risk of progression toward invasive cancer increases with the lesions' grade (Ostor 1993), thus, biomarkers specifically associated with disease progression, allowing for a correct triage must improve the cervical cancer screening programs and the early detection of people at risk. Therefore, in order to be useful, the biomarkers must meet the following criteria: (1) they must be differently expressed in normal and high-risk tissues; (2) they should be synthesised in a well defined stage of carcinogenesis; (3) both the marker and its assay must be acceptable sensitive, specific and accurate; (4) they should be easily measured; (5) they should be correlated with a decrease in the cancer incidence rate (Follen and Schottenfeld, 2001). The inherent variability in interpretation between individuals has led to wide ranges in diagnostic precision between practices, but the advent of immunohistochemistry and the more recent discovery of new genes and their functions have resulted in the identification of cellular proteins that are differently expressed in tumours (Nucci et al., 2003).

3.1 Cell cycle regulation markers

The loss of cell-cycle control by HPV oncoproteins directly or indirectly interacting with the host genes (Giannoudis et al., 2000) leads to accelerated proliferation mirrored by an increased number of cells expressing specific markers. Among cyclins and cyclin dependent kinases (CDKs) that governed cell cycle, p53, Rb and CDK inhibitors (p15, p16, p18, p19, p21, p27) play a special role by arresting the cell cycle until damaged DNA is completely repaired. Therefore, the cell cycle regulators may shed light on the understanding of HPV-mediated cervical carcinogenesis (Conesa-Zamora et al., 2009).

The roles played by cyclins and CDKs in distinct phases of the cell cycle, suggest that they could be used as markers for cell proliferation in cervical malignancy (Skomedal et al., 1999).

The ability of HPV oncoproteins to disrupt growth regulatory proteins may have effects on the cyclin-dependent kinase inhibitors linked to the G1- and G2- checkpoints. As mentioned before, cell cycle deregulation in cervical carcinogenesis is by far linked to p53 and pRb. The degradation of p53 tumour-suppressor gene by E6 may result in accumulation of damaged DNA. By contrast with other cancers where p53 appears to be down-regulated by point mutations, in cervical cancer p53 expression seems to be increased; the levels of p53 in high-grade SIL (HSIL) and cervical carcinoma is higher than in low-grade SIL (LSIL) and normal cervix. There are authors who reported higher p53 expression in cervical biopsy specimens from patients without HPV infection or who where infected with low-risk HPV (Tsuda et al., 2003). Conflicting results on this topic have been published: some studies showed a significant correlation of p53 expression with CIN 3 or carcinoma compared with normal cervix or LSIL (Bahnassy et al., 2007) whereas others showed no significant association. These results suggest that the absence of p53 immunostaining might be due to the capacity of some hrHPVs to down-regulate in different extent the p53 expression, probably via E6-induced ubiquitination. Over-expression of p53 does not seem to be related to HPV oncoprotein action, as some authors noted higher expression of p53 protein in early lesions. These data support the hypothesis of a partially protective role of the wild-type p53 in the early stages of cervical lesions (Vassallo et al., 2000) and is correlated with the observation that high levels of p53 expression are detected mostly in low-grade SILs (LSILs) and lrHPV-associated lesions (Kurvinen et al., 1996). Thus, p53 might function as a molecular marker for the risk of the progression of HPV-associated SILs. Øvestad et al, (2011) reported that CIN2–3 lesions regressed if higher epithelial pRb and p53 levels were present. Therefore, they proposed p53 and pRB as biomarkers. One paper noted that in HPV-positive or –negative low CIN or ASCUS, in the majority of cases, p53 was overexpressed in the basal cell layer, thus presenting a positive response to viral infection or to the lesion (Cenci et al., 2005). A paper reported that the majority of CIN showed absent to focal staining while most of the invasive carcinoma showed regional to diffuse staining. A greater expression of p53 in the malignant cervical neoplasms than in the pre-malignant cervical lesions was noted, suggesting that p53 overexpression is not an early phenomenon in cervical cancer (Tan et al., 2007). p53 control the G1 transition to S phase and its abrogation affect the expression of p16, p21 and p27 cyclin inhibitors. p21, p27 and p57 CDK inhibitors inhibit the cyclin/CDK2, CDK4 complexes and causes G1 arrest. The levels of these proteins are of prognostic significance in cervical oncogenesis. p27 might be inactivated early in carcinogenesis by E7 hrHPV and may precede tumor invasion (Zur Hausen, 1994).

p16 is a tumor suppressor protein belonging to the family of INK4 cyclin-dependent-kinase inhibitors whose increased expression has been associated with HPV-infected dysplastic and neoplastic epithelium of the cervix. p16 expression is the result of negative feedback on functional inactivation of pRb by E7 HPV (Zur Hausen 1994). p16 protein normally acts like a negative regulator of cellular proliferation, but its inhibitory action is not efficient in the case of proliferating hrHPV infected cells (Dray et al., 2005). Most studies confirm p16 overexpression in all HSIL lesions but also in some normal epithelium of cervix at both protein (von Knebel Doeberitz et al., 2002) and messenger levels (Bleotu et al., 2009). On the other hand, p16 is not expressed in cervicitis nor is in squamous metaplasic epithelium (in the absence of CIN stages) (Hu et al., 2005). Still, other studies proved that p16 high level was found in cervical glandular epithelium and also in metaplasic epithelium. Therefore immunohistochemical analysis of p16 is considered a powerful tool in the identification of HPV-mediated premalignant and malignant lesions of the uterine cervix. Cytoplasm predominant localization of p16 seems to be related to the increasing histological grade of cervical lesion (Horn et al., 2006). Yıldız et al. found strong and full thickness staining for p16 in the cervix epithelium in HSIL lesions and weak and basal/rare staining in LSIL. All hrHPV-positive cases were p16-positive, but no statistically significant relationship between HPV infection and the intensity and distribution of p16 was found (Yıldız et al., 2007). Depending on the positive cells distribution, there have been recognised four patterns of p16 staining which correlate to the lesion's grade (Kostopoulou et al., 2011).

Cyclins such as cyclin D1 are subjected to molecular alterations that characterize cervical carcinoma. Cyclin D1 forms a complex with CDK4 or CDK6 to carry out the phosphorylation of pRb. The phosphorilation of pRb leads to the release of the transcriptional factor E2F which, in turn, induces the expression of proteins required for S phase. Since D type cyclins and E7 HPV possess similar binding regions for pRb and pRb related pocket proteins, inactivation of pRb either by the cyclin/CDK complexes in G1 or by interaction with the E7 hrHPV may result in a decreased expression of cyclin D1. There are controversial results on the role of cyclin D1 in cervical carcinogenesis and clinical outcome (Goia et al., 2010). Although some studies reported no correlation between the expression of D1 cyclin and dysplasia (Goia et al., 2010) some authors associated overexpression of cyclin D1 with a poor prognosis in cervical carcinoma (Bae et al., 2001). An increase in cyclin D1 expression was observed from CIN 3 to invasive carcinoma as a consequence of the inability of overexpressed p16 to inactivate CDK4/6, the partner of cyclin D1. The authors suggested that the immunohistochemical expression of cyclin D1 might be a marker in cervical cancer progression only if restricted beyond to the lower third layer (Conesa-Zamora et al, 2009).

Moreover, cytoplasmic staining is more noticeable in the basal and parabasal layers, suggesting a recently acquired alteration related to a high-grade dysplasia and the progression of the disease (Baldin et al., 1993). A significant increase in the cytoplasmic staining associated with an increasing degree of dysplasia was reported by Carreras et al. (2007) due to the fact that the number of cells in the S phase increases in severe lesions. This finding gives support to the cytoplasmic expression of p16 in lesions of higher grade since p16 is the inhibitor partner of cyclin D1 and they often appear together (Zhao M., et al., 2006). The relationship between cyclin D1 expression and an increasing degree of dysplasia was not as remarkable as that seen for p16 but was statistically significant.

Cyclin B1 complexes solely CDK1 (cdc2) to form the mitosis-promoting factor, which regulates the G2-M transition and is the primary regulator of mitosis. p53 was shown to prevent the G2-M transition by decreasing cyclin B levels. Some authors reported significantly cyclin B1 expression in invasive cervical cancer than in normal cervical tissue (Zhao P., et al., 2006).

Cyclin E is expressed and associated with CDK2 near the G1-S boundary. Cyclin E hyperexpression is related to pRB inactivation by E7HPV but can not be correlated with hrHPV types. Recent studies have shown that cyclin E antigen correlates with the presence of HPV in atypical squamous epithelial cells. The association is stronger in LSIL, thus recommending this potential biomarker as a useful tool in distinguishing between benign/reactive changes from preneoplastic squamous atypia (Weaver et al., 2000). Much more common in cervical lesions *versus* non-neoplastic epithelium, cyclin E sensitivity may hamper its use as a marker (Crum, 2000). Other authors consider cyclin E together with p16 as the most sensitive tools for LSIL and HSIL detection respectively (Keating et al., 2001). In ThinPrep samples, cyclin E and p21 expression seems to correlate better with HSIL (Moore et al., 2005). The Cyclin E/CDK2 complex phosphorylates p27, tagging it for degradation, thus promoting expression of **cyclin A** with progression toward the S phase. A close association between hrHPV and cyclin A1 was noted (Goia et al, 2010). This could be explained by its complex up-regulation by both E7 and E6 oncoproteins, making cyclin A active in both S phase and late G2 phase of the cell cycle. Cyclin A1 might be a useful marker of cell proliferation most notably orchestrated by the capability of E7 to abrogate the inhibitory activity of p21CIP1/WAF1/SDI1 on CDK and proliferating cell nuclear antigen-dependent DNA replication necessary for the G1-S transition (Erlandsson, F. et al, 2006). Studies on cyclin A as prognostic marker are limited.

Immunohistochemistry investigation of several cell markers (cyclin D1, cyclin E, CDK4, p53, mdm-2, p21, p27, p16, Rb and Ki-67) revealed that aberrations involving p27, cyclin E, CDK4 and p16 are early events in HPV 16 and 18-associated cervical carcinoma, whereas cyclin D1 and p53 pathway abnormalities are considered late events. Therefore, the authors considered that immunohistochemical tests for p16 and cyclin E could be useful in early diagnosis of cervical carcinoma (Bahnassy et al., 2007).

E7 HPV binds to and blocks the function of p21 and p27 in a p53-independent manner (Zehbe et al., 1999). Both p21 and p27 are involved in cell cycle arrest through binding to G1 phase cyclin-CDK complexes. E7 hrHPV modulates the cytoplasmic localization of p27 and inhibits p21 function. Some studies showed that p21 immunoreactivity seems to be significantly correlated with high grade stage of cervical disease. The protein was reported to be significantly increased in CIN3 and *in situ* carcinoma. On the other hand, p27 was reported to decrease from normal cases to carcinoma (Cheung et al., 2001). On the other hand, Huang et al. (2010) reported that p21 expression decreased in HPV 18 positive carcinomas. The fact that aberrant expression of p27, cyclin E and p16 are early events in carcinogenesis (while p21 occur late in cervical carcinogenesis) might be of interest for early diagnostic and for monitoring patients with cervical dysplasia (Bahnassy et al, 2007). No established relationship was found between p27 expression and cell proliferation in cervical cancer (Kumar & Verma, 2006).

3.2 Proliferation markers

Those cells with high proliferative activity that allow the accumulation of transforming mutations are more likely to be associated with premalignant and malignant tissues. The proliferative aspects distribution in specific layers (basal vs. parabasal vs. superficial) might indicate growth-regulatory mechanisms; thus the relation between proliferation and growth deregulation is of interest (Heatley, 1998). Proliferation in the normal cervix, in cervical intraepithelial neoplasia and in invasive cervical carcinomas can be assessed by a range of techniques requiring technologies of varying sophistication and accessibility, considered in four broad groups (Heatley, 1998): (l) mitotic counts on routinely processed histological sections and cytological smears; (2) *in vivo* or *in vitro* incorporation of tritiated thymidine in actively proliferating cells, by injection into the cervix and by incubation with fresh tissue, respectively; (3) immunohistochemical techniques for Ki-67 labelling index and AgNOR counts; (4) flow cytometry.

In the normal cervix, mitotic activity (quantified in routinely processed histological sections and cytological smears or by tritiated thymidine incorporation) is usually confined to the basal and parabasal layers, but in CIN the numbers and height of mitotic figures within the epithelium increases. The presence of mitotic figures is part of routine diagnosis and biomarker value is discussed as a whole.

Flow cytometry DNA content analysis on minced biopsy specimens (Melsheimer et al. 2004) or smear (Tong et al., 2009) allow the association between aneuploidy and dysplasia degree. lrHPV types tend to be associated with polyclonal lesions whereas hrHPV types are associated with monoclonal lesions (Park et al, 1996). Ploidy appears to be a measurable biomarker and a good predictor of the biological behaviour with a better predictive value than the histopathologic characteristics (Follen and Schottenfeld, 2001). It is considered that in advanced dysplastic lesions, aneuploidy precedes HPV integration, further supporting the notion that integration of viral genomes is the consequence and not the cause of chromosomal instability and transformation (Melsheimer et al. 2004). Therefore, an increased aneuploid DNA value together with the increase in grades of cervical dysplasia are specific prognostic markers of malignancy (Kashyap & Das, 1998); flow cytometric analysis of DNA ploidy may be a potential means providing a strategic diagnostic tool for early detection of cervical cancer (Melsheimer et al. 2004). The combination of DNA ploidy (determined by cytometric test) with HPV screening and cytology is an optimal method to detect progressive lesions since it has the highest sensitivity and specificity (Singh et al. 2008).

Some proliferating molecules were investigated by immunohistochemistry like biomarkers in cervical precursor lesions: PCNA, Ki67, ICBP90, etc.

Ki-67 is a nonhistone protein expressed in the nucleus during the whole cell cycle, except for the early phases of G0 and G1. It constitutes a marker for proliferating cells and was associated with severe dysplasia and cervical cancer (Sarian et al., 2006*)*. Ki-67 stains positive in the parabasal, basal and intermediate layers of condylomas, in the basal and parabasal layers of CIN; in addition, cells positive for Ki-67 staining are identified in intermediate and superficial layers of the squamous epithelium. Ki-67 expression correlates positively with histologic grade and distinguishes non-diagnostic atypia from SIL. The grade and pattern of Ki-67 expression in precursor lesions are still topics of debate (Vijayalakshmi et al., 2007*)*. Even Ki-67 is not as specific as p16 for precancerous lesions, its immunohistochemical diffuse pattern is associated with a severe lesion. A lot of studies were conducted in order to establish the objective, reproducible, and reliable use of Ki-67 in the classification of dysplastic changes in cervical epithelium. Expression of Ki-67 (MIB-1) in the upper layers/superficial layers of the epithelium corroborated with more than 15% of basal cells positive for MIB-1 staining can be used to distinguish condyloma from inflammation or squamous metaplasia (Mittal and Palazzo, 1998). Ki-67 evaluation can be also a valuable adjunct in the distinction of CIN from normal or benign cervical squamoepithelial lesions (Kruse et al., 2002; Keating et al., 2001). MIB-1 expression in the basal and the upper-third layer proved useful in grading SIL with equivocal mitotic index (Popiolek et al., 2004). Immature squamous metaplasia can be MIB-1 cluster positive, but this false-positive case showed a special staining pattern, different from CIN: 1) MIB-1 staining in the nuclei is not diffuse (as in CIN) but clumped; 2) positive nuclei are somewhat less densely packed than in CIN (Kruse et al., 2002). Noteworthy is that the presence of a cluster of at least two MIB-1-positive nuclei (MIB-C) in the upper two thirds of the epithelial thickness is a highly sensitive and specific marker to discriminate between normal epithelium and low-grade squamous intraepithelial lesion (Pirog et al., 2002). Cauterized dysplastic/condylomatous epithelium showed significantly greater expression of MIB-1 than cauterized normal epithelium, being a good marker (Mittal 1999).

Recent studies showed that two cell cycle-related proteins, minichromosome maintenance protein-2 (MCM2) and topoisomerase II-α (TOP2A) are overexpressed in cervical cancer. **Minichromosome maintenance protein 2** drives the formation of pre-replicative complexes in G1 phase; overexpression of MCM2 provides the link between oncogenic HPV infection and the molecular event of cervical dysplasia (Rihet et al, 1996). **DNA TOP IIA** is a nucleic enzyme that plays an important role in DNA replication, transcription, recombination, condensation, and segregation through interaction with the double-helix DNA (Ofner et al, 1994). **ProEx C** is a cocktail of two monoclonal antibodies that targets the expression of these two proteins (MCM2 and TOP II A) and its increased expression is associated with HSIL lesions. The ProExC signal is intense, diffuse and comprises the entire thickness of the epithelium in HSIL, with a variable pattern of the staining in LSIL, and is usually negative in reparative or reactive immature squamous metaplasias (Pinto et al., 2010). ProEx C positive expression seems to be more specifically associated with SIL than Ki-67 positive expression (Conesa-Zamora et al, 2009). ProExC immunostaining, when compared with p16 immunostaining, have similar specificity for CIN 2+ and higher specificity for CIN 3+ but lower sensitivity for CIN 2+ and CIN 3+ (Guo et al., 2011). Some reports suggested that ProExC can be more selective and informative for the progression of low-grade (CIN1) and moderate-grade (CIN2) lesions than Ki67 (Beccati et al., 2008).

ICBP90 protein is a member of a nuclear proteins family with DNA-binding properties involved in DNA replication. ICBP90 detection, used as a proliferation marker (Hopfner R, et al, 2000), gives information only concerning the number of cells that entered the cycle without any indication on the duration of the cycle. ICBP90 like Ki67 was linked to the development of an HSIL. 97.6% of HSILs positively stained for ICBP90; thus confirms it as a useful proliferation marker (Lorenzato et al., 2005). If an hrHPV type was present, the association of a suspect DNA profile with a positive proliferation marker could predict the presence of HSIL in a very accurate way. On the other hand the association of a suspect DNA profile with the presence of ICBP90-positive cells and MIB-1 in the upper two thirds of the epithelium could help to discriminate between an LSIL and an HSIL with high PPV, (Lorenzato et al., 2005).

3.3 Markers of epithelial organization and differentiation

The life cycle of human papillomaviruses (HPVs) is tightly linked to the differentiation program of the host's stratified epithelia that it infects. Viral infection induces changes in squamous differentiation, which is reflected by the pattern of cytokeratin polypeptide expression. By studying this pattern in relation with the presence of the virus, it was obtained an indication on the influence the virus has in individual cells, on the cellular differentiation. For example, E1-E4 contributes to different processes in both the early and late stages of the virus life cycle (Nakahara et al., 2005). The viral E1-E4 protein contributes to the replication of the viral genome as a nuclear plasmid in basal cells. Expression of the HPV-16 E1–E4 protein in human keratinocytes results in the total collapse of the cytokeratin matrix, but nuclear lamins and tubulin and actin networks are unaffected (Doorbar et al., 1991). On the other hand, the presence of the skin-type cytokeratins CK1 and CK10 in condylomata accuminata derived from anogenital skin (HPV 6 and HPV 11 positive) was decreased, whereas CK13 and to a lesser degree CK4 appeared increased (Mullink et al., 1991).

HPV infection may alter the differentiation status of the epidermis leading to a major expression of K14 in the basal and suprabasal layers (like in HPV infected normal epithelium), up to the more superficial layers (like in epidermodysplasia verruciformis, EV) (Barcelos & Sotto, 2009). Comparing the morphologic distribution of cytokeratins 13 and 14 and involucrin in naturally occurring low-grade SILs and high-grade SILs infected with a variety of HPV types, Southern et al., (2001) observed that: (1) the absence of cytokeratin 14 expression is associated with high-risk HPV infection and occurs more frequently in high-grade SILs; and (2) dedifferentiation, with loss of cytokeratin 13 or involucrin expression occurs only in high-grade lesions. Also, it was noted that in most LSILs infected with lrHPVs, cytokeratin 14 expression was present in all epithelial layers, with fewer lesions; the expression confined to the basal/parabasal layers with focal loss of expression. By contrast, only in few cases (11%) of LSILs infected with hrHPVs, cytokeratin 14 expressions was present in all epithelial layers; most of these lesions showed cytokeratin 14 expression confined to the basal/parabasal layers (56%), with a number of lesions showing focal loss of expression (33%) (Southern et al 2001). Loss/reduction of cytokeratin 14 protein expression level is associated with transformation but not immortalization because in HPV16 immortalized keratinocytes downregulation of cytokeratin 14 occurred only at a transcriptional level (the protein level remaining normal) (Bowden et al, 1992). In epidermodysplasia verruciformis CK1/10 showed retarded or negative expression and e-cadherin is diminished in superficial koilocytotic cells' foci, more superficially in EV. Positive staining for K16 and K4 was observed in normal HPV infected epithelium as in EV (Barcelos & Sotto, 2009).

Regauer & Reich (2007) found the following profile for the CK17: when antibodies against CK17 were used, the columnar endocervical epithelium showed no staining; basal keratinocytes in ectocervical glycogenated squamous epithelium have inconsistently, focally and weakly CK17 expression in cytoplasm; the proliferating cells of immature squamous metaplasia stain positive for CK17 in the subcolumnar reserve cells and in the proliferating basal and suprabasal cells, and negative for columnar cells; the mature metaplastic epithelium presents decreased or even lack of CK17 expression; high-grade dysplasia show concomitant staining of both CK17 and p16. They sustain a mutually exclusive immunohistochemical profile of CK17 and p16 that allows the separation of immature metaplasia with or without reactive atypia (characterized by strong, uniform CK17 staining of the proliferating cells with concomitant p16 negativity) from CIN III (characterised by strong diffuse staining of p16 in all dysplastic proliferating cells). The dual expression of CK17 and p16 in atypical squamous lesions with metaplastic features can sustain the hypothesis that CIN III alternatively may develop via HPV infection of metaplastic cells.

Considering all these aspects, we can say that in order to establish the correct diagnostic, all potential markers involved in epithelial reorganization and differentiation must be synchronic evaluated with other proliferating markers.

Plasma membrane expression of caveolin-1 (Cav-1), a constituent of lipid rafts and regulator of cell signalling, increases by the E5 HPV16 oncoprotein through the C-terminal 10 amino acids of E5. Moreover, E5 induces a 23- to 40-fold increase in the lipid raft component, ganglioside GM1, on the cell surface and mediates a dramatic increase in caveolin-1/GM1 association, a potential mechanism for immune evasion by the papillomaviruses (Suprynowicz et al., 2008). This phenomenon is very important in productive infection, in production of viral progen. But, an inverse relationship between Cav-1 expression and transformation has been clearly established. Cav-1 levels are reduced in transformed cells and forced reexpression of Cav-1 could abrogate anchorage-independent growth in transformed cells (Williams & Lisanti, 2005). In HPV transformed cells, caveolin-1 is downregulated and its expression is reduce by E6 HPV (Razani et al, 2000). In a small percentage of cervical cancer tumors caveolin-1 silencing occurs via promoter methylation (Chan et al., 2003; Dueñas-González et al, 2005).

E-cadherin is a transmembrane protein with a cytoplasmic domain connected to the actin cytoskeleton through association with cytoplasmic proteins, α-, β-, and γ-catenins (Piepenhagen & Nelson, 1993; Hinck et al, 1994). E-cadherin is essential for cell-to-cell junction and for cellular adhesion, being responsible for cellular interconnection, segregation of cell types, differentiation, epithelial polarization, cell stratification, signaling, cell motility and proliferation. Loss of E-cadherin function or expression has been implicated in cancer progression and metastasis. Down-regulation of E-cadherin was closely associated with progressive CIN and cell proliferation (Branca et al., 2006a) in HPV-positive tissue but not in the HPV-negative tissue (Samir et al., 2011). E-cadherin downregulation result in an increased cellular motility and metastasis.

Tissue transglutaminase 2 (TG2), member of calcium dependent enzymes family (Peng et al., 1999), is a cytosolic protein that catalyzes the formation of a covalent bond between the gamma carboxamide group of peptide bound to glutamine residue and the primary amino group of a wide variety of proteins leading to their post-translation modification (Boehm et al., 2002). TG2 induce polyamination of retinoblastoma protein, protecting it from caspase-mediated cleavage (Boehm et al., 2002), but also of HPV E7 disruption (the interaction of HPV E7 and pRb is a major step for cervical carcinogenesis) (Jeon et al. 2003).

TG2 levels in CIN1 are high, reflecting cellular response to inflammation and HPV infection and facilitating cell survival by its interaction with proteins involved in cell proliferation and cell death. In CIN2 and CIN3, the immunoreactivity for TG2 remains at moderately high levels, but typical for these cases, as compared with CIN1, it appears to be specifically expressed into nucleus. These nuclear translocations of TG2 in the high-grade CIN were associated to cell survival or anti-apoptotic phenotype, and therefore aid the progression or persistence of the CIN lesion. TG2 is a potentially useful marker for low-grade dysplasia or CIN1 lesions because there are clear differences between normal and CIN1 epithelium. On the other hand, TG2 represents one potential biomarker due to the nuclear/nucleo-cytoplasmic staining of TG2 in high-grade dysplasia (CIN2/3); that type of staining is not observed in normal cervical epithelium or generally in CIN1 lesions (Gupta et al., 2010).

3.4 Transcription factors and cell signalling pathway

Transcription factors are the principal modulators of gene expression and are involved in various processes controlling normal and transformed cell behaviour. Viral transcription is known to be positively regulated by glucocorticoid hormones via the up-stream regulatory region, which may partly explain its contributing effect to the transformation (Gloss et al, 1987; Mittal et al, 1993). However, in the complex picture of cervical cancer, hormone actions represent only one cofactor of HPV transformation. Thus, whatever the mechanism leading to carcinogenicity, there is a complex activation of transcription factors.

Previous studies demonstrated a functional involvement of the AP1 transcription factor in HPV-induced cervical carcinogenesis. Transcriptional activation of HPV in a keratinocyte-specific manner, depend on specific interaction between several nuclear factors and specific sites from LCR of certain HPV genotype. AP1 appears to be a common regulator of various HPV types expression, which act directly or through additional HPV type-specific that cooperate with AP1 to achieve full activation of virus gene expression (Butz & Hoppe-Seyler, 1993; Mack & Laimins, 1991; Kyo et al., 1995; Chan et al., 1990; Chong et al., 1991). Transcriptional regulation of HPV16 is activated also by NF1, TEF- 1, TEF-2 and Oct1 factors (Chan et al., 1990; Chong et al., 1991; Ishiji et al., 1992).

In HPV productive infection, E6/E7 transcripts were found to be expressed in most cellular layers with a reduced level of expression in the differentiated cells. E6/E7 expression was shown to correlate with AP1 factors distribution, suggesting that AP1 plays a significant role in the expression of viral oncogenes in uterine cervix differentiating epithelia. Co-expression of two proliferation inductors, AP1 and E6/E7, in undifferentiated cell layers might create a positive regulatory loop, contributing to the maintenance of initial HPV infection and subsequent activation in basal and suprabasal cellular layers (Kyo et al., 1997).

Aiming to obtain information about alterations in the expression of AP1 family members, de Wilde et al. (2008) found that, starting from immortal stages, c-Fos, Fra-2 and JunB expression became up regulated towards tumorigenicity while Fra-1, c-Jun, Notch1, Net and CADM1 became down regulated. They established that if the onset of deregulated expression of various AP1 family members became already manifest during the immortal state, a shift in AP1 complex composition appeared as a late event associated with tumorigenicity (de Wilde et al., 2008).

Nuclear factor-kappa B (NF-kB) is a ubiquitously expressed transcription factor, which has an important role in intracellular regulation of immune response, inflammation, and cell cycle regulation (Nair et al., 2003; Niederberger & Geisslinger, 2010; Hayden & Ghosh, 2011). NF-κB is one of the targets through which HPVs could interfere with the transcriptional control in cervical carcinogenesis (Spitkovsky et al., 2002; Fontaine et al., 2000). The oncogenic HPVs action on NF-kB through several ways: 1) there is a functional NF-kB binding site within the HPV16 LCR (long control region), at position 7554–7563, acting as an effective repressor of HPV transcription (Fontaine et al., 2000); 2) involvement of viral oncogene: hrHPV E7 inhibits NF-kB activation and nuclear translocation and prevents its binding to the responsive DNA elements, e.g. the LCR of hrHPV. On the other hand, hrHPV E6 inhibits NF-kB (p65)-dependent transcriptional activity within the nucleus, thus further contributing to the escape of hrHPV from the transcriptional control of NF-kB (Spitkovsky et al., 2002; Nees et al., 2001). Thus, NF-kB is one of the targets through which these HPVs could interfere with the transcriptional control in cervical carcinogenesis.

Using immunohistochemistry it was demonstrated that NF-kB is constitutively activated in high-grade CIN (Nair et al., 2003). In term of stain pattern, the intensity of cytoplasmic NF-kB expression increased along with the increasing grade of CIN, being most frequent in invasive carcinomas. There was no detectable nuclear NF-kB expression in the normal cervix or CIN1 and CIN2 lesions; an intense nuclear expression appears very rare, even in CIN3 and cervical cancer and is related to hrHPV (Branca et al., 2006b). Like biomarker, increased/normal cytoplasmic NF-kB expression can distinguish CIN with high specificity, but low sensitivity. On the other hand, the nuclear expression suffers from lower sensitivity. Studies accomplished by Branca et al, (2006b) clearly demonstrated that neither cytoplasmic nor nuclear NF-kB staining is a significant predictor of the clearance/persistence of hrHPV types after treatment of CIN.

The ERK/MAPK cascade has been reported to be activated in cervical cancer cell lines both by hrHPV and by some low-risk HPV types. In normal squamous epithelium of the cervix as well as in metaplastic squamous cells, Branca et al (2004) found weak cytoplasmic ERK1 expression confined mostly to the parabasal layers. Intranuclear staining is detected in CIN lesions that increase in both intensity and extent towards higher grade CIN lesions.

ERK1 expression showed poor specificity for predicting hrHPV, and do not have a practical value as a predictor of hrHPV in cervical cancer and its precursors. Although E5 HPV seems to mediate overexpression and activation of the ERK/MAPK signalling cascade, multiple other mechanisms that mediate the activation of ERK/MAPK pathways might be involved. Despite the fact that ERK1 expression seems to be an early marker of cervical carcinogenesis, it is not a specific marker of hrHPV in CIN and cervical cancer, and does not predict disease outcome in the latter.

3.5 Apoptotic markers

Apoptosis or programmed cell death is initiated by two types of biological signals: (1) extrinsic - the specific ligands activate their receptors (Fas-Fas ligand interaction) and (2) intrinsic - mitochondrial pathway used in response to non-specific stimuli (such as alteration of DNA, radiation and osmotic stress), leading to release of cytochrome c. Both paths lead to the activation of caspase 3.

In HPV infected cells, inhibition of apoptosis may be a mechanism to promote viral persistence (Kanodia, 2007). HPVs exhibit several mechanisms for overcome the apoptotic program. E6 binding to p53 stimulates p53 degradation thus preventing p53-dependent apoptosis of infected cells. On the other hand, it suppresses FasL E5 mediated apoptosis and is associated with reduction to half of the Fas expression.

Fas (APO-1/CD95) system regulates diverse physiological and pathological mechanisms for apoptosis. Interaction between Fas ligand and Fas receptor induces cell death, mechanism that could help to destroy HPV-infected keratinocytes. Facilitated cellular proliferation (Das et al., 2000), through reduced Fas mediated apoptosis has been described in cervical carcinogenesis by immunohistochemistry (Reesink-Peters et al., 2005) and polymerase chain reaction (Das et al., 2000). On the other hand, the paracrine overproduction of Fas-L could facilitate tumour progression by inducing apoptosis of the immune cells usually expressing Fas in their membrane, such as CD8 and natural-killer cells. During HPV induced cervical carcinogenesis two Fas-related mechanisms may be taken into consideration: (a) suppression of apoptosis in infected keratinocytes by downregulation of Fas-R expression; and (b) active immunosuppression by Fas-L overproduction by tumor cells (Das et al., 2000; Griffith et al., 1995). Granular cytoplasmic and membranous Fas-R stains are identified by immunohistochemistry in the normal cervix, and their loss has been reported in approximately 50% of squamous intraepithelial lesion (SIL) and SCC (Jones & Munger, 1996; Lerma et al., 2008). Fas-R expression by tumor cells seems to be unrelated to the stage or quantity of the lymphoid infiltrate and it is a constitutive event independent of tumor progression (Lerma et al., 2008). Fas L immunostaining in tumor cells is directly correlated with the tumor stages: 36.4% in stage I, 50% in stage II, and 75% in stage III, and inversely correlated with the presence of a florid lymphoid infiltrate. This suggest that Fas-L production by tumor cells results in decreased lymphoid cell reaction and might be a defence mechanism of the tumor against host's immunity (Lerma et al., 2008).

Bcl2 protein is localized in the mitochondrial membrane, the endoplasmic reticulum and in the nucleus. Bcl2 is an oncoprotein blocking cell apoptosis that can be induced by the absence of growth factors, alterations in DNA, viral infection, lymphokines action, cytostatic drug or radiation therapy. Its overexpression permits the malignant transformation of the cells and extends the survival potential of malignant cells.

The prognostic value in predicting lesion progression is disputed. Guimarães et al., (2005) found by immunohistochemical techniques that expression of Bcl2 in HPV-infected cervical biopsies is not useful for predicting the progression of HPV-related SIL. On the other hand, Singh et al., (2009) noted cytoplasmic expression of Bcl2 protein in cervical dysplasia, a various intensity of immunoreactivity between different cytological grades of cervical smears and an association with the presence of HPV16/HPV18.

Follow-up data revealed that cases with high-risk HPV and co-induced expression of apoptosis-regulatory proteins presented a trend to progressive disease (Sing et al., 2009). These data confirm the observations of Fonseca-Moutinho et al., (2004), that Bcl2 is an independent factor in defining low risk of progression for CIN 3 and co-expression of estrogen receptor, progesterone receptor, and Bcl2 may be a useful tool in identifying the CIN 3 lesions with low risk of progression toward cervical cancer. Bcl2 has a more important value in cancer, the ratio of Bcl2 to Bax expression determining the survival or the death following an apoptotic stimulus. In order to establish a new predictor of the outcome of radiotherapy for human cervical carcinoma, Harima et al., (1998) established that the increased Bcl2 expression after radiotherapy is correlated with poor survival, while increased Bax expression after radiotherapy is correlated with good survival; these findings suggest that the levels of Bax and Bcl2 expression after radiotherapy are useful prognostic markers in patients with human cervical carcinoma (Harima et al., 1998). Some studies confirm that evaluation of Bax and Bcl2 expressions provide independent prognostic information for the clinical course of the disease and therefore could be developed as prognostic indicators for cervical cancer: Bax expression was associated with good survival while Bcl2expression was associated with poor survival, and combination of Bcl2+/Bax+ was significantly associated with poorer disease free survival (Wootipoom et al., 2004).

3.6 Markers of chromosomal stability

Cells that escape from senescence by gene inactivation continue to divide and suffer telomeres loss reaching the second proliferative block, stage 2 of mortality (M2); this is characterized by massive cell death caused by critical shortness of telomeres and telomeres dysfunction. The telomerase is a RNA-dependent DNA-polymerase that synthesizes telomeres DNA and provides molecular bases for unlimited proliferative potential. Telomerase activity is absent in most normal somatic cells but present in more than 90% of tumor cells and immortalized cells *in vitro* (Kim et al., 1994). Regarding cervical neoplasia, it is not clear whether telomerase is activated during the progression of this disease or whether HPV16 infection activates directly telomerase *in vivo*. Most studies on cervical tissue or cervical swabs indicate telomerase activation only after progression to intraepithelial lesion (Nowak, 2000). Taken together, *in vitro* and *in vivo* studies suggest that infection with HPV16 and the concomitant expression of E6 is associated with telomerase activation. Cervical lesions containing hrHPV in early stages does not present telomerase activity or present it at low levels (Nowak, 2000). Some results show that telomerase activity appears only when E6 is expressed at elevated levels. The hTERT expression (telomerase catalytic subunit) is in agreement with E6 hrHPV role in telomerase activation, but this association lost its significance due to strong association between hTERT and stage of intraepithelial lesion. One feasible explanation may be done by the recent experiments concerning the E6/ E7 dynamics and telomerase expression along with the progressive grades (Peitsaro et al., 2004). The initially high levels of E6 decrease dramatically, while hTERT mRNA expression and telomerase activity increase by 10 and respectively 4 fold. This means that the telomerase activation by E6 HPV is an early event and selection of clones with increased telomerase activity will lead to tumor progression and this intimate association with gradual lesions hides hTERT association with E6 hrHPV. Taking into account that HPV infections have been associated with cervical cancer, telomerase activity may be a central mechanism by which HPV infections can lead to malignant transformation of cervical mucosa. Immunohystochemical studies on biopsy specimens have shown that normal epithelium is completely negative for hTERT or presents a profile scoring positive cells in parabasal layer. More positive cells were observed in the squamous metaplasia epithelium and sometimes in suprabasal metaplasia proliferating cells. Positive immunostaining was nuclear and limited to a few cells and stromal immunoreactivity was strictly associated to lymphocytes having constitutive hTERT expression. CIN lesions and cancer present a different pattern: hTERT-positive nuclei are present in all the layers of epithelium, but occasional cytoplasm expression can appear (Branca et al., 2006c). Paradoxically, there was a decrease in the nuclear staining intensity of hTERT in squamous cell carcinomas (Frost et al., 2000; Yan et al., 2004) with an increase in cytoplasm staining (Jarboe et al., 2002). Disturbance of the normal translocation mechanisms of hTERT to the nucleus, associated with cervical mucosa malignant transformation may be responsible for these differences in the expression pattern. Although it has been demonstrated that the loss of hTERT immunostaining may be associated with the deregulation of normal translocation mechanisms of hTERT to the nucleus, some authors suggest another mechanism involved in a reduced hTERT expression in human cancers: inactivation at the transcription level (Bleotu et al, 2010). The heterogeneity of both sensitivity and specificity in telomerase detection seen between different studies is due to: sample size (smear/lavage versus cervical biopsy), contamination with blood or necrotic cells (including telomerase inhibitors, which can lead to false-negative results) (Wang et al., 2004) or haemoglobin (a powerful inhibitor of PCR reaction). False positive results in strong inflammatory reactions may occur due to inflammatory infiltration.

More recently, some **epigenetic modifications** were associated with cervix HPV infection. Modifications encompass three types of changes: chromatin modifications, DNA methylation and genomic imprinting, each of which is altered in cancer cell.

Generally, HPV infections are followed by epigenetic changes such as methylation of viral genes or host genome. The pattern of HPV genes methylation varies depeding with the viral life cycle, the presence of disease and possibly the viral type. The *de novo* methylation of HPV DNA could be a host defence mechanism or a strategy that the virus uses to maintain a long-term infection, or both. Aberrant methylation of CpG islands in the promoter regions of tumour suppressor genes (TSG) is one of several epigenetic changes which contribute to carcinogenesis (Kumar & Verma, 2006). Viral oncogenes can induce tumor suppressor gene methylation following activation of DNA methyltransferases. For some genes, the prevalence of methylated forms increases with disease severity; for others, methylated forms are only detected in women with invasive disease. In a recent paper, aberrant DNA methylation was found as an early event in carcinogenesis and as an additional molecular marker for the early diagnosis. Among all studied genes, three were found as potential biomarkers of cervical cancer risk (hypermethylation of CDH13, DAPK1 and TWIST1 promoters) (Missaoui et al., 2011).

Aberrant methylation of the p16 gene occurs early within tumor cell populations. p16 is more frequently methylated in advanced tumors (Wong et al., 1999) thus suggesting that its reactivation could have therapeutic value. In a study performed on 62 cases of squamous cell carcinomas, Cheung et al showed that promoter methylation of PTEN was found in 58% of patients with persistent disease while those who died of the disease had a significantly higher percentage of PTEN methylation. Thus, PTEN was considered an important significant predictor for both total and disease-free survival after controlling age, pathologic grade and clinical stage (Cheung et al., 2004). Another studied gene was E-cadherin which methylation frequency in cervical cancer varies between 28 and 80.5% (Widschwendter et al., 2004a). It appears that E cadherin methylation have prognostic significance, cases with no promoter methylation having a better outcome in univariate and multivariate analyses. New studies are focused on identification of the methylation status of several genes present in the serum or plasma of patients with cervical cancer with regard to their prognostic significance.

In a study on 93 serum samples using the methyLight technique MYOD1 promoter methylation was strongly associated with shorter, disease-free and overall survival (Widschwendter et al., 2004b). Data suggesting that methylation of gene promoters in patients with cervical cancer is a common phenomenon have been reported. Strong correspondence between DAPK, p16, and MGMT genes methylation in serum and in primary tumors was noted thus allowing the discovery of a potential biomarker in sera. It has been found that parallel testing of HPV and PAX1 methylation in cervical swabs confers an improved sensitivity than HPV testing alone (80% vs. 66%) without compromising specificity (63% vs. 64%) for HSIL/SCC (Yang et al., 2003; Lai et al., 2008). When PAX1 methylation marker is tested alone, the specificity for HSIL/SCC is 99%. These data encourage further studies to identify a set of methylated genes that would have prognostic significance as surrogate markers.

Although the causal relationship between hrHPV infection and cervical cancer is demonstrated, HPV infection alone is not sufficient to induce the malignant transformation. Other genetic alterations, such as miRNAs, are required. MicroRNAs (miRNAs) are ~22 nt single-stranded, non-coding RNAs that generally negatively regulate their target mRNAs at a posttranscriptional level. The different expression of miRNAs in cervical cancer cells or tissues as compared with normal controls has been reported, and candidate miRNAs functioning as oncogenes (including miR-21, miR-127, miR-146a, miR-199a) and tumor suppressors (including miR-34a, miR-143, miR-145, miR-200a, miR-218) in cervical cancer carcinogenesis have been suggested (Lee et al., 2011). Using TaqMan MicroRNA Arrays, McBee and colab (McBee, et al, 2011) found that 18 miRNAs were overexpressed and 2 underexpressed (miRs-218 and 433). Only five miRNAs (miR-21, miR-135b, miR- 223, and miR-301b) may have the potential to be used as markers for progression from dysplasia toward invasive cervical disease. Some miRNAs might be down regulated in cervical HPV infection through methylation (Botezatu et al., 2011).

3.7 Markers of immune recognition

HPV presents some features that allow a specific immune behaviour: bypass the immune response, persist in the lower genital tract, induce and promote the progression of cervical cancer. These characteristics are related to (i) preferential localization of intraepithelial HPV infection, (ii) the absence of viral infection on the impact keratinocytes, (iii) the ability of HPV to interfere with innate immunity, and (iv) the expression of late proteins antigens responsible for generating antibody response. The virus uses some mechanisms to evade immune system: (1) it maintain slow infection levels so that only a low amount of virus is exposed to the immune system; (2) it exploits the redundancy of genetic code; (3) it mimics host proteins; (4) it modulates the antigen presentation; (5) interfere with IFN; (6) inhibition of cytokines and chemokine profile; (7) distortion of adhesion molecules; (8) modulation of adhesion molecules; (9) prevention of apoptosis; (10) inhibition of APC migration.

Several studies have analyzed immunohistochemically different sub-types of immune cells in tumor tissue biopsies (TCD4, TCD8, TCD3, BCD20, CD45, CD57, CD68, etc.). The immune response to cervical neoplasia varies with the extension of the disease. In SIL, typically associated with persistent HPV infection and high viral load, the lymphocyte subpopulations percentages estimated by image analysis were 41% for CD4, 45% for CD8, 7% for CD20, and 7% for CD56 (Kobayashi et al. 2004). Most researchers revealed the essential role intra-and peri-tumor cells play in the favourable development of cervical cancer, suggesting that certain survival predictors in cervical cancer relapse may be involved (Nedergaard et al., 2007, 2008). Such predictors are: inflammatory infiltrate (role in promoting long-term survival), low CD3 (role in predicting relapse), high CD8 cell density (involved in cervical cancer favourable prognosis) and low CD4 cell (involved in advanced stages of disease) (Nedergaard et al., 2007, 2008; Bell et al., 1995; Bethwaite et al., 1996; Chao et al., 1999).

Cytokine profile distortion leads to inappropriate immune response, which may have immunosuppressive effects (failure to eliminate infection in host). HPV infections are focal and detection of systemic cytokine serum levels are not associated with the clearance or persistence of HPV infection (Hong et al., 2010).

Evaluation of cytokines may predict high-risk HPV clearance or persistence in untreated patients with mild dysplasia or less. Among HPV-infected women, IFN-gamma is significantly associated with E6, E7 HPV16 and high-risk HPV viral load in the uterine cervix. Thus, increased intralesional IFN-gamma may be considered a prognostic marker for oncogenic potential of high-risk HPV (Song et al., 2007). The multivariate logistic regression analysis showed that IFN-gamma-positive results were significantly associated with clearance of high-risk HPV after 12 months of follow-up, suggesting that intralesional IFN-gamma may be a prognostic marker for clearance of high-risk HPV (Song et al., 2008).

Most studies regarding cytokine profiles in HPV associated cancers indicate that Th2 cytokines correlate with progression toward invasive tumors (Bais et al., 2005). So, cervical tumors infiltrating lymphocytes have predominantly Th2/Tc2 polarity and regional lymph nodes seem to have a high proportion of T cells. However, this is due to the tumor rather than to the mechanisms of circumvention used by HPV. Comparing the cytokine profiles in cervical secretions of normal cervicitis, presenting or not HPV DNA, it were described high levels of IL-10 in HPV + samples (Azar et al., 2004). The early increase of IL-10 in cervical lesions can induce the inhibition of immune response against HPV infection. These data suggest that the cytokine profile distortion to an immunosuppressive profile can be induced by HPV and can cause the development of cancerous lesions (Kanodia et al., 2007). Several cytokines have been shown to reduce HPV transcription; this repression involves TGF-β, interleukin 1 and TNF-α (H. zur Hausen, 2002). TNF-α repression is lost during malignant conversion.

4. Conclusions

HPV associated cancer still remains a cause of death in women. Epidemiological studies and laboratory data confirmed that persistent infections with high risk human papillomaviruses (hrHPV) cause virtually all cases of invasive cervical cancer. Cofactors and additional molecular events are essential for the transformation of cervical epithelial cells. These events imply cell changes that can be quantified in order to evaluate the correct status of the disease. An ideal marker should be easy to assay in a not invasively collected sample and should have a good sensitivity, specificity, positive predictive value (PPV) and negative predictive value (NPV). To investigate the cancer risks associated with HPV infection, sensible tools to asses the risk hierarchysation are requested to be developed, since the cytological assessment alone is not sufficient to classify cervical dysplasia. Sometimes, in order to discriminate between productive and transforming infection, a combination of biomarkers is required. Such combination will allow a correct risks hierarchysation. Although there are many studies focused on new potential biomarker for cervical cancer, until now few are validated by the scientific community and health care units.

5. Acknowledgements

Romanian National Grants CEEX 119; PN2-41030; PN2-41081.

6. References

Anton, G.; Peltecu, G.; Socolov, D.; Cornitescu, F.; Bleotu C.; Sgarbura Z.; Teleman S.; Iliescu D.; Botezatu A.; Goia C.D.; Huica I.; Anton A.C. (2011). Type-specific human papillomavirus detection in cervical smears in Romania. APMIS, 119, 1-9.

Azar, K.K.; Tani, M.; Yasuda, H.; Sakai, A.; Inoue, M.; Sasagawa, T. (2004) Increased secretion patterns of interleukin-10 and tumor necrosis factor-alpha in cervical squamous intraepithelial lesions. Hum. Pathol., 35, 1376-1384.

Bae, D.S.; Cho, S.B.; Kim YJ, et al. (2001). Aberrant expression of cyclin D1 is associated with poor prognosis in early stage cervical cancer of the uterus. Gynecol Oncol., 81, 341–347.

Bahnassy, A.A.; Zekri, A.R.; Saleh, M.; Lotayef, M.; Moneir, M.; Shawki, O. (2007). The possible role of cell cycle regulators in multistep process of HPV-associated cervical carcinoma. BMC Clin Pathol. 24;7:4. doi:10.1186/1472- 6890-7-4.

Bais, A.G.; Beckmann, I.; Lindemans, J.; Ewing, P.C.; Meijer, C.J.; Snijders, P.J.; Helmerhorst, T.J. (2005). A shift to a peripheral Th2-type cytokine pattern during the carcinogenesis of cervical cancer becomes manifest in CIN III lesions. J. Clin. Pathol., 58, 1096-1100.

Baldin, V.; Lukas, J.; Marcote, M.J.; et al. (1993). Cyclin D1 is a nuclear protein required for cell cycle progression in G_1. Genes Dev, 7, 812–821.

Barcelos, C.A.N. & Sotto M.N. (2009). Comparative analysis of the expression of cytokeratins (1, 10, 14, 16, 4), involucrin, filaggrin and e-cadherin in plane warts and epidermodysplasia verruciformis plane wart-type lesions. J Cutan Pathol. 36(6), 647-654.

Beccati, M.D.; Buriani, C.; Pedriali. M.; Rossi. S.; Nenci, I.; Quantitative detection of molecular markers ProEx C (minichromosome maintenance protein 2 and topoisomerase IIa) and MIB-1 in liquid-based cervical squamous cell cytology. Cancer 2008; 114: 196-203

Bell, M.C.; Edwards, R.P.; Partrige, E.E.; Kuykendall, K.; Conner, W.; Gore, H.; Turbat-Herrara, E.; Crowley-Nowick, P.A. (1995). CD8+ T lymphocytes are recruited to neoplastic cervix, J Clin Immunol., 15(3), 130–136.

Bernard, H.U.; Burk, R.D.; Chen, Z.; van Doorslaer, K.; Hausen, H.; de Villiers, E.M. (2010). Classification of papillomaviruses (PVs) based on 189 PV types and proposal of taxonomic amendments, Virology, 401, 70-79.

Bethwaite, P.B.; Holloway, L.J.; Thornton, A.; Delahunt, B. (1996). Infiltration by immunocompetent cells in early stage invasive carcinoma of the uterine cervix: a prognostic study, Pathology, 28(4), 321–327.

Bleotu, C.; Botezatu, A.; Goia, C.D.; Socolov, D.; Cornițescu, F.; Teleman, S.; Huică, I.; Iancu, I.; Anton, G. (2009) P16INK4A--A possible marker in HPV persistence screening. Roum Arch Microbiol Immunol. 68(3), 183-189.

Bleotu, C.; Botezatu, A.; Goia, C.D.; Socolov, D.; Dragomir, L.; Popa, E.; Cornitescu, F.; Teleman, S.& Anton, G. (2010), hTERT expression as a potential diagnostic marker, Romanian Biotechnological Letters, Vol. 15, No.1, pp. 4922-4930

Botezatu, A.; Goia, C.D.; Iancu, I.V.; Huica, I.; Plesa, A.; Socolov, D.; Ungureanu, C.; Anton, G. (2011). Quantitative analysis of the relationship between microRNA-124a,-34b and -203 gene methylation and cervical oncogenesis. Mol Med Report. 4 (1), 121-128.

Branca, M.; Ciotti, M.; Santini, D.; Di Bonito, L.; Benedetto, A.; Giorgi, C.; Paba, P.; Favalli, C.; Costa, S.; Agarossi, A.; Alderisio, M.; Syrjänen, K. (2004). Activation of the ERK/MAP Kinase Pathway in Cervical Intraepithelial Neoplasia Is Related to Grade of the Lesion but Not to High-Risk Human Papillomavirus, Virus Clearance, or Prognosis in Cervical Cancer, Am J Clin Pathol., 122(6), 902-911.

Branca, M.; Giorgi, C.; Ciotti, M.; Santini, D.; Di Bonito, L.; Costa, S.; Benedetto, A.; Bonifacio, D.; Di Bonito, P.; Paba, P.; Accardi, L.; Mariani, L.; Syrjänen, S.; Favalli, C.; Syrjänen, K.; HPV-Pathogen ISS Study Group., (2006a) Down-regulation of E-cadherin is closely associated with progression of cervical intraepithelial neoplasia (CIN), but not with high-risk human papillomavirus (HPV) or disease outcome in cervical cancer. Eur J Gynaecol Oncol., 27(3), 215-23

Branca, M.; Giorgi, C.; Ciotti, M.; Santini, D.; Di Bonito, L.; Costa S.; Benedetto, A.; Bonifacio, D.; Di Bonito, P.; Paba, P.; Accardi, L.; Mariani, L.; Ruutu, M.; Syrjanen, S.; Favalli, C.; Syrjanen, K. & HPVstudy group. (2006b), Upregulation of nuclear factor-kb (NF-kB) is related to the grade of cervical intraepithelial neoplasia, but is not an independent predictor of high-risk human papillomavirus or disease outcome in cervical cancer, Diagn Cytopathol, 34, 555–563.

Branca, M., Giorgi, C., Ciotti, M., Santini, D., Di Bonito L., Costa, S., Benedetto A., Bonifacio, D., Di Bonito, P., Paba, P., Accardi, L., Mariani, L., Ruutu, M., Syrjanen, S., Favalli, C., Syrjanen, K., (2006c), Upregulation of telomerase (hTERT) is related to the grade of cervical intraepithelial neoplasia, but is not an independent predictor of high-risk human papillomavirus, virus persistence, or disease outcome in cervical cancer, Diagnostic Cytopathology, 34, 739-748.

Boehm, J.E.; Singh, U.; Combs C et al (2002) Tissue transglutaminase protects against apoptosis by modifying the tumor suppressor protein p110. Rb J Biol Chem., 277, 20127–20130.

Bowden, P.E.; Woodworth, C.D.; Doniger, J., et al: (1992). Down-regulation of keratin 14 gene expression after v-Ha-ras transfection of human papillomavirus-immortalised human cervical epithelial cells. Cancer Res., 52, 5865-5871.

Butz, K. & Hoppe-Seyler, F. (1993). Transcriptional control of human papillomavirus (HPV) oncogene expression: composition of the HPV type 18 upstream regulatory region. J Virol, 67, 6476-6486.

Carreras, R.; Alameda, F.; Mancebo, G.; et al. (2007). A study of Ki-67, c-erbB2 and cyclin D-1 expression in CIN-I, CIN-III and squamous cell carcinoma of the cervix. Histol Histopathol., 22, 587–592.

Cenci, M.; Pisani, T.; French, D.; Alderisio, M.; Vecchione, A. (2005). pRb2/p130, p107 and p53 Expression in precancerous lesions and squamous cell carcinoma of the uterine cervix Anticancer Res. 25, 2187-2192.

Chan, W.K.; Chong, T.; Bernard, H.U. & Klock, G. (1990). Transcription of the transforming genes of the oncogenic human papillomavirus type- 16 is stimulated by tumor promoters through AP1 binding sites. Nucleic Acids Res, 18, 763-769.

Chan, T.F.; Su, T.H.; Yeh, K.T.; Chang, J.Y.; Lin, T.H.; Chen, J.C.; Yuang, S.S.; Chang, J.G. (2003). Mutational, epigenetic and expressional analyses of caveolin-1 gene in cervical cancers. Int J Oncol, 23, 599-604.

Chao HT, Wang PH, Tseng LY, Lai CR, Chiang SC, Yuan CC, Lymphocyte-infiltrated FIGO Stage IIB squamous cell carcinoma of the cervix is a prominent factor for disease-free survival, Eur J Gynaecol Oncol, 1999, 20(2):136–140.

Cheung, T.H.; Lo, K.W.K.; Yu, M.M.Y.; Yim, S.F.; Poon, C.S.; Chung, T.K.H.; Wong, Y.F. (2001). Aberrant expression of $p21^{WAF1/CIP1}$ and $p27^{KIP1}$ in cervical carcinoma Cancer Lett., 172, 93-98.

Cheung, T.H.; Lo, K.W.; Yim, S.F.; Chan, L.K.; Heung, M.S.; Chan, C.S.; Cheung, A.Y.; Chung, T.K.; Wong, Y.F. (2004). Epigenetic and genetic alternation of PTEN in cervical neoplasm. Gynecol Oncol, 93, 621-627.

Chong, T.; Apt, D.; Gloss, B.; Isa, M. & Bernard, H.U. (1991). The enhancer of human papillomavirus type 16: binding sites for the ubiquitous transcriptional factors Oct-1, NFA, TEF-2, NF1 and AP1 participate in epithelial cell-specific transcription. J Virol, 65, 5933-5943.

Crum, C.P. (2000). Contemporary Theories of Cervical Carcinogenesis: The Virus, the Host, and the Stem Cell, Mod Pathol., 13(3), 243–251.

Conesa-Zamora, P.; Doménech-Peris, A.; Orantes-Casado, F.J.; Ortiz-Reina S.; Sahuquillo-Frías, L.; Acosta-Ortega, J.; García-Solano, J.; Pérez-Guillermo, M. (2009). Effect of human papillomavirus on cell cycle–related proteins p16, Ki-67, cyclin D1, p53, and ProEx C in precursor lesions of cervical carcinoma: a tissue microarray study, Am J Clin Pathol., 132, 378-390.

Das, H.; Koizumi, T.; Sugimoto, T.; Chakraborty, S.; Ichimura, T.; Hasegawa, K.; Nishimura, R. (2000). Quantitation of Fas and Fas ligand gene expression in human ovarian, cervical and endometrial carcinomas using real-time quantitative RT-PCR. Br J Cancer 82, 1682–1688.

de Sanjosé, S.; Diaz, M.; Castellsagué, X.; Clifford, G.; Bruni, L.; Muñoz, N.; Bosch, F.X. (2007). Worldwide prevalence and genotype distribution of cervical human papillomavirus DNA in women with normal cytology: a meta-analysis. Lancet Infect Dis., 7, 453–459.

de Wilde, J.; De-Castro, A.J.; Snijders, P.J.F.; Meijer, C.J.L.M.; Rösl, F.; Steenbergen, R.D.M. (2008). Alterations in AP-1 and AP-1 regulatory genes during HPV-induced carcinogenesis, Analytical Cellular Pathology 30, 1, 77-87.

Dirac, A.M. & Bernards R. (2003). Reversal of senescence inmouse fibroblasts through lentiviral suppression of p53. J Biol Chem, 278, 11731–11734.

Doorbar, J.; Ely, S.; Sterling, J.; McLean, C.; Crawford, L. (1991). Specific interaction between HPV-16 E1-E4 and cytokeratins results in collapse of the epithelial cell intermediate filament network, Nature 352, 824 - 827.

Dray, M.; Russell, P.; Dalrymple, C.; Wallman, N.; Angus, G.; Leong, A.; Carter, J.; Cheerala, B. (2005). p16 (INK4a) as a complementary marker of high-grade intraepithelial lesions of the uterine cervix. I: Experience with squamous lesions in 189 consecutivecervical biopsies. Pathology, 37, 112-124.

Dueñas-González, A.; Lizano, M.; Candelaria, M.; Cetina, L.; Arce, C.; Cervera, E. (2005). Epigenetics of cervical cancer. An overview and therapeutic perspectives, Molecular Cancer, 4, 38 doi:10.1186/1476-4598-4-38.

Duggan, M.A.; Akbari, M.; Magliocco, A.M. (2006) Atypical immature cervical metaplasia: immunoprofiling and longitudinal outcome. Hum. Pathol, 37, 1473-1481.

Erlandsson, F.; Martinsson-Ahlzén, H.S.; Wallin, K.L.; Hellström, A.C.; Andersson, S. & Zetterberg, A. (2006). Parallel cyclin E and cyclin A expression in neoplastic lesions of the uterine cervix. British Journal of Cancer, vol. 94, pp. 1045–1050

Egawa K., (2003) Do human papillomaviruses target epidermal stem cells? Dermatology., 207(3), 251-254.

Fehrmann, F. & Laimins, L.A. (2003) Human papillomaviruses: targeting differentiating epithelial cells for malignant transformation. Oncogene, 22, 5201–5207.

Ferlay, J.; Shin, H.R.; Bray, F.; Forman, D.; Mathers, C.; Parkin, D.M. (2010). Estimates of worldwide burden of cancer in 2008: GLOBOCAN 2008. Int J Cancer, 127, 2893-2917.

Follen, M. & Richards-Kortum, R. (2000). Emerging technologies and cervical cancer. J Natl Cancer Inst., 92, 363-365.

Follen, M. & Schottenfeld, D. (2001). Surrogate endpoint biomarkers and their modulation in cervical chemoprevention trials, Cancer, 91, 1758–1776.

Fontaine, V.; van der Meijden, E.; de Graaf, J.; Schegget, J.; Struyk, L. (2000). A functional NF-kB binding site in the human papillomavirus type 16 long control region. Virology, 272, 40–49.

Fonseca-Moutinho, J.A.; Cruz, E.; Carvalho, L.; Prazeres, H.J.; de Lacerda, M.M.; da Silva, D.P.; Mota, F.; de Oliveira, C.F. (2004). Estrogen receptor, progesterone receptor, and bcl-2 are markers with prognostic significance in CIN III. Int J Gynecol Cancer, 14, 911-920.

Frost, M., Bobak J.B, Gianani, R., Kim, N., Weinrich, S., Spalding D.C., Cass L.G., Thompson, L.C., Enomoto, T., Uribe-Lopez, D., Shroyer K.R. (2000). Localization of telomerase hTERT protein and hTR in benign mucosa, dysplasia, and squamous cell carcinoma of the cervix. Am. J. Clin. Pathol., 114, 726–734.

Geng, L.; Connolly, D.C.; Isacson, C.; Ronnett, B.M.; Cho, K.R. (1999). Atypical immature metaplasia (AIM) of the cervix: is it related to high-grade squamous intraepithelial lesion (HSIL)? Hum. Pathol., 30, 345-351.

Giannoudis, A. & Herrington, C.S. (2000). Differential expression of p53 and p21 in low grade cervical squamous intraepithelial lesions infected with low, intermediate, and high hisk human papillomavirus, Cancer, 89, 1300–1313.

Giroglou, T.; Florin, L.; Schäfer, F.; Streeck, R.E.; Sapp, M. (2001). Human papillomavirus infection requires cell surface heparan sulfate. J. Virol., 75, 3, 1565-1570.

Gloss, B.; Bernard, H.U.; Seedorf, K.; Klock, G.; (1987). The upstream regulatory region of the human papilloma virus-16 contains an E2 protein-independent enhancer which is specific for cervical carcinoma cells and regulated by glucocorticoid hormones. EMBO J 6. 3735-3743.

Goia, C.D.; Iancu, I.V.; Socolov, D.; Botezatu, A.; Lazaroiu, A.M.; Huica, I.; Plesa, A.; Anton, G. (2010). The expression of cell cycle regulators in HPV - induced cervical carcinogenesis, Romanian Biotechnological Letters, 4, 15, 5377-5388.

Griffith, T.S.; Brunner, T.; Fletcher, S.M.; Green, D.R.; Ferguson, T.A. (1995). Fas ligand-induced apoptosis as a mechanism of immune privilege. Science, 270, 1189–1192.

Guimarães, M.C.; Gonçalves, M.A.; Soares, C.P.; Bettini, J.S.; Duarte, R.A.; Soares, E.G. (2005). Immunohistochemical expression of p16INK4a and bcl-2 according to HPV type and to the progression of cervical squamous intraepithelial lesions. J Histochem Cytochem., 53, 4, 509-516.

Guo, M.; Baruch, A.C.; Silva, E.G.; Jan, Y.J.; Lin, E.; Sneige, N.; Deavers, M.T. (2011). Efficacy of p16 and ProExC Immunostaining in the Detection of High-grade Cervical Intraepithelial Neoplasia and Cervical Carcinoma, Am J Clin Pathol, 135, 212-220.

Gupta, R.; Srinivasan, R.; Nijhawan, R.; Suri, V. (2010). Tissue transglutaminase 2 as a biomarker of cervical intraepithelial neoplasia (CIN) and its relationship to p16INK4A and nuclear factor κB expression, Virchows Arch, 456, 45–51.

Gustafsson, L.; Pontén, J.; Zack, M.; Adami, H.O. (1997). International incidence rates of invasive cervical cancer after introduction of cytological screening. Cancer Causes Control., 8, 755–763.

Harima, Y.; Harima, K.; Shikata, N.; Oka, A.; Ohnishi, T. & Tanaka, Y. (1998). Bax and Bcl-2 expressions predict response to radiotherapy in human cervical cancer, J Cancer Res Clinical Oncol, 124 (9)

Hayden, M.S. & Ghosh S. (2011) NF-κB in immunobiology, Cell Res, 21, 2, 223-244.

Heatley, M.K. (1998). What is the value of proliferation markers in the normal and neoplastic cervix? Histol Histopathol, 13, 249–254.

Hinck, L.; Nathke, I.S.; Papkoff, J.;et al (1994) Dynamics of cadherin/ catenin complex formation: novel protein interactions and pathways of complex assembly. J Cell Biol 125:1327–1340.

Hong, J.H.; Kim, M.K.; Lee, I.H.; Kim, T.J.; Kwak, S.H.; Song, S.H.; Lee, J.K. (2010). Association between serum cytokine profiles and clearance or persistence of high-risk human papillomavirus infection: a prospective study. Int J Gynecol Cancer, 20, 6, 1011-1016.

Hopfner, R.; Mousli, M.; Jeltsch, J.M.; Voulgaris, A.; Lutz, Y.; Marin, C.; Bellocq, J.P.; Oudet, P.; Bronner, C. (2000). ICBP90, a novel human CCAAT binding protein, involved in the regulation of topoisomerase II a expression. Cancer Res, 60, 121- 128.

Horn, L.C.; Lindner, K.; Szepankiewicz, G.; Edelmann, J.; Hentschel, B.; Tannapfel, A.; Bilek, K.; Liebert, U.G.; Richter, C.E.; Einenkel, J.& Leo, C. (2006). p16, p14, p53, and cyclin D1 expression and HPV analysis in small cell carcinomas of the uterine cervix, Int J Gynecol Pathol., 25, 2, 182-186.

Hu, L.; Guo, M.; He, Z.; Thornton, J.; McDaniel, L.S. & Hughson, M.D. (2005). Human papillomavirus genotyping and p16INK4a expression in cervical intraepithelial neoplasia of adolescents. Mod. Pathol., 18, 267-273.

Huang, L.W.; Seow, K.M.; Lee, C.C.; Lin, Y.H.; Pan, H.S.& Chen, H.J. (2010). Decreased p21 expression in HPV-18 Positive Cervical Carcinomas, Pathol. Oncol Res, 16, 1, 81-86.

Hung, C.F.; Monie, A.; Weng, W.H. &Wu, T.C. (2010). DNA vaccines for cervical cancer,Am. J. Transl. Res, ;2, 1, 75-87.

Ishiji, T.; Lace, M.J.; Parkkinen, S.; Anderson, R.D.; Haugen, T.H.; Cripe, T.P.; Xiao, J.H.; Chambon, P. & Turek, L.P. (1992). Transcriptional enhancer factor (TEF-1) and its cell-specific co-activator activate human papillomavirus-16 E6 and E7 oncogene transcription in keratinocytes and cervical carcinoma cells. EMBO J, 11, 2271-2281.

Jarboe, E.A.; Liaw, K.L.; Thompson, L.C.; Heinz, D.E.; Baker, P.L.; Mcgregor, J.A. , Dunn, T.; Woods, J.E. & Shroyer, K.R. (2002) Analysis of telomerase as a diagnostic biomarker of cervical dysplasia and carcinoma. Oncogene, 21, 664–673.

Jeon, J.H.; Choi,. KH.; Cho, S.Y.; Kim, C.W.; Shin, D.M.; Kwon, J.C.; Song, K.Y.; Park, S.C.; Kim, I.G. (2003) Transglutaminase 2 inhibits Rb binding of human papillomavirus E7 by incorporating polyamine. EMBO J 22:5273–5282

Jones, D.L. & Munger K (1996) Interactions of the human papillomavirus E7 protein with cell cycle regulators. Semin Cancer Biol vol. 7 pp. 327–337.

Kalantari, M,; Calleja-Macias, I.E.; Tewari, D.; Hagmar, B.; Lie. K.; Barrera-Saldana, H.A.; Wiley, D.J. & Bernard, H.U. (2004) Conserved methylation patterns of human papillomavirus type 16 DNA in asymptomatic infection and cervical neoplasia. J Virol. vol 78, pp. 12762-12772.

Kanodia, S.; Fahey, L.M, & Kast W.M.(2007), Mechanisms used by human papillomaviruses to escape the host immune response, Curr. Cancer Drug Targets, vol 7, pp. 79-89.

Kashyap, V.& Das, B.C. (1998), DNA aneuploidy and infection of human papillomavirus type 16 in preneoplastic lesions of the uterine cervix: correlation with progression to malignancy. Cancer Lett vol.123, pp. 47–52.

Keating, J. T.; Cviko, A.; Riethdorf, S.; Riethdorf, L.; Quade, B. J.; Sun, D.; Duensing, S.; Sheets. E. E.; Munger, K.& Crum, C. P. (2001) Ki-67, Cyclin E, and p16 INK4 are complimentary surrogate biomarkers for Human Papilloma Virus-related cervical neoplasia, American Journal of Surgical Pathology, vol 25 no. 7, pp. 884-891.

Kim, N.W.; Piatyszek, M.A.; Prowse, K.R.; Harley, C.B.; West, M.D.; Ho, P.L.; Coviello, G.M.; Wright W.E.; Weinrich, S.L.& Shay, J.W.(1994) Specific association of human telomerase activity with immortal cells and cancer. Science, vol 266, pp. 2011–2015,

Kobayashi, A.; Greenblatt, R.M.; Anastos, K.; Minkoff, H.; Massad, L.S.; Young, M.; Levine, A.M.; Darragh, T.M.; Weinberg, V.& Smith-McCune KK (2004) Functional attributes of mucosal immunity in cervical intraepithelial neoplasia. Cancer Res. Vol 64, pp.6766–6774

Kostopoulou, E.; Samara, M.; Kollia, P.; Zacharouli, K.; Mademtzis, I.; Daponte, A.; Messinis, I.E.; Koukoulis, G. (2011).Different patterns of p16 immunoreactivity in cervical biopsies: correlation to lesion grade and HPV detection, with a review of the literature.Eur J Gynaecol Oncol., 32, 1, 54-61.

Kruse, A.J.; Baak, J.P.A.; Helliesen, T.; Kjellevold, K.H.; Bol, M.G.W.; Janssen, E.A.M. (2002). Evaluation of MIB-1-positive cell clusters as a diagnostic marker for cervical intraepithelial neoplasia, Am J Surgical Pathol, 26, 11, 1501–1507.

Kumar, D. & Verma, M. (2006). Molecular markers of cervical squamous cell carcinoma, CME J Gynecol. Oncol, 11, 41-60.

Kurvinen, K.; Syrjanen, K.; Syrjanen, S. (1996) p53 and bcl-2 proteins as prognostic markers in human papillomavirus- associated cervical lesions, J Clin Oncol, 14, 2120-2130.

Kyo, S., Tam, A. & Laimins, L. A. (1995). Transcriptional activity of human papillomavirus type 31b enhancer is regulated through synergistic interaction of AP1 with two novel cellular factors. Virology 211, 184-197.

Kyo, S.; Klumpp, D.J.; Inoue, M.; Kanaya, T.; Laimins, L.A. (1997). Expression of AP1 during cellular differentiation determines human papillomavirus E6/E7 expression in stratified epithelial cells, J Gen Virol, 78, 401–411.

Lai, H.C.; Lin, Y.W.; Huang, T.H.M.; Yan, P.; Huang, R.L.; Wang, H.C.; Liu, J.; Chan, M.W.Y.; Chu, T.Y.; Sun, C.A.; Chang, C.C.; Yu, M.H.; (2008). Identification of novel DNA methylation markers in cervical cancer, Int. J. Cancer, 123, 161–167

Lee, J.W.; Kim, B.G.; Bae, D.S. (2011). MicroRNAs in cervical carcinoma, microRNAs in Cancer Translational Research, 189-199, DOI: 10.1007/978-94-007-0298-1_8

Lerma, E.; Romero, M.; Gallardo, A.; Pons, C.; Muñoz, J.; Fuentes, J.; Lloveras, B.; Catasus, L.; Prat, J. (2008). Prognostic significance of the Fas-receptor/Fas-ligand system in cervical squamous cell carcinoma, Virchows Arch, 452, 65–74.

Longworth, M.S. & Laimins, L.A. (2004). Pathogenesis of human papillomaviruses in differentiating epithelia. Microbiol Mol Biol Rev, 68, 362–372.

Lorenzato, M.; Caudroy, S.; Bronner, C.; Evrard, G.; Simon, M.; Durlach, A.; Birembaut, P.; Clavel, C.; (2005). Cell cycle and/or proliferation markers: what is the best method to discriminate cervical high-grade lesions?, Human Pathol, 36, 1101- 1107.

Mack, D.H. & Laimins, L.A. (1991). A keratinocyte-specific transcription factor, KRF-1, interacts with AP1 to activate expression of human papillomavirus type 18 in squamous epithelial cells. PNAS, 88, 9102-9106.

McBee, W.C.; Gardiner, A.S.; Edwards, R.P.; Lesnock, J.L.; Bhargava, R.; Marshall Austin, R.; Guido, R.S.&Khan, S.A. (2011). MicroRNA analysis in human papillomavirus (HPV)-associated cervical neoplasia and cancer. Journal of Carcinogenesis and Mutagenesis, vol 1, 114, doi:10.4172/2157- 2518.1000114

Melsheimer, P.; Vinokurova, S.; Wentzensen. N.; Bastert G., & von Knebel Doeberitz M. (2004). DNA aneuploidy and integration of human papillomavirus type 16 e6/e7 oncogenes in intraepithelial neoplasia and invasive squamous cell carcinoma of the cervix uteri, Clin Cancer Res, 10, 9, 3059–3063.

Missaoui, N.; Hmissa, S.; Trabelsi, A.; Traoré, C.; Mokni, M.; Dante, R.; Frappart, L. (2011). Promoter hypermethylation of CDH13, DAPK1 and TWIST1 genes in precancerous and cancerous lesions of the uterine cervix, Pathology - Research and Practice, 207, 1, 37-42.

Mittal, R.; Pater, A.; Pater, M.M. (1993). Multiple human papillomavirus type 16 glucocorticoid response elements functional for transformation, transient expression, and DNA-protein interactions. J Virol, 67, 5656-5659.

Mittal, K.; & Palazzo, J. (1998). Cervical condylomas show higher proliferation than do inflamed or metaplastic cervical squamous epithelium. Mod Pathol., 11, 780–783.

Mittal, K. (1999). Utility of MIB-1 in evaluating cauterized cervical cone biopsy margins. Int J Gynecol Pathol.;18, 3, 211-214.

Molijn, A.; Kleter ,B.; Quint, W.; van Doorn, L.J. (2005). Molecular diagnosis of human papillomavirus (HPV) infections, J. Clin. Virol., 32S, S43-S51.

Moore, G.D.; Lear, S.C.; Wills-Frank, L.A.; Martin, A.W.; Snyder, J.W.; Helm, C.W. (2005). Differential expression of cdk inhibitors p16, p21cip1, p27kip1, and cyclin E in cervical cytological smears prepared by the ThinPrep method. Diagn Cytopathol., 32, 2, 82-87.

Mullink, H.; Jiwa, N.M.; Walboomers, J.M.; Horstman, A.; Vos, W.; Meijer, C.J. (1991). Demonstration of changes in cytokeratin expression in condylomata accuminata in relation to the presence of human papilloma virus as shown by a combination of immunohistochemistry and in situ hybridization. Am J Dermatopathol., 13, 6, 530-537.

Nair, A.; Venkatraman, M.; Maliekal, T.T.; Nair, B. &, Karunagaran D. (2003). NF-kB is constitutively activated in high-grade squamous intraepithelial lesions and squamous cell carcinomas of the human uterine cervix. Oncogene, 22, 50–58.

Nakahara, T.; Peh, W.L.; Doorbar, J.; Lee, D.; Lambert, P.F. (2005). Human papillomavirus type 16 E1circumflexE4 contributes to multiple facets of the papillomavirus life cycle. J Virol. 79, 20, 13150-13165.

Narita, M.; Nunez, S.; Heard, E.; Narita, M.; Lin. A.W.; Hearn, S.A.; Spector, D.L.; Hannon, G.J.; Lowe, S.W. (2003). Rb-mediated heterochromatin formation and silencing of E2F target genes during cellular senescence. Cell, 113, 703–716.

Nedergaard, B.S.; Ladekarl, M.; Thomsen, H.F.; Nyegaard, J.R.; Nielsen, K. (2007). Low density of CD3+, CD4+ and CD8+ cells is associated with increased risk of relapse in squamous cell cervical cancer, Br J Cancer, 97, 8, 1135–1138.

Nedergaard, B.S.; Ladekarl, M.; Nyengaard, J.R.; Nielsen, K. (2008). A comparative study of cellular immune response in patients with stage IB cervical squamous cell carcinoma. Low number of several immune cell subtypes are strongly associated with relapse of disease within 5 years, Gynecol Oncol, 108, 1, 106–111.

Nees, M.; Geoghegan, J.M.; Hyman, T.; Frank, S.; Miller, L.; Woodworth, C.D. (2001). Papillomavirus type 16 oncogenes downregulate expression of interferon-responsive genes and upregulate proliferation-associated and NF-kB-responsive genes in cervical keratinocytes. J Virol, 75, 4283–4296.

Niederberger, E.& Geisslinger, G. (2010) Analysis of NF-kappaB signaling pathways by proteomic approaches. Expert Rev Proteomics. 7, 2, 189-203. Nucci, M.R.; Castrillon, D.H.; Bai, H.; Quade, B.J.; Ince, T.A.; Genest, D.R.; Lee, K.R.; Mutter, G.L.; Crum, C.P. (2003). Biomarkers in diagnostic obstetric and gynecologic pathology: a review. Adv Anat Pathol. 10, 2, 55-68.

Nowak, J.A. (2000).Telomerase, cervical cancer, and human papillomavirus. Clin. Lab. Med., 20, 369–382.

Ostor, AG. (1993). Natural history of cervical intraepithelial neoplasia: a critical review, Int J Gynecol Pathol, 12, 2, 186–192.

Ozaki, S.; Zen, Y.; Inoue, M. (2011). Biomarker expression in cervical intraepithelial neoplasia: potential progression predictive factors for low-grade lesions, Human Pathol, 42, 1007–1012.

Øvestad, I.T.; Gudlaugsson, E.; Skaland, I.; Malpica, A.; Munk, A.C.; Janssen, E.A.M.; Baak, J.P. (2011). The impact of epithelial biomarkers, local immune response and human papillomavirus genotype in the regression of cervical intraepithelial neoplasia grades 2–3. J Clin Pathol, 64, 303-307.

Park, T.W.; Richart, R.M.; Sun, X.W.; Wright, T.C.Jr. (1996). Association between human papillomavirus type and clonal status of cervical squamous intraepithelial lesions, J Natl Cancer Inst, 88, 355–358.

Peng, X.; Zhang, Y.; Zhang, H.; et al (1999) Interaction of tissue transglutaminase with nuclear transport protein importin-alpha3. FEBS Lett, 446, 35–39

Peitsaro, P.; Ruutu, M.; Syrjanen, S.; Johansson, B., (2004).Divergent expression changes of telomerase and E6/E7 mRNA, following integration of human papillomavirus type 33 in cultured epithelial cells. Scand. J. Infect. Dis., 36, 302–304.

Piepenhagen, P.A. & Nelson, W.J. (1993). Defining E-cadherin associated protein complexes in epithelial cells: plakoglobin, β-catenin and γ-catenin are distinct components. J Cell Sci, 104, 751–762.

Pinto, A.P.; Crum, C.P.; Hirsch, M.S. (2010). Molecular markers of early cervical neoplasia, Diagnostic Histopathology, 16, 445-454.

Pirog, E.C.; Baergen, R.N.; Soslow, R.A.; Tam, D.; DeMattia, A.E.; Chen, Y.T.; Isacson, C. (2002). Diagnostic accuracy of cervical low-grade squamous intraepithelial lesions is improved with MIB-1 immunostaining. Am J Surg Pathol. 26, 1, 70-75.

Popiolek, D.; Ventura, K.; Mittal, K. (2004). Distinction of low-grade squamous intraepithelial lesions from high-grade squamous intraepithelial lesions based on quantitative analysis of proliferative activity. Oncol Rep., 11, 3, 687-691.

Razani, B.; Altschuler, Y.; Zhu, L.; Pestell, R.; Mostov, K.E.; Lisanti, M.P. (2000). Caveolin-1 expression is down-regulated in cells transformed by the human papilloma virus in a p53-dependent manner. Replacement of caveolin-1 expression suppresses HPV-mediated cell transformation. Biochemistry, 39, 13916–13924.

Regauer, S. & Reich, O. (2007) CK17 and p16 expression patterns distinguish (atypical) immature squamous metaplasia from high-grade cervical intraepithelial neoplasia (CIN III), Histopathology, 50, 629–635. DOI: 10.1111/j.1365-2559.2007.02652.x

Reesink-Peters, N.; Hougardy, B.M.; van den Heuvel, F.A.; Ten Hoor, K.A.; Hollema, H.; Boezen, H.M.; de Vries, E.G.; de Jong, S.; van der Zee, A.G. (2005). Death receptors and ligands in cervical carcinogenesis: an immunohistochemical study. Gynecol Oncol, 96, 705–713.

Rihet, S.; Lorenzato, M.; Clavel C. (1996). Oncogenic human papillomaviruses and ploidy in cervical lesions. J Clin Pathol, 49, 892- 896.

Samir, R.; Asplund, A.; Tot, T.; Pekar, G.; Hellberg, D. High-Risk HPV Infection and CIN Grade Correlates to the Expression of c-myc, CD4+, FHIT, E-cadherin, Ki-67, and p16INK4a. J Low Genit Tract Dis. 2011

Sarian, L.O.; Derchain, S.F.; Yoshida, A.; et al. (2006). Expression of cyclooxygenase-2 (COX-2) and Ki67 as related to disease severity and HPV detection in squamous lesions of the cervix. Gynecol Oncol., 102, 537–541

Schiffman, M.; Wentzensen, N.; Wacholder, S.; Kinney, W.; Gage, J.C.; Castle, P.E. (2011) Human papilomavirus testing in the prevention of cervical cancer, JNCI, 103, 368-83.

Sinal. S.H.& Woods, C.R. (2005). Human papillomavirus infections of the genital and respiratory tracts in young children". Seminars in pediatric infectious diseases, 16, 306–316.

Singh, M.; Srivastava, S.; Singh, U.; Mathur, N.; Shukla, Y. (2009). Co-expression of p53 and Bcl-2 proteins in human papillomavirus-induced premalignant lesions of the uterine cervix: correlation with progression to malignancy. Tumour Biol. 30(5-6):276-285.

Singh, M.; Mehrotra, S.; Kalra, N.; Singh, U. & Shukla, Y.(2008). Correlation of DNA Ploidy with Progression of Cervical Cancer, J Cancer Epidemiol. 2008; Article ID 298495, 7 pages, doi:10.1155/2008/298495

Skomedal, H.; Kristensen, G.B.; Lie, A.K.; Holm, R. (1999). Aberrant expression of the cell cycle associated proteins TP53, MDM-2, P21, P27, cdK4, cyclin D1, RB, and EGFR in cervical carcinomas, Gynecol Oncolo., 73, 223–228.

Snijders, P.J.F.; Steenbergen, R.D.M.; Heideman, D.A.M.; Meijer, C.J.L.M. (2006). HPV-mediated cervical carcinogenesis:concepts and clinical implications, J Pathol, 208, 152-164.

Spitzer, M.; Apgar, B.S. & Brotzman G.L. (2006). Management of histologic abnormalities of the cervix, Am Fam Physician, 73, 1, 105–112.

Spitkovsky, D.; Hehner, S.P.; Hofmann, T.G.; Moller, A.; Schmitz, M.L. (2002). The human papillomavirus oncoprotein E7 attenuates NF-kB activation by targeting the NF-kB kinase complex. J Biol Chem, 277, 25576–25582.

Song, S.H.; Lee, J.K.; Seok, O.S. Saw, H.S. (2007). The relationship between cytokines and HPV-16, HPV-16 E6, E7, and high-risk HPV viral load in the uterine cervix. Gynecol Oncol., 104, 3, 732-738.

Song, S.H.; Lee, J.K.; Lee, N.W.; Saw, H.S.; Kang, J.S.; Lee, K.W. (2008) Interferon-gamma (IFN-gamma): a possible prognostic marker for clearance of high-risk human papillomavirus (HPV). Gynecol Oncol., 108, 3, 543-548.

Southern, S.A.; McDicken, I.W.; Herrington, C.S. (2001). Loss of cytokeratin 14 expression is related to human papillomavirus type and lesion grade in squamous intraepithelial lesions of the cervix. Hum Pathol., 32, 12, 1351-1355.

Suprynowicz, F.A.; Disbrow, G.L.; Krawczyk, E.; Simic, V.; Lantzky, K & Schlegel, R. (2008). HPV-16 E5 oncoprotein upregulates lipid raft components caveolin-1 and ganglioside GM1 at the plasma membrane ofcervical cells, Oncogene, 27, 1071-1078.

Tan, G.C.; Sharifah, N.A.; Salwati, S.; Hatta, A.Z.; Shiran, M.S.; Ng, H.O. (2007). Immunohistochemical study of p53 expression in premalignant and malignant cervical neoplasms. Medicine & Health, 2, 2, 125-132. ISSN 1823-2140

Tong, H.; Shen, R.; Wang, Z.M.; Kan, Y.J.; Wang, Y.Q.; Li, F.S.; Wang, Z.H.; Yang, J.; Guo, X.R.; the Mass Cervical Cancer Screening regimen group (macreg), (2009). DNA ploidy cytometry testing for cervical cancer screening in China (DNACIC Trial): a prospective randomized, controlled trial, Clin Cancer Res, 15, 20, 6438–6445.

Tsuda, H.; Hashiguchi, Y.; Nishimura, S., et al. (2003). Relationship between HPV typing and abnormality of G_1 cell cycle regulators in cervical neoplasm. Gynecol Oncol., 91, 476–485.

Vassallo, J.; Derchain, S.F.; Pinto, G.A.; Martinez, E.Z.; Syrjänen, K.J.; Andrade, L.A.; (2000). High risk HPV and p53 protein expression in cervical intraepithelial neoplasia Int J Gynaecol Obstet. 71, 1, 45-48.

Vijayalakshmi, N.; Selvaluxmi, G.; Majhi, U., et al. (2007). Alterations found in pl6/Rb/cyclin D1 pathway in the dysplastic and malignant cervical epithelium. Oncol Res.16, 527–533.

von Knebel Doeberitz, M. (2002). New markers for cervical dysplasia to visualise the genomic chaos created by aberrant oncogenic papillomavirus infections. Eur. J. Cancer, 38, 2229-2242.

Wang, S.Z.; Sun, J.H.; Zhang,W, Jin, SQ, Wang, HP, . Jin, IS, Qu, P. , Liu, Y. , Li, M. Telomerase activity in cervical intraepithelial neoplasia. Chin. Med. J., 117, 202–206, (2004)

Weaver, E.J.; Kovatisch, A.J.; Biboo, M. (2000). Cyclin E expression in early cervical neoplasia in ThinPrep specimens, Acta Cytologica, 44, 3, 301-304.

Wentzensen, N. & von Knebel Doeberitz, M. (2007). Biomarkers in cervical cancer screening, Disease Markers 23, 315–330 315.

Widschwendter, A.; Ivarsson, L.; Blassnig, A.; Muller, H.M.; Fiegl, H.; Wiedemair, A.; Muller-Holzner, E.; Goebel, G.; Marth, C.; Widschwendter, M.; (2004 a), CDH1 and CDH13 methylation in serum is an independent prognostic marker in cervical cancer patients. Int J Cancer, 109, 163-166.

Widschwendter, A.; Muller, H.M.; Fiegl, H.; Ivarsson, L.; Wiedemair, A.; Muller-Holzner, E.; Goebel, G.; Marth, C.; Widschwendter, M. (2004b) DNA methylation in serum and tumors of cervical cancer patients. Clin Cancer Res, 10, 565-571.

Williams, T.M. & Lisanti, M.P. (2005). Caveolin-1 in oncogenic transformation, cancer, and metastasis , Am J Physiol Cell Physiol, 288, C494–C506,.

Wong, Y.F.; Chung, T.K.; Cheung, T.H.; Nobori, T.; Yu, A.L.; Yu, J.; Batova, A.; Lai, K.W.; Chang, A.M. (1999). Methylation of p16INK4A in primary gynecologic malignancy. Cancer Lett, 136, 31-235

Woodman, C.B.J.; Collins, S.I.; Young, L.S. (2007) The natural history of cervical HPV infection, Nature, 7, 11-22.

Wootipoom, V.; Lekhyananda, N.; Phungrassami, T.; Boonyaphiphat, P.; Thongsuksai, P. (2004) Prognostic significance of Bax, Bcl-2, and p53 expressions in cervical squamous cell carcinoma treated by radiotherapy. Gynecol Oncol., 94, 3, 636-642.

Wright, T.C.Jr.; Cox, J.T.; Massad, L.S.; Carlson, J.; Twiggs, L.B.; Wilkinson, E.J. (2003). 2001 consensus guidelines for the management of women with cervical intraepithelial neoplasia, Am J Obstet Gynecol, 189, 1, 295–304.

Yan, P.; Benhattar, J.; Seelentag, W.; Stehle, J.C.; Bosman, F.T. (2004). Immunohistochemical localization of hTERT protein in human tissues. Histochem. Cell Biol., 121, 391–397.

Yang, H.J.; Liu, V.W.; Wang, Y.; Chan, K.Y.; Tsang, P.C.; Khoo, U.S.; Cheung, A.N.; Ngan, H.Y. (2003). Detection of hypermethylated genes in tumor and plasma of cervical cancer patients. Gynecol Oncol, 93, 435-440.

Yıldız, I.Z.; Usubütün, A.; Fırat, P.; Ayhan, A.; Küçükali, T. (2007). Efficiency of immunohistochemical p16 expression and HPV typing in cervical squamous intraepithelial lesion grading and review of the p16 literature, Pathology-Research and practice, 203, 445-449.

Zehbe, I.; Ratsch, A.; Alumni-Fabbroni, M. (1999). Overriding of cyclin-dependent kinase inhibitors by high and low risk human papillomavirus types: evidence for an in vivo role in cervical lesions. Oncogene, 18, 2201–2211.

Zhao, P.; Mao, X.; Talbot, I.C. (2006). Aberrant cytological localization of p16 and CDK4 in colorectal epithelia in the normal adenoma carcinoma sequence. World J Gastroenterol. 12:6391–6396.

Zhao, M.; Kim, Y.T.; Yoon, B.S.; Kim, S.W.; Kang, M.H.; Kim, S.H.; Kim, J.H.;. Kim, J.W.; Park, Y.W. (2006). Expression profiling of Cyclin B1 and D1 in Cervical Carcinoma, Exp Oncol 28, 1, 44–48.

zur Hausen, H. (1994). Molecular pathogenesis of cancer of the cervix and its causation by specific human papillomavirus types. Curr Top Microbiol Immunol.186, 131–156.

zur Hausen, H. (2002). Papillomaviruses and cancer: from basic studies to clinical application. Nat. Rev. Cancer, 2, 342-350.

6

Cervical Cancer Treatment in Aging Women

Kenji Yoshida[1], Ryohei Sasaki[1], Hideki Nishimura[1],
Daisuke Miyawaki[1] and Kazuro Sugimura[2]
[1]Division of Radiation Oncology
[2]Department of Radiology
Kobe University Graduate School of Medicine, Hyogo
Japan

1. Introduction

In Japan, the elderly population has been rapidly increasing, and the "aging society" is currently considered one of the nation's most important social concerns. According to statements by the Ministry of Health, Labour, and Welfare, the average life spans of men and women in 2008 were 79 and 86 years, respectively, and that of women in Japan is the longest in the world (Ministry of Health, Labour, and Welfare, 2009). The percentage of the elderly population in Japan will continue to increase. With the growing aging society, the number of elderly patients with various malignancies has been increasing. However, the rate of cancer in younger patients has also been increasing, due to changes in lifestyles, such as the increased popularity of Western food, viral infections, and genetic factors. In Japan, malignant neoplasms demonstrate the highest mortality rate, surpassing cerebrovascular and heart diseases since 1981, and lung cancer has demonstrated the highest mortality rate among every malignancy in both men and women.

Cervical cancer affects a wide age demographic, but, recently, the prevalence of disease among young women has been emphasized. It is well known that the most common cause of cervical cancer is human papilloma virus (HPV). Sexual relationships in younger women with little knowledge of sexually transmitted diseases appear to be an important factor contributing to the prevalence of HPV infection. In Japan, the most commonly afflicted age group is women in their late 30s to early 40s. Cervical cancer is one of the most common forms of cancer women aged ≤ 39 years old. The prevalence rate decreases for women aged 50 to 60 years and increases again for women in their 70s. As a result of the aging society and re-increase of prevalence rate, the number of elderly patients with cervical cancer has been increasing in Japan. The number of elderly patients with cervical cancer in the Western counties with aging societies has also been increasing as in Japan. We should remember that a 77-year-old cervical cancer patient, for example, may live for 10 to 20 additional years if the disease is cured and that these elderly patients should be treated with radical modalities similar to those used on young patients to achieve successful outcome. However, treatment modalities should be selected carefully because of the high likelihood of toxicity from the treatment and concurrent medical problems, such as hypertension, diabetes mellitus, dementia, cerebral infarction, and other cancers. In the daily clinical setting, the opportunities for treating elderly patients with several concurrent medical problems are increasing.

The basic treatment modality for cervical cancer is a surgical approach or radiotherapy (RT). In general, surgery is performed for patients with early-stage cervical cancers. RT can be performed for the patients with early- to advanced-stage cervical cancer. Additionally, in the previous reports, the treatment results of surgery and RT for early-stage cervical cancer were similar (Landoni et al., 1997; Perez et al., 1995 and Yamashita et al., 2005). Furthermore, RT appears to be a less invasive modality compared to surgery. These facts indicate that RT is a more appropriate treatment for the elderly patient population.

The aim of this chapter is to discuss the treatment modalities for elderly patients with cervical cancer with a focus on RT based on the knowledge from our experience and previous reports.

2. Details of a standard RT method, including recommendations for elderly patients with cervical cancer and a review of treatment outcomes

Selecting a treatment modality for elderly patients, cautious evaluation of their general condition, clinical staging, and concurrent medical problems are important because they usually do not tolerate treatment-related toxicity as well as do young patients. Inadequate treatment may result in lethal toxicity. Generally, RT is thought to be one of the most suitable modalities for preserving quality of life, and, therefore, RT is important for elderly patients. In this section, the general knowledge of clinical manifestations and pretreatment evaluation of elderly patients are described. Subsequently, the details of a standard RT method for cervical cancer, including recommendations for elderly patients, are illustrated, and the treatment outcomes of RT for elderly patients with cervical cancer are discussed.

2.1 Clinical manifestations and pretreatment evaluation

The most frequent and important clinical manifestation of cervical cancer is irregular vaginal bleeding. Other important clinical manifestations include bleeding during sexual activity, increase of vaginal discharge and lower-back pain. For advanced disease, the bleeding sometimes becomes severe, and blood transfusions are usually performed. Severe bleeding may have lethal results in elderly patients.

Clinical staging is generally performed according to the International Federation of Gynecology and Obstetrics (FIGO) stages (Creasman, 1995). However, thoracic to pelvic computed tomography (CT) or pelvic magnet resonance imaging (MRI) must be performed in both elderly and younger patients. Additionally, positron emission tomography (PET) scans should also be performed, if possible. These imaging procedures are useful for clinical staging and are important for the determination of the treatment modality. Similarly, pretreatment evaluation, including concurrent medical problems and performance status, is also important because elderly patients usually do not tolerate treatment-related toxicity as well as do younger patients. Using these methods, adequate treatment modalities for elderly patients can be determined.

2.2 Standard RT method for cervical cancer, including recommendations for elderly patients

According to the Clinical Practice Guideline in Oncology from the National Comprehensive Cancer Network (NCCN) guidelines (National Comprehensive Cancer Network, 2011), RT is recognized to be important in the definitive treatment. For FIGO stage IA2 disease, radical hysterectomomy (RH) + pelvic lymph node dissection (PLND) ± para-aortic lymph node sampling, or intracavitary brachytherapy (ICBT) ± pelvic RT, or radical trachelectomy + PLND ± para-aortic lymph node sampling is recommended. In addition, for FIGO stage IB1 or IIA1, RH + PLND ± para-aortic lymph node sampling, or pelvic RT + ICBT, or radical trachelectomy for tumors ≤ 2 cm (stage 1B1) + PLND ± para-aortic lymph node sampling is recommended. These recommendations indicate that RT can be used in early-stage diseases, and its importance increases in advanced-stage diseases. In other words, RT can be used to treat cervical cancer at any stage, and it is the most important treatment modality for elderly patients.

External beam radiotherapy (EBRT) combined with ICBT is the standard RT method for cervical cancer. For EBRT, patients were initially treated with whole-pelvic RT using a box field. The gross tumor, whole uterus, pelvic lymph nodes, parametria and uterosacral ligaments must be included in the RT field. Additionally, a sufficient vaginal margin from the gross disease (at least 3 cm) is necessary. In X-ray films, the superior limit is the upper border of the 5th lumber, and the inferior limit is the lower border of the obturator foramen for the anterior/posterior RT field. For the lateral RT field, the anterior limit is approximately 0.5 cm behind the pubic joint, and the posterior limit should involve the entire sacrum. In Japan, a centrally shielded field using an anterior/posterior opposed field is applied just before the starting ICBT subsequent to whole-pelvic RT to reduce the doses for organs at risk, especially the rectum and bladder. The daily fraction size of EBRT is approximately 1.8 to 2.0 Gy in general. The total dose of pelvic RT is 45.0 to 50.4 Gy. Although standard EBRT for cervical cancer is performed using a 3D technique, while a new RT method, which is known as intensity modulated radiotherapy (IMRT), has been expanding in many institutions. IMRT achieves the dose reduction of organs at risk, such as the rectum, bladder, colon, and small intestine, in the pelvic RT. Dose reduction for these organs will provide certain benefits, especially for elderly patients.

ICBT using a distinctive dose prescription point known as "Point A" is performed to boost the primary tumor and is an indispensable procedure in the RT of cervical cancer. Traditionally, low-dose rate ICBT (LDR-ICBT) was usually used, but high-dose rate ICBT (HDR-ICBT) using a 192-iridium remote afterloading system has become favored over LDR-ICBT. In Japan, most patients are treated with HDR-ICBT, and it is performed 3 to 5 times at 1-week intervals during EBRT. Generally, the single fraction size of HDR-ICBT ranges from 5.0 to 6.0 Gy, and the total dose is 15.0 to 29.0 Gy. Patients with higher stage diseases are usually treated with higher doses of whole-pelvic RT and lower doses of ICBT. Patients with lower-stage diseases are usually treated with higher doses of ICBT and lower doses of whole-pelvic RT. It is also important to reduce the doses for organs at risk in ICBT as well as EBRT. When performing ICBT, we should consider that toxicity from overdose to the rectum and bladder may lead to lethal results for elderly patients with cervical cancer. The doses for the rectum and bladder are evaluated according to the recommendation of ICRU Report 38 in most institutions (International Commission on Radiation Units and Measurements, 1985); however, these recommendations are based on the use of 2D treatment planning using X-ray films. Recently, 3D treatment planning systems for brachytherapy using CT or MRI, which are known as image-guided brachytherapy (IGBT), have been gradually expanding similarly to IMRT. Using this technique, the doses for the rectum and bladder are calculated more accurately compared to past treatment methods, and a more adequate dose distribution for the gross tumor will be achieved. In the near future, IGBT will be the preferred method in the treatment planning of brachytherapy. In the treatment of elderly patients, RT induced toxicity must be reduced as much as possible. The standard definitive RT methods and doses for cervical cancer in Japan according to stage (tumor size) are described in Table 1 (Japan Society of Obstetrics and Gynecology, The Japanese Society of Pathology, Japan Radiological Society, 1997).

stage (tumor size)	EBRT (Gy)		HDR-ICBT (Gy / fractions)
	whole pelvis	cenrally-shielded	
I	0	45-50	29 / 5
II (small)	0	45-50	29 / 5
II (large)	20	30	23 /4
III (small to middle)	20-30	20-30	23 /4
III (large)	30-40	20-25	15-20 /3-4
IVA	30-50	10-20	15-20 /3-4

EBRT: External beam radiotherapy, HDR-ICBT: High dose rate intracavitary brachytherapy

Table 1. Standard definitive RT methods and doses according to stage (tumor size)

A boost to the primary tumor by EBRT is an alternative method for elderly patients because they are usually in poor condition, due to concomitant medical problems, and these patients may not be tolerant of ICBT. To reduce the irradiated volume, retreatment planning based on newly obtained CT scans should be performed just before the start of the boost. In our institution, the most commonly used dose is 10.0 Gy in 5 fractions. ICBT alone for small tumors is also a treatment choice for elderly patients who cannot continue long-term hospitalization because of dementia or other mental problems. Additionally, pelvic RT with smaller fields, reducing the dose of ICBT, and other efforts should be performed to avoid severe toxicity for elderly patients with poor performance statuses.

A boost to the gross lymph node involvement on CT or MRI is often performed because the lymph node usually cannot be controlled by 50 Gy of pelvic RT. Although the boost to the lymph node involvement is important for cure, it may be too aggressive for elderly patients. Therefore, indication should be determined with caution. Patients with poor performance statuses from the beginning of RT, patients who experienced severe acute toxicity, or patients with multiple lymph node involvement (3 or more) should be excluded. Similar to the boost to the primary tumor by EBRT, retreatment planning based on newly obtained CT should be performed just before the start of the boost. In our institution, the most commonly used dose is 10.0 Gy in 5 fractions. Using IMRT will provide higher safety for elderly patients when the boost to the primary tumor or lymph node involvement is performed.

Para-aortic lymph node involvement is an evidence of advanced disease. For these patients, extended-field RT including the entire pelvis and the para-aortic region is sometimes performed. Extended-field RT is an aggressive modality for elderly patients. Treatment delay will often occur, and some patients cannot complete RT. Moreover, patients with advanced disease usually demonstrate poor performance status. Therefore, extended-field RT does not seem to be suitable for elderly patients. Palliative RT should be recommended for elderly patients with para-aortic lymph node involvement, while excluding patients in quite good condition.

2.3 Treatment outcomes of definitive RT for elderly patients with cervical cancer

Several reports have examined the treatment results of RT for elderly patients with cervical cancer. As for Japanese papers, Sakurai et al. retrospectively evaluated 380 patients with cervical cancer treated with definitive RT between 1970 and 1994 (Sakurai et al., 2000). Of the 380 patients, 215 were younger than 70 years, 124 were 70 to 79 years, and 41 were 80 years or older. All of the patients were treated with EBRT combined with LDR-ICBT. They reported that the 5-year overall survival (OS) rate in the youngest (younger than 70 years), intermediate (70 to 79 years), and oldest (80 years or older) groups were 58%, 50%, and 33%, respectively. The 5-year OS rate in the oldest group was significantly worse than that of the youngest group. They also reported that the 5-year cause-specific survival (CSS) rate in the youngest, intermediate, and oldest groups were 68%, 70%, and 65%, respectively. The CSS rates were not significantly different among the 3 groups. For the chronic complications, Grade 3 or 4 occurred in 6.5% of the youngest, 11.3% of the intermediate, and 7.3% of the oldest group. No significant differences were observed in those complications among the 3 groups. They concluded that EBRT combined with LDR-BT proved to be highly effective and safe for elderly patients with cervical cancer. Ikushima et al. retrospectively evaluated 727 patients treated with definitive RT between 1970 and 1994 (Ikushima et al., 2007). In this report, 727 patients were also divided into 3 groups. Patients aged ≤ 64 years (n = 337) was defined as the younger group (YG), patients aged 65 - 74 years (n = 258) were defined as the young-old group (YOG), and patients aged ≥ 75 years (n = 132) composed the older group (OG). EBRT combined with LDR-ICBT was the basic treatment. However, 16 of 337 patients in the YG, 7 of 258 in the YOG, and 10 of 122 in the OG were not treated with LDT-ICBT. The 5- and 10-year OS rates were 59% and 49% in the YG, 68% and 51% in the YOG, and 49% and 30% in the OG, respectively. The differences in the 5- and 10-year OS rates between the OG and other groups were significant. The 5- and 10-year disease-specific survival (DSS) rates were 60% and 52.5% in the YG, 75.7% and 67.8% in the YOG, and 65.9 % and 56.7% in the OG, respectively. In this study, the 5- and 10-year DSS rates in the YG were worse compared to the other groups, and the differences between the YG and the YOG were significant. Grade 2-4 late radiation morbidity in the bladder and/or rectum occurred in 22% of the YG, 31% of the YOG, and 8% of the OG. Grade 3-4 morbidity did not occur in the OG. They concluded that age was not a significant prognostic factor, and, in the management of cervical cancer, advanced age was not a contraindication to radical RT. We also retrospectively evaluated 40 patients aged ≥ 75 years who were treated with RT between 2000 and 2009 (9 were treated between 2000 and 2005, and 31 were treated between 2006 and 2009). In our study, 35 patients were treated with definitive RT, and 5 were treated with surgery + adjuvant RT (Yoshida et al., 2011). Among the 35 patients treated with definitive RT, 31 were treated with EBRT combined with HDR-ICBT. Of the remaining 4 patients, 3 were treated with EBRT alone and 1 with HDR-ICBT alone because of their medical condition. Of the initial 40 patients, 38 completed the treatment as planned, 1 completed with a delay, due to concomitant heart disease, and 1 could not complete the treatment because of acute toxicity. The 3-year OS and DSS rates for all of the patients were 58% and 80%, respectively, with a median follow-up of 20 months. Both acute and late toxicity were evaluated in our study. Grade 3 acute toxicity occurred in 5 patients. Of the 3 patients, 3 were treated with surgery + adjuvant RT. Grade 4 toxicity did not occur. Grade 3 late toxicity occurred in 2 patients. Of the two patients, one was treated with surgery + adjuvant RT, and the other was treated with BERT + HCR-ICBT with concurrent chemotherapy. Although the median follow-up was shorter, and a smaller number of patients were evaluated, our results were consistent with 2 large Japanese studies. We concluded that definitive RT for elderly patients was generally effective and safe, but aggressive treatment, such as surgery + adjuvant RT, concurrent chemoradiation, or a combination of these modalities, should be performed with caution.

Studies from other countries have also reported results regarding elderly patients with cervical cancer treated with RT. Mitchell et al. retrospectively analyzed 398 patients treated with RT between 1975 and 1993. Patients were divided into nonelderly (ages 35-69, n = 338) and elderly (ages ≥ 70, n = 60) groups (Mitchell et al., 1998). The basic RT method was a combination of EBRT and LDR-ICBT. However, 12.9% of the nonelderly group and 31.7% of the elderly group did not receive RT. The 5-year OS rates were 58.0% in the nonelderly group and 46.4% in the elderly group. The difference in the OS rate between the 2 groups was significant. However, the 5-year CSS rates were 76.3% in the nonelderly group and 84.1% in the elderly group. Unlike the OS rate, the CSS rate in the elderly group was better than in the nonelderly group, but this difference was not significant. The frequency and severity of acute and chronic toxicity were similar in both groups, and they concluded that definitive RT was effective and also well tolerated in elderly cervical cancer patients. Chen et al. described 295 patients treated with definitive RT between 1992 and 1997 and focused on HDR-ICBT (Chen et al., 2003). Patients were divided into 2 groups. Patients under 70 years of age (n = 179) were defined as a younger group, and patients aged 70 years or older (n = 79) were included in an older group. They used whole-pelvic RT with a total dose of 45-50 Gy in 20-25 fractions over 4-5 weeks. A boost for patients with FIGO IIB-IVA bilateral parametrial disease was performed up to 54-58 Gy using central shielding. After the completion of whole-pelvic RT, HDR-ICBT was performed at 1-week intervals. The standard dose to Point A for three insertions (before July 1995) was 7.2 Gy or 6.0 Gy (after July 1995). The authors noted that the Point A dose was decreased to 5.0 Gy for all 79 patients in the older group. Survival was calculated according to age and clinical stage. The 5-year respective OS for the older and younger groups were 82% and 85% for stage IB, 65% and 65% for IIA, 61% and 71% for 2 IIB, and 35% and 59% for 3 IIIA-B, respectively. No significant differences were observed. The respective 5-year CSS rates for the older and younger groups were 100% and 95% for IB, 85% and 75% for IIA, 78% and 72% for IIB, and 42% and 61% for IIIA-B, respectively. No significant differences were observed. As for the complications, only 3 patients developed acute Grade 3-4 gastrointestinal complications (2 in the older and 1 in the younger group). Twelve (15%) patients in the older group and 14 (7.8%) in the younger group developed late Grade 3-4 rectal complications, while 7 (8.9%) patients in the older group and 10 (5.6%) patients in the younger group developed Grade 3-4 small bowel complications. No significant difference was observed between the 2 groups for Grade 3-4 complications. The authors concluded that a combination of EBRT and HDR-ICBT was effective and tolerable for elderly patients.

The results in these reports indicated that there were no significant differences in the CSS (DSS) rates between the elderly and younger patients. Although several papers noted that the OS rate in elderly patients was significantly worse than the younger patients, this result was due to the increase of death from other causes in the elderly population and was expected. Toxicity due to RT was similar in both elderly and younger patients in all of the reports. Therefore, definitive RT, especially a combination of EBRT and ICBT, was equally effective for elderly patients and younger patients. Using IMRT, IGBT, or both, further reduction of treatment-related toxicity will be achieved with excellent treatment outcomes. In the near future, a combination of IMRT and IGBT will be the standard method of definitive RT for elderly patients with cervical cancer.

3. Surgical approaches for elderly patients

A surgical approach for elderly patients with cervical cancer is controversial. Conization of the cervix for FIGO stage 0 cancer is well tolerable, even for elderly patients, but the standard surgical approach, RH and PLND, appears to be invasive. Wright et al. retrospectively analyzed 1582 patients with cervical cancer who were treated between 1986 and 2003 (Wright et al., 2005). Of the 1582 patients, 1385 were aged < 70 years, and 197 were aged ≥ 70 years. Surgery (including RH, modified RH, extrafascial hysterectomy, or trachelectomy) was performed for 753 of 1385 (54.4%) patients aged < 70 years and was performed for 32 of 197 (16.2%) patients aged ≥ 70 years. However, RT or chemoradiation (CRT) was performed for 605 of 1385 (43.7%) patients aged < 70 years and was performed for 156 of 197 (79.1%) patients aged ≥ 70 years. They stressed that younger patients were more likely to undergo surgery, and older patients were more likely to receive RT. There are several reports about RH for cervical cancer concerning age. Fuchtner et al. (1992) compared 45 women older than 65 years treated with RH and 90 women less than 65 years treated similarly (Fuchtner et al., 1992). Although transfusions were required more frequently in the elderly patients, there were no significant differences in survival or complications. They concluded that age alone should not be a contraindication for RH in elderly patients with cervical cancer. Geisler et al. examined 62 patients aged over 65 years who underwent RH and a lymphadenectomy between 1965 and 1998 (Geisler et al., 2001). These patients were matched with 124 patients aged 50 years or younger who underwent the same procedure. Although the period of the postoperative hospital stay was longer in the elderly group than the younger group, there were no significant differences in the percentages of intraoperative and postoperative complications. They concluded that radical hysterectomy is a safe surgical procedure in a select population of patients aged 65 years or over. Mousavi et al. retrospectively evaluated 22 patients aged 60 years and above who underwent a Wertheim RH between 1999 and 2005, comparing 128 matched cases under 60 years who underwent the same procedure during the same period (Mousavi et al., 2008). There were no operative mortalities in either group, and there was no significant difference in morbidity between the 2 groups. The mean postoperative hospital stay was significantly longer in the older patients. They concluded that Wertheim RH is a safe surgical procedure in the selected population of patients aged 60 years and older. From the results of these reports about RH, the authors emphasized that it was a safe treatment modality for elderly patients. However, they defined "elderly" as "60 years and above" or "over 65 years." On the other hand, in the reports about RT, "elderly" was defined as "over 70 years" or "75 years or older." In recent years, "elderly" generally includes patients aged 75 years or older or at least over 70 years. Therefore, patients defined as elderly in reports about RH were considered to be "middle aged." Therefore, whether RH is safe for elderly patients aged "over 70 years" or "75 years or older" remains unclear.

Patients treated with RH + PLND with pathological risk factors, such as lymph node metastasis, lymphatic, vascular, or deep stromal invasion, should receive postoperative adjuvant RT. RH + PLND and adjuvant RT is considered an aggressive treatment and, generally, treatment-related toxicities, such as adhesive intestinal obstruction, or lymphatic edema of the lower extremities, increases compared to surgery or RT alone. Kashima et al. evaluated 149 patients with cervical cancer treated with RH or combined with postoperative RT between 1990 and 2004 (Kashima et al., 2010). Of the 149 patients, 41 were over 60 years, and 105 were under 59 years. The complications were significantly higher in the elderly patients and especially in those treated with RH combined with postoperative RT. In our study, 5 patients aged ≥ 75 years were treated with surgery (RH + PLND) and adjuvant RT. Three of the 5 patients experienced Grade 3 acute toxicity and 1 of the 5 patients experienced Grade 3 late toxicity. The results of these reports indicated that surgery and adjuvant RT were not safe for elderly patients. If adjuvant RT is necessary for elderly patients, IMRT may be used to limit severe toxicity.

Overall, the standard surgical approach RH + PLND is generally safe for patients aged over 60 or 65 years. However, the safety of RH + PLND for patients aged over 70 or 75 years is still unclear. Surgery and adjuvant RT must be performed with careful evaluation of pretreatment clinical staging, concurrent medical problems, and performance status for these age groups because severe life-threatening treatment-related toxicity may occur. More large-scale studies should be performed to confirm the safety of surgical approaches, including adjuvant RT for elderly patients.

4. Concurrent CRT for elderly patients

Concurrent CRT for elderly patients should also be discussed. Generally, in the treatment of cervical cancer, concurrent CRT is recommended, especially for locally advanced disease (Eifel et al., 2004; Rose et al, 1999; Whitney et al, 1999 and Pearcey et al., 2002). Weekly cisplatin (CDDP) is the most frequently used regimen. Concurrent CRT is also regarded as important for elderly patients because stage III-IVA disease usually cannot be cured by definitive RT alone. Therefore, CRT should be considered if the elderly patient is in good condition. Goodheart et al. retrospectively evaluated 96 patients treated with definitive RT between 1997 and 2001 (Goodheart et al., 2008). In their report, patients were divided into 2 groups: nonelderly (< 65, n = 69) and elderly (≥ 65, n = 27). Chemotherapy administration was considered when the performance status and laboratory values were acceptable. Most of the patients were administered weekly CDDP. In the nonelderly group, 54 of 78 (78%) patients were treated with CRT, and, in the elderly group, 15 of 27 (56%) patients were treated with CRT. The 5-year CSS rates in the CRT and RT group were 68.5% and 49.7%, respectively. The 5-year CSS rates in the nonelderly and elderly groups were 61.6% and 70.8%, respectively. Multivariate analyses showed a survival advantage for the administration of chemotherapy in addition to RT, and complication rates between the 2 groups were similar. They concluded that CRT was associated with improved survival in elderly patients who had adequate performance status with no excess treatment-related morbidity when compared to younger patients. Kunos et al. also examined 335 patients with locally advanced cervical cancer treated with CRT using weekly CDDP (Kunos et al., 2009). Patients were also divided into 2 groups: age < 55 years (n = 232) and age ≥ 55 years (n = 103). In their report, the survival of patients aged 55 or older was similar to that of the younger patients. The severity and frequency of treatment-related sequelae were also similar. These authors emphasized that CRT for elderly patients was effective and safe, but they defined "elderly" as "≥ 65 years" or "≥ 55 years", in accordance with the reports about RH. These age groups are usually not defined as "elderly." Therefore, whether concurrent CRT is safe for elderly patients aged over 70 years or 75 years or older remains unclear.

However, to achieve further improvement in survival outcomes for elderly patients with cervical cancer, especially locally advanced disease, CRT is a necessary modality. After performing large and prospective studies, concurrent CRT for selected patients aged ≥ 70 or 75 years may provide excellent outcomes with acceptable toxicity. Published reports about elderly patients with cervical cancer are described in Table 2.

Authors (year)	No. of elderly patients (years)	Modality	Treatment results
Mitchell. (1998)	60 (≥ 70)	RT	OS rate: 46% (5-y) CSS rate: 58% (5-y)
Sakurai. (2000)	41 (≥ 80)	RT	OS rate: 33% (5-y) CSS rate: 65% (5-y)
Lindegaard. (2000)	114 (≥ 70)	RT	
Geisler. (2001)	62 (≥ 65)	Surgery	
Chen. (2003)	79 (≥ 70)	RT	
Brun. (2003)	31 (≥ 75)	Surgery, RT	OS rate: 42% (5-y)
Wright. (2005)	197 (≥ 70)	Surgery, RT, CRT	
Ikushima. (2007)	132 (≥ 75)	RT	OS rate: 49% (5-y) CSS rate: 66% (5-y)
Goodheart. (2008)	27 (≥ 65)	CRT	OS rate: 44% (5-y) CSS rate: 71% (5-y)
Magne. (2009)	113 (> 70)	Surgery, RT	OS rate: 89% (3-y)
Kunos. (2009)	103 (≥ 55)	CRT	OS rate: 56 % (5-y)
Yoshida. (2010)	40 (≥ 75)	RT	OS rate: 58%, (3-y) CSS rate: 80% (3-y)
Kashima. (2010)	41 (≥ 60)	Surgery ± adjuvant RT	

RT: Radiotherapy, CRT: Concurrent chemoradiation, OS: Overall survival, CSS: Cause specific survival

Table 2. Published reports about elderly patients with cercical cancer

5. Conclusions

Selection of treatment modalities for elderly patients with cervical cancer is often limited compared to younger patients, but definitive RT, a combination of EBRT and ICBT is effective and safe. Indications for a surgical approach with or without adjuvant RT or concurrent CRT are still unclear because these aggressive modalities may cause severe treatment-related toxicity, especially for elderly patients. However, for locally advanced disease, CRT is an effective treatment. Therefore, large and prospective studies using CRT for patients aged at least ≥ 70 years with cervical cancer are needed. For RT, new techniques, such as IMRT, IGBT or a combination of both, may help to reduce the RT-induced toxicity in both definitive and adjuvant treatment. In the near future, IMRT combined with IGBT with or without new chemotherapeutic regimens will be the standard cervical cancer treatment in aging women.

6. References

Abridged life tables for Japan 2009, Ministry of Health, Labour and Welfare (2010). http://www.mhlw.go.jp/english/database/db-hw/lifetb09/index.html

Brun, JL.; Stoven-Camou, D.; Trouette, R.; Lopez, M.; Chene, G. & Hocké, C. (2003). Survival and prognosis of women with invasive cervical cancer according to age. *Gynecol Oncol.* Vol. 91(2), pp. 395-401, ISSN 0090-8258

Chen, SW.; Liang, JA.; Yang, SN. & Lin, FJ. (2010). High dose-rate brachytherapy for elderly patients with uterine cervical cancer. *Jpn J Clin Oncol.* Vol. 33(5), pp. 221-8, ISSN 0368-2111

Creasman, WT. (1995). New gynecologic cancer staging. *Gynecol Oncol.* Vol. 58(2), pp. 157-8, ISSN 0090-8258

Eifel, PJ.; Winter, K.; Morris, M.; Levenback, C.; Grigsby, PW.; Cooper, J.; Rotman, M.; Gershenson, D. & Mutch DG. (2004). Pelvic irradiation with concurrent chemotherapy versus pelvic and para-aortic irradiation for high-risk cervical cancer: an update of radiation therapy oncology group trial (RTOG) 90-01. *J Clin Oncol.* Vol. 22(5), pp. 872-80, ISSN 0732-183X

Fuchtner, C.; Manetta, A.; Walker, JL.; Emma, D.; Berman, M. & DiSaia, PJ. (1992). Radical hysterectomy in the elderly patient: analysis of morbidity. *Am J Obstet Gynecol.* Vol. 166(2), pp. 593-7, ISSN 0002-9378

Geisler, JP. & Geisler, HE. (2001). Radical hysterectomy in the elderly female: a comparison to patients age 50 or younger. *Gynecol Oncol.* Vol. 80(2), pp. 258-61, ISSN 0090-8258

Goodheart, M.; Jacobson, G.; Smith, BJ. & Zhou, L. (2008). Chemoradiation for invasive cervical cancer in elderly patients: outcomes and morbidity. *Int J Gynecol Cancer.* Vol. 18(1), pp. 95-103, ISSN 1048-891X

Ikushima, H.; Takegawa, Y.; Osaki, K.; Furutani, S.; Yamashita, K.; Kawanaka, T.; Kubo, A.; Kudoh, T. & Nishitani, H. Radiation therapy for cervical cancer in the elderly. *Gynecol Oncol.* Vol. 107(2), pp. 339-43, ISSN 0090-8258

International Commission on Radiation Units and Measurements (1985). Dose and volume specification for intracavitary therapy in gynecology. ICRU report 38. ICRU, Washington,USA.

Japan Society of Obstetrics and Gynecology, the Japanese Society of Pathology, Japan Radiological Society (1997). The General Rules for Clinical and Pathological Management of Uterine Cervical Cancer, October 1997 (The second Edition). ISBN 4307300734, Tokyo, Japan.

Kashima, K.; Yahata, T.; Fujita K. & Tanaka, K. (2010). Analysis of the complications after radical hysterectomy for stage IB, IIA and IIB uterine cervical cancer patients. *J Obstet Gynaecol Res.* Vol. 36(3), pp. 555-9, ISSN 1341-8076

Kunos, C.; Tian, C.; Waggoner, S.; Rose, PG. & Lanciano, R. (2009). Retrospective analysis of concomitant Cisplatin during radiation in patients aged 55 years or older for treatment of advanced cervical cancer: a gynecologic oncology group study. *Int J Gynecol Cancer.* 2009 Vol. 19(7), pp. 1258-63, ISSN 1048-891X

Landoni, F.; Maneo, A.; Colombo, A.; Placa, F.; Milani, R.; Perego, P.; Favini, G.; Ferri, L. & Mangioni, C. (1997). Randomised study of radical surgery versus radiotherapy for stage Ib-IIa cervical cancer. *Lancet*. Vol. 350(9077), pp. 535-40, ISSN 0140-6736

Lindegaard, JC.; Thranov, IR. & Engelholm SA. (2000). Radiotherapy in the management of cervical cancer in elderly patients. *Radiother Oncol.* Vol. 56(1), pp. 9-15, ISSN 0167-8140

Magné, N.; Mancy, NC.; Chajon, E.; Duvillard, P.; Pautier, P.; Castaigne, D.; Lhommé, C.; Moric, P. & Haie-Meder C. (2009). Patterns of care and outcome in elderly cervical cancer patients: a special focus on brachytherapy. *Radiother Oncol.* Vol. 91(2), pp. 197-201, ISSN 0167-8140

Mitchell, PA.; Waggoner, S.; Rotmensch, J. & Mundt AJ. (1998). Cervical cancer in the elderly treated with radiation therapy. *Gynecol Oncol.* Vol. 71(2), pp. 291-8, ISSN 0090-8258

Mousavi, A.; Karimi Zarchi, M.; Gilani, MM.; Behtash, N.; Ghaemmaghami, F.; Shams, M. & Irvanipoor, M. (2008). Radical hysterectomy in the elderly. *World J Surg Oncol.* Vol. 6:38, ISSN 1477-7819

National Comprehensive Cancer Network (2011). NCCN Clinical Practice Guidelines in Oncology-Cervical Cancer-Version1. 2011. http://www.nccn.org/professionals/physician_gls/pdf/cervical.pdf

Pearcey, R.; Brundage, M.; Drouin, P.; Jeffrey, J.; Johnston, D.; Lukka, H.; MacLean, G.; Souhami, L.; Stuart G. & Tu, D. (2002). Phase III trial comparing radical radiotherapy with and without cisplatin chemotherapy in patients with advanced squamous cell cancer of the cervix. *J Clin Oncol.* Vol. 20(4), pp. 966-72, ISSN 0732-183X

Perez, CA.; Grigsby, PW.; Camel, HM.; Galakatos, AE.; Mutch, D. & Lockett, MA. (1995). Irradiation alone or combined with surgery in stage IB, IIA, and IIB carcinoma of uterine cervix: update of a nonrandomized comparison. *Int J Radiat Oncol Biol Phys.* Vol. 31(4), pp. 703-16, ISSN 0360-3016

Rose, PG.; Bundy, BN.; Watkins, EB.; TClarke-Pearson, DL. & Insalaco S. (1999) Concurrent cisplatin-based radiotherapy and chemotherapy for locally advanced cervical cancer. *N Engl J Med.* Vol. 340(15), pp. 1144-53, ISSN 0028-4793

Sakurai, H.; Mitsuhashi, N.; Takahashi, M.; Yamakawa, M.; Akimoto, T.; Hayakawa, K.; & Niibe, H. (2000). Radiation therapy for elderly patient with squamous cell carcinoma of the uterine cervix. *Gynecol Oncol.* Vol. 77(1), pp. 116-20, ISSN 0090-8258

Whitney, CW.; Sause, W.; Bundy, BN.; Malfetano, JH.; Hannigan, EV.; Fowler, WC Jr.; Clarke-Pearson, DL. & Liao, SY. (1999). Randomized comparison of fluorouracil plus cisplatin versus hydroxyurea as an adjunct to radiation therapy in stage IIB-IVA carcinoma of the cervix with negative para-aortic lymph nodes: a Gynecologic Oncology Group and Southwest Oncology Group study. *J Clin Oncol.* Vol, 17(5), pp. 1339-48, ISSN 0732-183X

Wright, JD.; Gibb, RK.; Geevarghese, S.; Powell, MA.; Herzog, TJ.; Mutch, DG.; Grigsby, PW.; Gao, F.; Trinkaus, KM. & Rader JS. (2005). Cervical carcinoma in the elderly: an analysis of patterns of care and outcome. *Cancer.* Vol. 103(1), pp. 85-91, ISSN 0008-543X

Yamashita, H.; Nakagawa, K.; Tago, M.; Shiraishi, K.; Nakamura, N.; Ohtomo, K.; Oda, K.; Nakagawa, S.; Yasugi, T. & Taketani Y. (2005). Comparison between conventional surgery and radiotherapy for FIGO stage I-II cervical carcinoma: a retrospective Japanese study. *Gynecol Oncol.* Vol. 97(3), pp. 834-9, ISSN 0090-8258

Yoshida, K.; Sasaki, R.; Nishimura, H.; Miyawaki, D.; Kawabe, T.; Okamoto, Y.; Nakabayashi, K.; Yoshida, S. & Sugimura K. (2011). Radiotherapy for Japanese elderly patients with cervical cancer: preliminary survival outcomes and evaluation of treatment-related toxicity. *Arch Gynecol Obstet.* Vol. 284(4), pp. 1007-14, ISSN 0932-0067

7

Cervical Cancer Prevention by Liquid-Based Cytology in a Low-Resource Setting

Mongkol Benjapibal and Somsak Laiwejpithaya
Department of Obstetrics and Gynecology,
Faculty of Medicine Siriraj Hospital,
Mahidol University, Bangkok
Thailand

1. Introduction

Cervical cancer is a major public health problem. Worldwide, it is the second most common cancer in women after breast cancer. Approximately 500,000 new cases of invasive cervical cancer have been diagnosed each year with more than 250,000 women dying of the disease. It is the most or second most common cancer among women in developing countries. In Thailand, a low-resource country, cervical cancer is the second most frequent cause of cancer in women, with nearly 10,000 new cases diagnosed and more than 5,200 dying from this disease each year (Ferlay et al., 2010). The incidence and mortality have declined during the last 50 years in developed countries because of increased availability of cervical cancer screening programs (Nieminen et al., 1995). However, cervical cancer continues to be a leading cause of cancer deaths in populations with a low socioeconomic level.

2. Cervical cancer screening

Screening is the use of methods to distinguish apparently unaffected people from those who may have a disease, or may develop it. It is a preliminary process to offer a diagnostic test and if required, treatment. Screening test is usually applied on a large scale and are generally offered to a population of people who have not sought medical attention on account of symptoms of the disease. The purpose of screening is to benefit the individuals being screened. Screening procedures are generally easier to perform and cheaper than diagnostic procedures. Although the screening test is harmless, it can cause anxiety and the subsequent investigations and treatment can be hazardous. Screening methods should provide the most attractive combination of negative predictive value (e.g., reassurance) and false positives that is attainable in a given setting and providers should ensure that a useful remedy is available for all individuals identified as being true positive.

The most widely used screening method for cervical cancer is conventional cytology (conventional Pap smear). Nowadays, conventional cytology is still considered a standard screening method worldwide, especially in developing countries. Conventional cytology has been being used as a standard screening method for cervical cancer in Siriraj Hospital since 1952. This cytological testing involves three major steps, i.e. collecting exfoliated cells from the cervix, spreading the cells onto a slide, and microscopically examining these cells after staining. Collection of specimens for conventional cytology is performed according to the standard vaginal-cervical-endocervical (VCE) smear technique. A wooden (Ayre's) spatula and a cotton swab are used to collect cells from the posterior fornix, portio vaginalis and endocervix. The collected cells are then spread onto a glass slide and immediately immersed in 95% ethanol for fixation. Despite the proven effectiveness of cervical cytology screening in reducing the incidence of cervical cancer, over the last decade the accuracy of cervical cytology has been questioned. Two large meta-analyses have indicated that although the specificity of conventional cervical cytology is high, its sensitivity is much lower than previously estimated (Fahey et al., 1995; Nanda et al., 2000). Errors due to poor sampling and partial transferring of the collected sample onto a glass slide, consequently producing a nonrepresentative specimen, may account for up to 62% of false negative results (Gay et al., 1985).

3. Siriraj liquid-based cytology

Liquid-based cytology (LBC) was introduced in the mid-1990s as a way to improve performance of the test. LBC can improve specimen quality by providing a standardized method of collecting cervicovaginal material, and dispersing cells in a thin layer with relatively free of inflammation (Austin et al.,1998; Mount et al.,2004; Vassilakos et al.,2002). This results in the decrease in incidence of unsatisfactory smears and increase in detection rate of cytologic abnormality (Bolick et al.,1998; Corkill et al.,1998; Diaz-Rosario et al.,1999; Dupree et al.,1998; Fremont-Smith et al.,2004; Papillo et al.,1998; Roberts et al.,1997). Besides, the leftover specimen for LBC can also be used for HPV DNA testing which is currently incorporated into the management guidelines and post-therapy surveillance of the patient in some institutes. Recently, a number of different LBC techniques are available worldwide. ThinPrep® and SurePath™ are prototypes of LBC technology. They have been approved by the Food and Drug Administration for cervical cancer screening in the USA and are the most commonly used LBC techniques (Bishop et al., 1998; Lee et al., 1997). LBC was introduced as a cervical cancer screening technique in Thailand in 1997. Nowadays there are at least three commercially available LBC in Thailand, e.g. ThinPrep®, SurePath™, and Liqui-Prep®. Despite of their reputation, these LBC are still not in general use because of their cost. In the year 2005, we have developed an alcohol-based preservative solution, Siriraj liquid-based solution, and applied a modified Saccomanno's technique for cells preparation in our institute, and named this technology as the "Siriraj liquid-based cytology" or "Siriraj-LBC". The collection of specimens for Siriraj-LBC is similar to that for conventional cytology, except that a special plastic spatula is used instead of the Ayre's spatula and cotton swab. The plastic spatula has an extended endocervical tip at one end and a rounded rectangular tip at the other end, and scores at 4 cm from each end to facilitate spatula breaking (Figure 1). Immediately after cell collection, both ends of the spatula are manually broken at the scores, and put into a 30 mL plastic bottle containing 10 mL of Siriraj liquid-based solution.

3.1 Processing of Siriraj-LBC

The cell specimens are collected in bottles containing Siriraj liquid-based solution and keep at room temperature until processing. Siriraj-LBC slides are prepared according to the following steps (Bales, 2006) : agitate the bottle of specimen on a vortex mixer for 10 sec, and

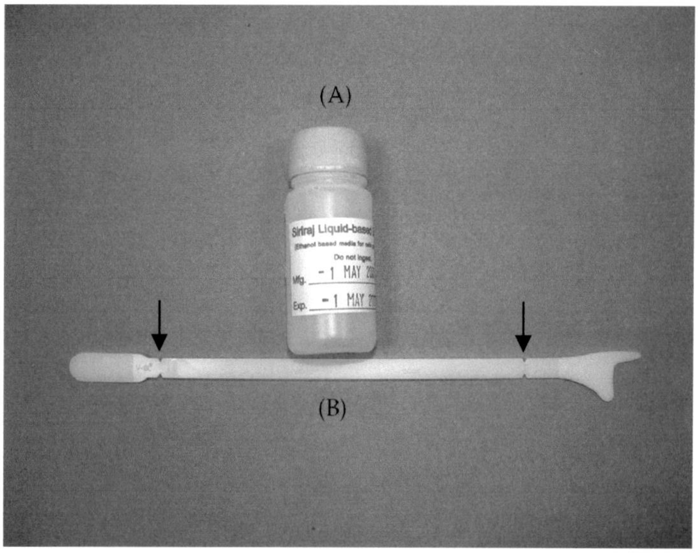

Fig. 1. Collecting devices for Siriraj-LBC: a 30-mL plastic bottle containing 10 mL of Siriraj liquid-based solution (A), and an extended-tip plastic spatula, arrow heads showing scores on the spatula (B)

pour the suspension into a 15-mL centrifuge test tube; centrifuge the specimen at 1000 g. for 10 min, and discard the supernatant; add Siriraj liquid-based solution (approximately 3 times of the sediment volume); agitate the test tube for 10 sec, aspirate 15-20 µL of the sample by using an auto-pipette, drop the sample onto a clean glass slide, smear the droplet to 2 cm in diameter, and let air dry at room temperature for 30 min; fix the slide in 95% ethanol for 20 minutes, and finally stain it with the routine Papanicolaou's staining technique (Figure 2).

3.2 Performance of Siriraj-LBC

Before a new screening or diagnostic tool is introduced into clinical use, it is necessary to evaluate its diagnostic performance. The best way for this evaluation is to compare the result from the new tool with that from the gold standard, revealing the performance parameters including sensitivity, specificity, positive predictive value (PPV), negative predictive value (NPV), false positive (FP), false negative (FN), and accuracy of the test. However, such parameters cannot be obtained in studies evaluating performance of cervical cytology methods because not all of the study population undergoes the gold standard testing, i.e. colposcopy or cervical histology. The gold standard is mostly lacking in the group of patients who have normal cervical cytology. Therefore, numerous studies have evaluated the comparative performance of the LBC methods and conventional cytology with respect to test positivity, i.e. the detection rate of squamous intraepithelial lesion (SIL). Most studies have utilized one to two types of study design, i.e. "split-sample" or "direct-to-vial" study. With "split-sample" study, it is difficult to ensure that the two cytology specimens are comparable, since the specimen for conventional cytology slide is collected before the specimen for LBC. Therefore, this design seems to lead inherently to bias against LBC. With "direct-to-vial" study, the result of LBC is compared with that of conventional smear from historical data of an identical population; however, it is not certain that the two

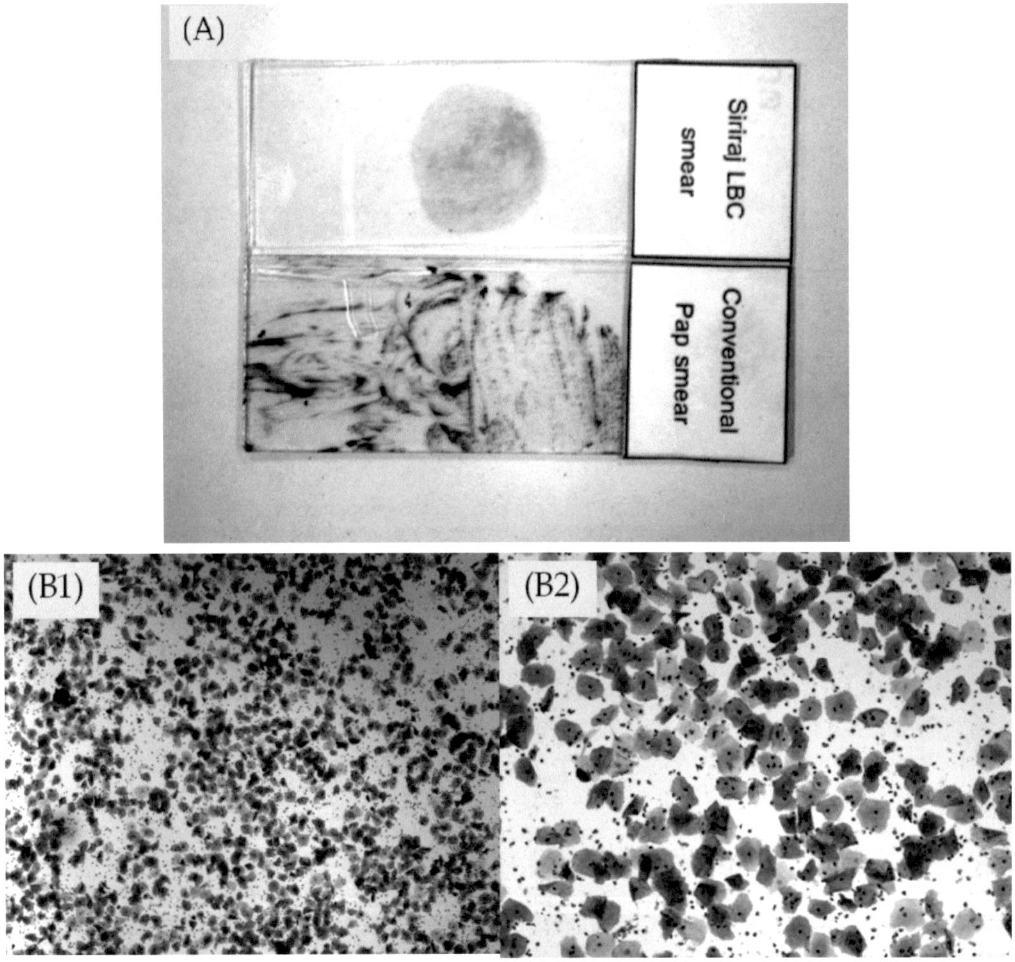

Fig. 2. Stained slides of Siriraj-LBC and conventional smears (A); micrographs of cervical cytology at low magnification: conventional smear (B1), Siriraj-LBC smear (B2)

populations are identical. The diagnostic performance of our home-made LBC has been evaluated in both the "split-sample" study and "direct-to-vial" study.

3.3 A split-sample study (Laiwejpithaya et al., 2008)

3.3.1 Study population and specimen processing

A cross-sectional study was carried out in the Gynecologic Cytology Unit, Department of Obstetric and Gynecology, Faculty of Medicine Siriraj Hospital, Mahidol University from January to February 2005. Study population were randomly selected from women attending for pelvic examination and cervical cancer screening at the Gynecologic Outpatient Department, Siriraj Hospital during the study period, excluding the women who had previously undergone any surgical procedures of the cervix, were pregnant or suspected of being pregnant, used any kinds of vaginal preparations within previous 24 hours, or denied to participate in the study. Specimens were collected for "split-sample" study by residents

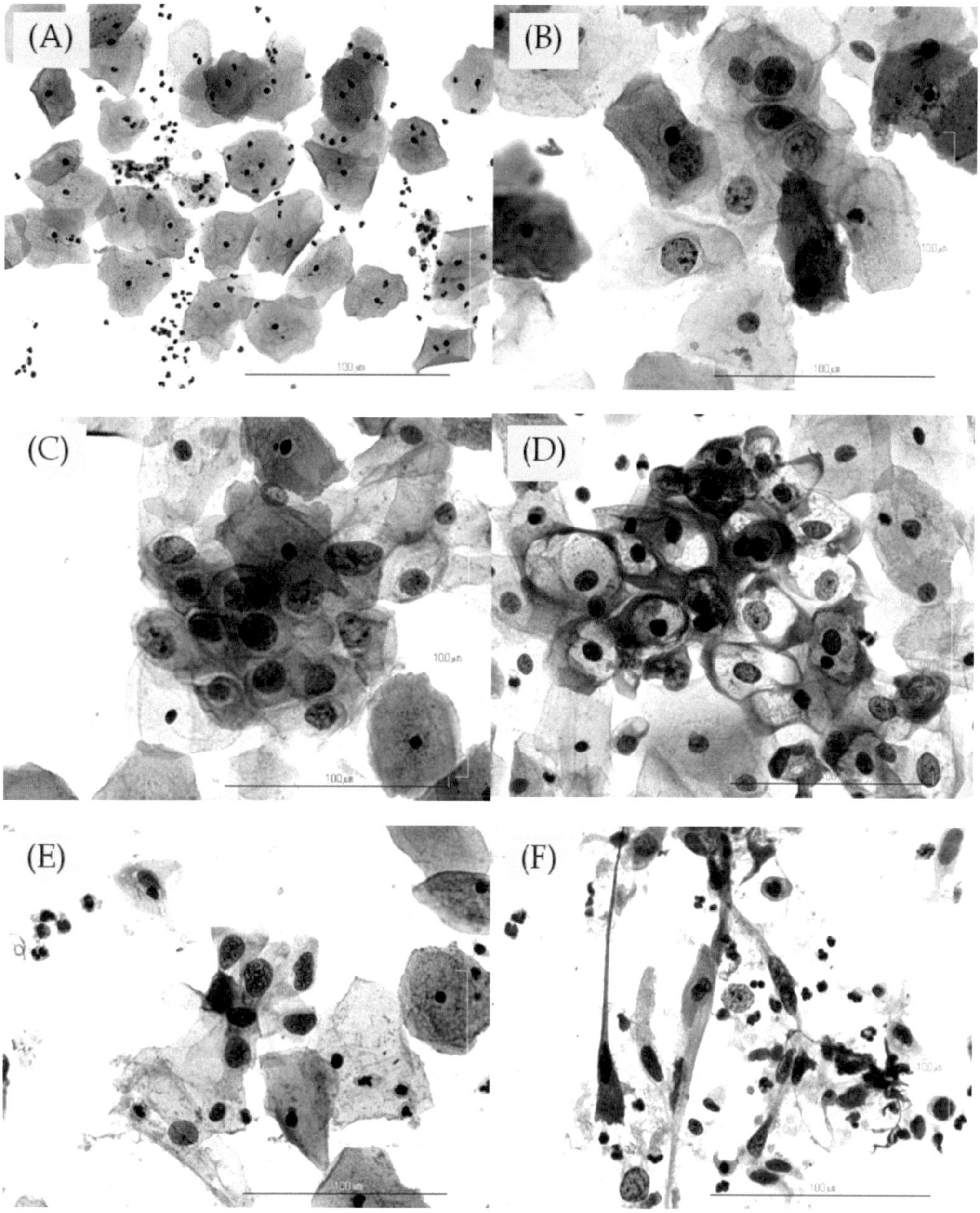

Fig. 3. Micrographs of cervical cytology using Siriraj-LBC at high magnification: normal (A), atypical squamous cells of undetermined significance (B), atypical squamous cells cannot exclude HSIL (C), low-grade squamous intraepithelial lesion with koilocytosis (D), high-grade squamous intraepithelial lesion (E), and squamous cell carcinoma (F)

or gynecologists who were staff members of the Department of Obstetrics and Gynecology. The collected cells were initially prepared for conventional cytology. Leftover cells in the collecting instruments were then collected for Siriraj-LBC by putting the instruments into a

30 mL plastic bottle containing 10 mL of Siriraj liquid-based solution. Specimens for both techniques were transported to the Gynecologic Cytology Unit, and processed by experienced technicians. All of the slides were screened by a team of cytotechnologists. The abnormal slides were reviewed and diagnosis made by an experienced cytopathologist. Examples of various abnormal cervical cells are shown in Figure 3. Evaluation of slides for conventional cytology and Siriraj-LBC was made in a blind fashion, i.e. the interpretations of the results from one technique were made without knowledge of those from the other technique. The cytological interpretation was made according to the Bethesda system 2001 as followed: negative for intraepithelial lesion or malignancy, reactive or reparative change, atypical squamous cells of undetermined significance (ASCUS), low-grade squamous intraepithelial lesion (LSIL), high grade squamous intraepithelial lesion (HSIL), atypical squamous cells cannot exclude HSIL (ASC-H), squamous cell carcinoma (SCC), atypical glandular cells (AGC), or adenocarcinoma (Solomon et al., 2002). Clinical management of abnormal cytology includes referral to colposcopy and treatment according to the guideline of Siriraj Hospital. The patients with cytology results of ASCUS or LSIL were suggested to have either colposcopy or repeat cervical cytology testing, and those with ASC-H, HSIL or more aggressive ones were referred to colposcopy.

3.3.2 Performance of cytology as a screening test

The performance of cytology was evaluated from detection rate of abnormal cervicovaginal cytology, and predictive values using colposcopy and/or histology as the gold standard. The data for calculating positive predictive value (PPV) were obtained from the patients who had abnormal results of Siriraj-LBC, and underwent operative procedures revealing histology. Those procedures included colposcopic directed cervical biopsy, loop electrosurgical excision procedure (LEEP), cold-knife conization, and hysterectomy. The data were presented in n (%), or odds ratio (OR) and 95% confidence interval (CI), as appropriate. Percentage of agreement was used to determine the diagnostic agreement between pairs of specimens evaluated by conventional cytology and Siriraj-LBC. Kappa and Spearman rho correlation coefficient were used to determine correlation of result between pairs of specimens. Chi-square test was used to compare frequency between the two cytology techniques. All tests were 2-sided, and a P value of less than 0.05 was considered statistically significant.

3.3.3 Results

There were 479 participants recruited during the study period. Their mean age was 41.6 ± 12.6 years. The Siriraj-LBC significantly increased overall detection rate of abnormal cytology compared to the conventional method, i.e. from 1.67% to 11.1%, $P < 0.001$ (Table 1). The data yielded a complete diagnostic agreement of 430 of 479 pairs of specimens (89.8%). Among these, HSIL was detected in both specimens in 2 cases and cancer in 1 case. There were 49 cases whose Siriraj-LBC revealed higher cytologic grading than the conventional cytology did; whereas, none of the conventional cytology showed the vise versa result. The highest disagreement was found in 18 cases which were interpreted as normal by conventional cytology, but as ASCUS by Siriraj-LBC. As a result, these two cytology techniques had minimal to fair correlation with a Kappa of 0.128 ($P < 0.001$) and a Spearman rho correlation coefficient of 0.394 ($P < 0.001$) (Table 2).

Table 3 reveals final diagnoses by colposcopy or histology in 45 patients with abnormal cytological diagnoses by Siriraj-LBC. In this specific group, the Siriraj-LBC had a positive

Finding	Conventional	Siriraj-LBC	P-value
Overall	8 (1.67)	53 (11.1)	<0.001
ASCUS	2 (0.42)	18 (3.76)	
ASC-H	1 (0.21)	7 (1.46)	
LSIL	2 (0.42)	15 (3.13)	
HSIL	2 (0.42)	10 (2.09)	
Cancer	1 (0.21)	3 (0.63)	

[Data are n (%). The data were analyzed using Fisher's exact test.]
From Laiwejpithaya, S.; Rattanachaiyanont, M.; Benjapibal, M.; Khuakoonratt, N.; Boriboonhirunsarn, D.; Laiwejpithaya, S.; Sangkarat, S.; & Wongtiraporn, W. (2008). Comparison between Siriraj liquid-based and conventional cytology for detection of abnormal cervicovaginal smears: A split-sample study. Asian Pacific J Cancer Prev, Vol.9, No.4, pp. 575-580.

Table 1. Detection Rates of Abnormal Cervical Cytology by Conventional Cytology and Siriraj-LBC

Siriraj-LBC	Conventional cytology					
	Negative	ASCUS	ASC-H	LSIL	HSIL	Cancer
Negative	**426**	0	0	0	0	0
ASCUS	18	**0**	0	0	0	0
ASC-H	7	0	**0**	0	0	0
LSIL	12	2	0	**1**	0	0
HSIL	6	0	1	1	**2**	0
Cancer	2	0	0	0	0	**1**

(Data are number of cases. Identical diagnoses are shown in bold; cases with negative diagnosis by conventional cytology but abnormal diagnoses by Siriraj-LBC are in red; Spearman rho correlation = 0.394, Kappa = 0.128, P <0.001.)
From Laiwejpithaya, S.; Rattanachaiyanont, M.; Benjapibal, M.; Khuakoonratt, N.; Boriboonhirunsarn, D.; Laiwejpithaya, S.; Sangkarat, S.; & Wongtiraporn, W. (2008). Comparison between Siriraj liquid-based and conventional cytology for detection of abnormal cervicovaginal smears: A split-sample study. Asian Pacific J Cancer Prev, Vol.9, No.4, pp. 575-580.

Table 2. Comparison of Cytological Diagnoses between Conventional Cytology and Siriraj-LBC in 479 Pairs of Samples

predictive value (PPV) of 71.1% whereas conventional cytology had PPV and negative predictive value (NPV) of 85.7% and 31.6%, respectively. None of the ASCUS had cervical lesions beyond CIN1. Seven cases of ASC-H was found in Siriraj-LBC but only one in conventional cytology; one in seven (14.28%) of ASC-H had cervical lesion of CIN2/3. The Siriraj-LBC did not miss any high grade cervical lesions (CIN2/3 or cancer) but over-diagnosed cancer in one case; whereas conventional cytology failed to detect 3/6 (50%) cases of CIN2/3 and 1/2 (50%) cases of cancer.

3.3.4 Discussion

The present study used the data of the year 2005 when the Siriraj-LBC was undergoing the development process. We found that the detection rate of abnormal cells in Siriraj-LBC (11.06%) was much higher than that in the conventional cytology (1.67%). Even though the "split-sample" study has potential bias against LBC, we were not encountered with this problem. It was possible that the specimen processing in the Siriraj-LBC, especially the

Cytology	Diagnoses by Colposcopy or Histology			
	Normal	CIN1/HPV	CIN2/3	Cancer
Conventional				
Negative	12	22	3	1[b]
ASCUS	1	1	0	0
ASC-H	0	0	1	0
LSIL	0	0	1	0
HSIL	0	1	1	0
Cancer	0	0	0	1[c]
Siriraj-LBC				
Negative	NA	NA	NA	NA
ASCUS	7	9	0	0
ASC-H	3	3	1	0
LSIL	1	8	0	0
HSIL	1	4	5	0
Cancer	1[a]	0	0	2[b,c]

(Cytological vs. histological diagnoses: [a]adenocarcinoma of endometrium vs normal, [b]adenocarcinoma of unknown origin vs. adenocarcinoma of peritoneum, and [c]adenocarcinoma of endometrium vs. squamous cell carcinoma. CIN = cervical intraepithelial neoplasia, HPV = human papilloma virus infection, NA = not applicable)
From Laiwejpithaya, S.; Rattanachaiyanont, M.; Benjapibal, M.; Khuakoonratt, N.; Boriboonhirunsarn, D.; Laiwejpithaya, S.; Sangkarat, S.; & Wongtiraporn, W. (2008). Comparison between Siriraj liquid-based and conventional cytology for detection of abnormal cervicovaginal smears: A split-sample study. Asian Pacific J Cancer Prev, Vol.9, No.4, pp. 575-580.

Table 3. Final Diagnoses by Colposcopy or Histology in 45 patients with Abnormal Cytological Diagnoses

agitation of collecting devices in the liquid-based solution would elude the entrapped cells into the solution, therefore more cells were collected into the solution, and then evenly sampling to put onto a glass slide. We found that the complete diagnostic agreement between our LBC and the standard cytology was in high level (89.77%). However, the Kappa and the correlation coefficient were not in that high level; this was due to the interesting fact that detection rate of abnormal cells was much higher in the Siriraj-LBC than in the conventional cytology. Our result was comparable with that of Park et al (2001) showing that the results of conventional cytology and LBC exactly agreed in 91.4% of cases.

The increase in detection rate raised the concern of increase in false positive cytology. In the present study, 45 cases of the abnormal cytology detected by Siriraj- LBC undergone gold standard testing. We found that the overall PPV in the Siriraj-LBC was less than that in the conventional cytology (71.1% vs. 85.7%). This implied that the Siriraj-LBC increase false positive result from 7.7% to 100.0%. In this specific group of patients with positive result by Siriraj-LBC, the conventional cytology had an astounding high false negative result of 81.2%. The false negative result of Siriraj-LBC was unknown because none of the patients with negative cytology undergone gold standard testing, despites, we assumed that the Siriraj-LBC would have less false negative result since none of the negative Siriraj-LBC had abnormal conventional cytology. However, we are aware that these numbers are not the real false negative and false positive rates, as the actual rates cannot be obtained due to the limitation of this kind of study.

The high false positive result by Siriraj-LBC caused only little concern. Considering that only HSIL or cancer needs further invasive investigation, e.g. conization and/or diagnostic curettage, two in 45 cases had risk of unnecessary further investigation if the Siriraj-LBC was used in place of conventional cytology; this risk returned with the benefit of detecting three more cases of CIN2/3 and one case of cancer which were cases with false negative result in the conventional cytology. Noteworthy, the missing cancer in conventional cytology was a case of peritoneal adenocarcinoma without lesion at the uterine cervix.

Our limited data showed that the conventional cytology had high false negative result where as the Siriraj-LBC had high false positive result. It is estimated that approximately two thirds of false negative result in the conventional cytology are caused by sampling error due to limited transfer of cells from the collecting device onto the slide (Gay et al., 1985). The false positive result in the Siriraj-LBC was due to the increase in all types of abnormal epithelial cells. This may be due to the misinterpretation of immature squamous metaplastic or atrophic cells to be abnormal cells because the morphologies of these cells are alike. Moreover these cells could be more easily detected in the Siriraj-LBC than in the conventional cytology because of the better quality of slide. However, we could not disregard the fact that our novice in the LBC field also contributed to this false positive. We expect to get better results of this technique in the future.

Our result was compatible with many previous reports. Nanda et al (2000) reviewed the accuracy of conventional and new methods of Papanicolaou (Pap) testing to detect cervical cancer and its precursors. Ninety-four studies of the conventional Pap test showed that, estimates of sensitivity and specificity varied greatly in individual studies. In the 12 studies with the least biased, estimates sensitivity ranged from 30-80% and specificity ranged from 86-100%. Guo et al (2005) evaluated the accuracy of a LBC test, ThinPrep®, by comparing concurrent LBC and cervical biopsy results of 782 patients who were referred for colposcopy because of previously abnormal conventional cytology. They found that concurrent LBC has high diagnostic accuracy for SIL. Besides, several studies showed that the detection rates of LSIL and HSIL are improved by LBC but the effect of LBC on the detection of ASC-US is uncertain (Limaye et al., 2003; Mount et al., 2004).

The results from Siriraj-LBC and conventional cytology have high diagnostic agreement and minimal to fair correlation. The Siriraj-LBC increases detection rate of abnormal cervicovaginal cells with probably decrease false negative but increase false positive from the baseline values by conventional cytology. Therefore the screening performance of Siriraj-LBC is not inferior to the conventional cytology and may be used as an alternative screening method for cervical cancer.

3.4 A direct-to-vial study (Laiwejpithaya et al., 2009)

3.4.1 Study population and specimen processing

The study was carried out in the Gynecologic Cytology Unit, Department of Obstetrics and Gynecology, Faculty of Medicine Siriraj Hospital, Mahidol University. Data were retrieved from the database of the Gynecologic Cytology Unit. The data of conventional cytology and

LBC were recruited from records of the years 2004 and 2006, respectively. The specimens for either conventional cytology or LBC were obtained from patients who had pelvic examination at the Gynecologic Outpatient Department of Siriraj Hospital during the relevant study periods. Specimens were collected by residents and staff members of the Department of Obstetrics and Gynecology. Collection of specimens for conventional cytology was performed according to the standard VCE smear technique. The collection of specimens for Siriraj-LBC was similar to that for conventional cytology, except that a special plastic spatula was used instead of the Ayre's spatula and cotton swab. All specimens were transported to the Gynecologic Cytology Unit, and processed by experienced technicians. All of the slides were screened by a team of cytotechnologists and the abnormal slides were reviewed and diagnosis made by an experienced cytopathologist. Clinical management of abnormal cytology includes referral to colposcopy and treatment according to the guideline of Siriraj Hospital as mentioned above.

3.4.2 Performance of cytology as a screening test

The performance of Siriraj-LBC was evaluated from the detection rate of abnormal cervical cytology, and predictive values using cervical histology as the gold standard. The data for calculating negative predictive value (NPV) were obtained from the patients who had normal results of pre-hysterectomy screening cervical cytology. The data for calculating positive predictive value (PPV) were obtained from the patients who had abnormal results of cervical cytology and underwent operative procedures revealing cervical histology. Those procedures included colposcopic directed cervical biopsy, loop electrosurgical excision procedure (LEEP), cold-knife conization, and hysterectomy. Normal cervical histology was considered when the cervical mucosa was clear from any neoplastic lesion, ignoring the histopathological result of endometrium. The data were presented as mean±standard deviation (SD), n (%), or % change, as appropriate. Data were analyzed using the t-test for continuous data or Chi-square test for categorical data. All tests were 2-sided, and a P-value of < 0.05 was considered statistically significant.

3.4.3 Results

There were 23,676 records of conventional Papanicolaou's smear and 25,510 records of Siriraj-LBC in the years 2004 and 2006, respectively. Almost all of the specimens came from Thai women. The mean age±SD of women in the years 2004 and 2006 were 40.67±12.54 and 42.66±12.21 years, respectively, which were not statistically different. Compared with the conventional smear, the Siriraj-LBC significantly increased overall detection rate of abnormal cytology by 110.23% (from 1.76% to 3.70%, $P < 0.001$), as it increased the detection rate of ASCUS, LSIL, HSIL, ASC-H, and malignant cells, but it did not significantly increase the detection rate of atypical glandular cells (AGC). The Siriraj-LBC significantly reduced the number of smears that were deemed poor quality by 73.44% (from 18.60% to 4.94%, $P < 0.001$), as it markedly decreased the smears with obscuring blood and inflammatory cells, thick smears (Fig. 1b and c), and the smears without transformation zone component. However, the Siriraj-LBC had a marked increase in scant cellular smears (Table 4).

The predictive value of Siriraj-LBC was better than that of conventional smear. The NPV of Siriraj-LBC was apparently higher than that of conventional cytology (96.33% vs. 92.74%, $P = 0.001$). The PPV of both methods was > 80%, which did not demonstrate any significant

	Siriraj-LBC (N= 25,510)	Conventional (N= 23,676)	% change	P
All abnormal cervical cells	944 (3.70)	417 (1.76)	+110.23	<0.001
ASCUS	251 (0.98)	100 (0.42)	+133.33	<0.001
LSIL	278 (1.09)	132 (0.56)	+94.64	<0.001
HSIL	213 (0.83)	94 (0.40)	+107.50	<0.001
ASC-H	117 (0.46)	41 (0.17)	+170.59	<0.001
AGC	25 (0.10)	16 (0.07)	+42.86	0.243
Malignant	60 (0.24)	34 (0.14)	+71.43	0.020
All poor quality slides	1261 (4.94)	4404 (18.60)	-73.44	<0.001
No transformation zone component	1094 (4.29)	3766 (15.91)	-73.04	<0.001
Scant cellular smears	153 (0.60)	51 (0.22)	+172.73	<0.001
Thick smears	2 (0.01)	212 (0.90)	-98.89	<0.001
Obscuring blood and inflammatory cells	12 (0.05)	375 (1.58)	-96.84	<0.001

[Note: Data are n (%). Percent change was the incremental (+) or decremental (_) rate of Siriraj-LBC comparing to the baseline rate of conventional cytology. The data were analyzed using Chi-square test.] From Laiwejpithaya, S.; Benjapibal, M.; Laiwejpithaya, S.; Wongtiraporn, W.; Sangkarat, S.; & Rattanachaiyanont, M. (2009). Performance and cost analysis of Siriraj liquid-based cytology: a direct-to-vial study. Eur J Obstet Gynecol Reprod Biol, Vol. 147, No.2, pp. 201-205.

Table 4. Detection rates of abnormal cervical cells and quality of slides using Siriraj liquid-based cytology (Siriraj-LBC, year 2006) and conventional Papanicolaou's smear (year 2004)

difference between the methods. The PPV for SCC was the highest; whereas that for abnormal glandular cell types was the lowest (Table 5). The cost of Siriraj-LBC was higher than that of the conventional cytology used in Siriraj Hospital but lower than that of the commercially available LBC in Thailand. When cost was estimated from the laboratory charge, it was found that the cost of Siriraj-LBC was 1.67, 0.50, and 0.30 times of those of the conventional cytology, Liqui-Prep®, and ThinPrep®, respectively (Table 6).

Cervical cytology	N	Cervical histology, n (%)		P
		Normal	Abnormal	
Normal				
Siriraj-LBC	1012	975 (96.33)(a)	37 (3.67)	0.001
Conventional	744	690 (92.74) (a)	54 (7.26)	
Overall abnormalitie				
Siriraj-LBC	277	47 (16.97)	230 (83.03)(b)	0.285
Conventional	167	22 (13.17)	145 (86.83)(b)	
ASCUS				
Siriraj-LBC	13	7 (53.85)	6 (46.15)(b)	0.342
Conventional	9	3 (33.33)	6 (66.67)(b)	

Cervical cytology	N	Cervical histology, n (%)		P
		Normal	Abnormal	
LSIL				
Siriraj-LBC	41	6 (14.63)	35 (85.37)(b)	0.597
Conventional	29	3 (10.34)	26 (89.66)(b)	
HSIL				
Siriraj-LBC	124	10 (8.06)	114 (91.94)(b)	0.301
Conventional	71	3 (4.23)	68 (95.77)(b)	
ASC-H				
Siriraj-LBC	33	4 (12.12)	29 (87.88)(b)	0.579
Conventional	23	4 (17.39)	19 (82.61)(b)	
SCC				
Siriraj-LBC	26	0 (0.00)	26 (100.00)(b)	0.183
Conventional	15	1 (6.67)	14 (93.33)(b)	
Abnormal glandular cell types (AGC+AIS+Adenocarcinoma)				
Siriraj-LBC	40	20 (50.00)	20 (50.00)(b)	0.464
Conventional	20	8 (40.00)	12 (60.00)(b)	

[Note: Data are n (% of the corresponding row). The data were analyzed using Chisquare test. Abnormal cervical histology meant cervical tissue specimen showing intraepithelial neoplasia, squamous cell carcinoma, or adenocarcinoma. (a) Negative predictive value; (b) positive predictive value; AGC, atypical glandular cells; AIS, adenocarcinoma in situ; ASCUS, atypical squamous cells of undetermined significance; ASC-H, atypical squamous cells cannot exclude HSIL; CI, confidence interval; LSIL, low grade squamous intraepithelial lesion; HSIL, high-grade squamous intraepithelial lesion; SCC, squamous cell carcino]

From Laiwejpithaya, S.; Benjapibal, M.; Laiwejpithaya, S.; Wongtiraporn, W.; Sangkarat, S.; & Rattanachaiyanont, M. (2009). Performance and cost analysis of Siriraj liquid-based cytology: a direct-to-vial study. Eur J Obstet Gynecol Reprod Biol, Vol. 147, No.2, pp. 201-205.

Table 5. Predictive values of cervical cytology using Siriraj liquid-based cytology (Siriraj-LBC, year 2006) and conventional Papanicolaou's smear (year 2004)

Costs	Thai baht	US dollars
Siriraj liquid-based cytology	150.00	4.55
Siriraj conventional cytology	90.00	2.72
Commercially available liquid-based cytology techniques		
Liqui-Prep®	300.00	9.09
ThinPrep®	500.00	15.15

From Laiwejpithaya, S.; Benjapibal, M.; Laiwejpithaya, S.; Wongtiraporn, W.; Sangkarat, S.; & Rattanachaiyanont, M. (2009). Performance and cost analysis of Siriraj liquid-based cytology: a direct-to-vial study. Eur J Obstet Gynecol Reprod Biol, Vol. 147, No.2, pp. 201-205.

Table 6. Costs of Siriraj liquid-based cytology, conventional cytology at Siriraj Hospital, and commercially available liquid-based cytology techniques in Thailand

3.4.4 Discussion

In the present direct-to-vial study, we compared the data of patients undergoing specimen collection for cervical cytology by the same physician group in two 12-month periods, targeting conventional Papanicolaou's smear in 2004 and Siriraj-LBC in 2006. As expected, the Siriraj-LBC increased detection of precancerous lesions of the uterine cervix. From our previous split-sample study conducted during the development of this technology in 2005, the Siriraj-LBC showed a tremendously increased detection rate of abnormal cytology of 565%, from 1.67% to 11.10%. However, the increase in the detection rate decreased to 100% in 2006 when the Siriraj-LBC was routinely used. The huge increase in 2005 was probably due to rigorous examination of slides during the development of the new technology. The increase in 2006 was less pronounced but still impressive even though the slides were routinely examined in the same manner as they were in 2004.

The increase in detection rate of Siriraj-LBC was probably due to the benefit of improved slide quality. Whereas 18.60% of our conventional smears had limited quality due to no endocervical or transformation zone component, obscuring blood and inflammatory cells, thick smear, or scant cellular smears, only 4.94% of the Siriraj-LBC had smears limited by these factors. Our results were in line with the experience of others (Bolick et al.,1998; Corkill et al.,1998; Diaz-Rosario et al.,1999; Dupree et al.,1998; Fremont-Smith et al.,2004; Papillo et al.,1998; Roberts et al.,1997). The improvement in the quality of slides in 2006 is likely to be due to the property of Siriraj- LBC itself rather than other factors, since the detection rate and quality of slides before 2005 had never reached those of the slides in 2006. Our 3-year retrospective data from 2002 to 2004 showed that our conventional smears had detection rates varying from 1.7% to 2.1%, and the poor quality smears varying from 18.6% to 32.6%.

The better detection rate of intraepithelial lesions is a common thread in studies on liquid-based cervical cytology. The increase in detection rates in previous studies varied from 12.0% to 106.8% (Bolick et al.,1998; Corkill et al.,1998; Diaz-Rosario et al.,1999; Dupree et al.,1998; Fremont-Smith et al.,2004; Papillo et al.,1998; Roberts et al.,1997). The reason for the wide range of this effect is not clear; but a wide range in detection rates of intraepithelial lesions by the conventional smear is also noted in the same studies, i.e. 1.1–2.7%. The increment seems higher in the studies with a low baseline detection rate using the conventional smear. In addition, this variation may represent regional or population-based differences, or different practice patterns. In our direct-to-vial study, Siriraj-LBC had a 100% increment for the detection of SIL from a baseline rate of 0.96% (LSIL = 0.56% and HSIL = 0.40%). The overwhelming diagnostic improvement of Siriraj-LBC, especially with respect to HSIL detection, would enhance the success of cervical cancer screening in our institute. Owing to the fact that the LBC slide makes it easier for a cytologist to find small numbers of abnormal cells, the percentages of ASCUS and ASC-H were also higher with Siriraj-LBC compared with the conventional method. The results were welcomed by the gynecologists who were chronically in fear of false negative results.

The increase in detection rate came with the concern of an increase in false positive cytology. From our cytology-histology paired data, Siriraj-LBC increased NPV without compromising PPV. This information implied that the Siriraj-LBC decreased false negative results, i.e. from 7.26% to 3.67% (P = 0.001) without affecting the overall false positive result, i.e. 13.17% vs.

16.97% (P = 0.285). However, we were aware that these numbers were not the real false negative and false positive rates, as the actual rates could not be obtained due to the limitations of this kind of study. The Siriraj-LBC displayed a higher false positive HSIL than the conventional method did, probably due to the morphological resemblance of immature squamous metaplastic or atrophic cells to HSIL. As these cells were easier to detect in the Siriraj-LBC than in the conventional smear, the higher false positive HSIL was not unexpected. However, as discussed in the split-sample study, we could not disregard the fact that our being novices in the LBC field could contribute to this false positivity. We expect to get better results using this technique in the future.

When the laboratory cost of the various cervical cytology techniques was calculated, we found that the cost of Siriraj-LBC was only 67% higher than that of the conventional cytology technique used in Siriraj Hospital and was lower than that of the commercially available LBC techniques in Thailand. However, we did not directly compare the diagnostic performance among the LBC techniques; therefore we did not know which LBC technology was the most cost-effective for our population. Nevertheless, because of its low cost and better performance than conventional cytology, Siriraj-LBC would be an accessible LBC technology for women of low-socioeconomic level. As a result, Siriraj-LBC has replaced the conventional cytology in Siriraj Hospital since 2006.

The Siriraj-LBC shows an impressive improvement in the detection rate of abnormal cervical cells. The Siriraj-LBC has an acceptable performance and quality which are within the same range as other previously reported LBC techniques. Therefore, the Siriraj-LBC may be considered a better option for cervical cancer screening than the conventional method and more economical than the commercially available LBC.

4. Conclusion

The diagnostic performance of our home-made LBC has been evaluated in both the "split-sample" study and "direct-to-vial" study and we have found that the screening performance of Siriraj-LBC was superior to that of conventional cytology. Our LBC does not require any expensive equipment; therefore its cost is much less than that of the commercial ones. Siriraj-LBC may be considered a better option for cervical cancer screening than the conventional method. For centers where conventional Pap smear does not perform well, the introduction of a low cost Siriraj-LBC may help to improve performance. We believe that the Siriraj-LBC will make a significant change in cervical cancer screening and patient management in our country.

5. References

Austin, R.; & Ramzy, I. (1998). Increased detection of epithelial cell abnormalities by liquid-based gynecologic cytology preparations: A review of accumulated data. Acta Cytol, Vol.42, No.1, pp. 178-184.

Bales, C. (2006). Laboratory techniques, In: Koss' diagnostic cytology and its histopathologic bases, L.G. Koss and M.R. Melamed, (Eds.), 569-622, Lippincott William & Wilkins, Philadelphia

Bishop, J.; Bigner, S.; Colgan, T.; Husain, M.; Howell, L.; McIntosh, K.; Taylor, D.; & Sadeghi, M. (1998). Multicenter masked evaluation of AutoCyte PREP thin layers with matched conventional smears. Including initial biopsy results. Acta Cytol, Vol.42, No.1, pp. 189–197.

Bolick, D.; & Hellman, D. (1998). Laboratory implementation and efficacy assessment of the ThinPrep cervical cancer screening system. Acta Cytol, Vol.42, No.1, pp. 209-213.

Corkill, M.; Knapp, D.; & Hutchinson, M. (1998). Improved accuracy for cervical cytology with the ThinPrep method and the endocervical brush-spatula collection procedure. J Lower Genital Tract Dis, Vol. 2, No. 1, pp. 12-16.

Diaz-Rosario, L.; & Kabawat, S. (1999). Performance of a fluidbased, thin-layer Papanicolaou smear method in the clinical setting of an independent laboratory and an outpatient screening population in New England. Arch Pathol Lab Med, Vol.123, No.?, pp. 817-821.

Dupree, W.; Suprun, H.; Beckwith, D.; Shane, J.; & Lucente, V. (1998). The promise and risk of a new technology: The Lehigh Valley Hospital's experience with liquid-based cervical cytology. Cancer, Vol.84, No.4, pp. 202-207.

Fahey, MT.; Irwig, L.; & Macaskill, P. (1995). Meta-analysis of Pap test accuracy. Am J Epidemiol, Vol.141, No.7, pp. 680-689.

Ferlay, J,; Shin, H.; Bray, F.; Forman, D.; Mathers, C.; & Parkin, D. (2010). In: *GLOBOCAN 2008*, Cancer Incidence and Mortality Worldwide: IARC CancerBase No. 10 [Internet]. Lyon, France: International Agency for Research on Cancer; 2010. Available from: http://globocan.iarc.fr

Fremont-Smith, M.; Marino, J.; Griffin, B.; Spencer, L.; & Bolick, D. (2004). Comparison of the SurePath liquid-based Papanicolaou smear with the conventional Papanicolaou smear in a multisite direct-to-vial study. Cancer, Vol.102, No.5, pp. 269-279.

Gay, J.; Donaldson, L.; & Goellner, J. (1985). False-negative results in cervical cytologic studies. Acta Cytol, Vol.29, No.6, pp. 1043-1046.

Guo, M.; Hu, L.; Martin, L.; Liu, S.; Baliga, M.; & Hughson, M. (2005). Accuracy of liquid-based Pap tests: comparison of concurrent liquid-based tests and cervical biopsies on 782 women with previously abnormal Pap smears. Acta Cytol, Vol.49, No.2, pp. 132-138.

Laiwejpithaya, S.; Rattanachaiyanont, M.; Benjapibal, M.; Khuakoonratt, N.; Boriboonhirunsarn, D.; Laiwejpithaya, S.; Sangkarat, S.; & Wongtiraporn, W. (2008). Comparison between Siriraj liquid-based and conventional cytology for detection of abnormal cervicovaginal smears: A split-sample study. Asian Pacific J Cancer Prev, Vol.9, No.4, pp. 575-580.

Laiwejpithaya, S.; Benjapibal, M.; Laiwejpithaya, S.; Wongtiraporn, W.; Sangkarat, S.; & Rattanachaiyanont, M. (2009). Performance and cost analysis of Siriraj liquid-based cytology: a direct-to-vial study. Eur J Obstet Gynecol Reprod Biol, Vol. 147, No.2, pp. 201-205.

Lee, K.; Ashfaq, R.; Birdsong, G.; Corkill, M.; McIntosh, K.; & Inhorn, S. (1997). Comparison of conventional Papanicolaou smears and a fluid-based, thin-layer system for cervical cancer screening. Obstet Gynecol, Vol.90, No.2, pp. 278–284.

Limayec, A.; Connor, J.; Huang, X.; & Luff, R. (2003). Comparison analysis of conventional Papanicolaou tests and a fluid-based thin-layer method. Arch Pathol Lab Med, Vol.127, No.2, pp. 200-204.

Mount, S.; Harmon, M.; Eltabbakh, G.; Uyar, D.; & Leiman, G. (2004). False positive diagnosis in conventional and liquid-based cervical specimens. Acta Cytol, Vol.48, No.3, pp. 363-371.

Nanda, K.; McCrory, D.; Myers, E.; Bastian, L.; Hasselblad, V.; Hickey, J.; & Matchar, D. (2000). Accuracy of the Papanicolaou test in screening for and follow-up of cervical cytologic abnormalities: a systematic review. Ann Intern Med, Vol.132, No.10, pp. 810-819.

Nieminen, P.; Kallio, M.; & Hakama, M. (1995). The effect of mass screening on incidence and mortality of squamous and adenocarcinoma of cervix uteri. *Obstet Gynecol*, Vol.85, No.6, pp. 1017-1021.

Papillo, J.; Zarka, M.; & St John, T. (1998). Evaluation of the ThinPrep Pap test in clinical practice: A seven-month, 16,314-case experience in northern Vermont. Acta Cytol, Vol.42, No.1, pp. 203-208.

Park, I.; Lee, S.; Chae, S.; Park, K.; Kim, J.; & Lee, H. (2001). Comparing the accuracy of ThinPrep Pap tests and conventional Papanicolaou smears on the basis of the histologic diagnosis: a clinical study of women with cervical abnormalities. *Acta Cytol*, Vol.45, No.4, pp. 525-531.

Roberts, J.; Gurley, A.; Thurloe, J.; Bowditch, R.; & Laverty, C. (1997). Evaluation of the ThinPrep Pap test as an adjunct to the conventional Pap smear. Med J Aust, Vol.167, No.9, pp. 466-469.

Solomon, D.; Davey, D.; Kurman, R.; Moriarty, A.; O'Connor, D.; Prey, M.; Raab, S.; Sherman, M.; Wilbur, D.; Wright, T Jr.; & Young, N. (2002). The 2001 Bethesda System: terminology for reporting results of cervical cytology. JAMA, Vol.287, No.16, pp. 2114-2119.

Vassilakos, P.; Carrel, S.; Petignat, P.; Boulvain, M.; & Campana, A. (2002). Use of automated primary screening on liquid-based, thin-layer preparations. Acta Cytol, Vol.46, No.2, pp. 291-195.

8

Microinvasive Carcinoma of the Cervix

Fernando Anschau, Chrystiane da Silva Marc,
Maria Carolina Torrens and Manoel Afonso Guimarães Gonçalves
Pontifícia Universidade Católica do Rio Grande do Sul,
Fundação Universitária de Cardiologia – Instituto de Cardiologia de Porto Alegre,
Faculdade Nossa Senhora de Fátima – Caxias do Sul
Brazil

1. Introduction

There is a minimally invasive nosological entity among cervical precursor lesions and frank invasive cancer. Initially described by Mestwerdt in 1947, cases of microinvasive carcinoma of the uterine cervix represent a group of patients with better prognosis with the possibility of needing less radical treatment.[1] Despite that microinvasion has been defined since the 1940s, the depth of invasion, as well as the lateral extension, are subjects of various classifications and certain controversy.

2. Definition

There is a continuum of knowledge about microinvasive cervical cancer from its initial landmark in 1947, which must be understood so that we can reflect on the information and approaches recommended by different authors.

The first conception of microinvasive squamous cell carcinoma of the cervix was presented by Mestwerdt in 1947, who strived to develop an early diagnosis of cervical carcinoma. In this first work, Mestwerdt cited that the discovery of 43 cases of microcarcinoma was possible with the combination of colposcopy and the iodine test with the standard histologic examination over a period of 9 ½ years. This author considered the attributes of microcarcinoma of cervix to be the following:

- Size still at the microscopic level.
- All originate from the squamous epithelium of the cervix to cervical canal up to its limit, but is still not associated with the surface.
- They show all the phases of atypia.
- Besides the complete structure of changes in all layers of the surface epithelium, where its construction is in the longer recognizable, there is simultaneous rupture of the basal membrane by glandular budding in the connective tissue.
- Also observed on the surface is invasion of lymphatic spaces and blood vessels.

The measurement of stromal invasion, always defined microscopically, should be done from the basement membrane. [1] In 1961, the International Federation of Gynecology and Obstetrics (FIGO) on proposing the classification cervical cancer, recommended the subdivision of stage I into IA and IB. Stage IA would be defined as early stromal invasion. in 1965, two groups published the problematization with respect to depth of invasion. Margulis and coworkers believed that the definition should include invasion of 5.0 mm of the stroma, while Ullery and coworkers considered invasion beyond the basement membrane of 3.0 mm.

Temporarily, we can refer to 1971 when FIGO introduced the term "occult cancer of the cervix" for stage IA. In 1973, Burghardt proposed the study of the volume of the lesion, believing that 500 mm^3 would be a better option for the definition in question.

Despite the above mentioned proposal by FIGO, there was still no clear criteria for minimal stromal invasion. In 1974, the Society of Gynecologic Oncologists (SGO) proposed a definition for microinvasion as a lesion that invaded below the basement membrane to a depth of 3 mm or less, with no evidence of invasion of the lymphovascular space. SGO believed that the horizontal dimension would not enter into the classification of microinvasion. Despite new classifications in 1971 and 1975, with the introduction of the term occult carcinoma, FIGO would return in the 1980s with a definition that considered the measurement of the depth of invasion in cervical cancer in stage I. The preoccupation with the depth and extension of the lesion can also be observed in the study of Averette and coworkers, which in 1976 led to expectations regarding lesions of up to 1 mm, and in the study of Sedlis and colleagues, who determined a maximal extension of 4 mm for the definition of microinvasive cancer. The new definition from FIGO in 1985 brought criteria for carcinomas referred to as pre-clinical, dividing them into two groups: IA1 with minimal stromal invasion and IA2 with invasion up to 5 mm and not exceeding 7 mm. Again, in referring to the FIGO classification, we observe the reiteration of not considering the influence of the invasion of the lymphatic space in the stage.

In 1994, FIGO presented the classification of cervical cancer that put together clear measurements for the invasion of the stroma in stages IA1 and IA2. This classification was revised in 2009, and the term microscopic cancer was proposed for stage IA. Therefore, all gross lesions, even if superficial, were considered stage IB. The invasion was limited to 5 mm in depth and 7 mm of extension. The involvement of the lymphovascular space continued to have no effect on staging, but did influence the treatment. The invasion of the stroma up to 3 mm in depth and 7 mm of extension characterized stage IA1, and invasion of the stroma between 3 mm and 5 mm in depth and 7 mm of extension, stage IA2. [2, 3]

Certainly one of the main factors involved in the definition of the depth of invasion and in the classification of microinvasion was the involvement of the lymphovascular space and consequently the possibility of lymph node metastasis in the pelvis and vaginal recurrence. The role of lymphovascular invasion and the possibility of lymph node metastasis are also the subject of many speculations about the treatment of microinvasive cervical carcinoma.

3. Diagnosis

Over the last years this early invasive carcinoma has become an increasingly important part of the problem of cervical cancer. The mounting frequency with which these diagnoses are made is directly related to the increased use of the Papanicolaou smear technique and use of large loop excision of the transformation zone.

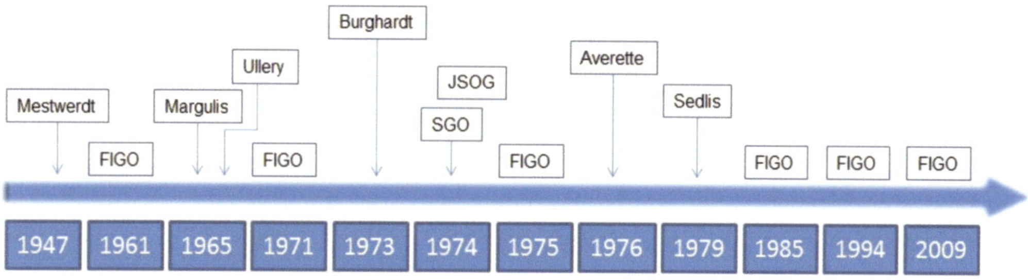

FIGO: International Federation of Gynecology and Obstetrics;
SOG: Society of Gynecologic Oncologists (USA);
JSOG: Japanese Society of Obstetrics & Gynecology;

Fig. 1. Evolution of the definition of microinvasive carcinoma of the cervix

Although definitive diagnosis of microinvasion must be done by histological evaluation of specimens obtained by conization or hysterectomy, some colposcopy signs could identify this situation. Reid pointed out some colposcopic and clinical warning signs of invasion:

- Friable areas, with easy bleeding upon touch
- Defined areas as colposcopically significant - with Reid index ≥ 5 - showing irregular surface
- Superficial ulcers with white epithelium at edges
- Atypical vessels
- Mosaic or rough dotted area at extreme, particularly when showing large and irregular intercapillary distance
- Groups of lesions with large extension and with characteristics of colposcopic lesion of high grade
- Colposcopic lesions of high grade type penetrating more than 5 mm in the endocervical canal
- Intra-epithelial cervical lesions of high grade on histology by biopsy in which the basement membrane cannot be clearly defined
- Cyotological evidence of squamous cell carcinoma or of adenocarcinoma *in situ*

Despite the efforts for colposcopic detection of microinvasive alterations, this diagnostic modality does not show a good predictive indicator of the severity of the cervical lesion and tends to underestimate microinvasive carcinoma. The colposcopic images, besides not being characteristic, are difficult to interpret and microinvasive lesions are often endocervical. Colposcopic signs are even more inconsistent when the focus of invasion is small and superficial.[4, 5, 6] There are no specific colposcopic findings of microinvasive carcinoma. The findings resemble cases of *in situ* and invasive carcinoma. Colposcopy is better at identifying pre-malignant or frank invasive disease than microinvasive lesions.

The determination of microinvasion should always be done by systematic histologic evaluation of a consistent sample of cervix, using serial sections in order to determine with precision the depth and extension of the invasion, besides the penetration of the lymphovascular space. Even with colposcopic lesion with guided biopsy of the cervix, sometimes there is no guarantee that the biopsied material is sufficient for defining the diagnosis. In the localization of the microinvasion, with the analysis of the conization specimens of the cervix, the focus of the microinvasion from the basement membrane of the epithelium is found at the following sites: the ectocervix besides the last gland in 11% of cases, inside the transformation zone in 71% of cases (22% on the surface of the epithelium and 49% in the depth or glandular crypts) and in the endocervical canal in 18% of cases. [7]

The whole extension of cervical cancer screening programs have led to an increase in the detection of microinvasion, as well as the dissemination of the utilization of a diathermy loop for excision of altered areas and resection of the transformation zone in the investigation of suspect cases.

The evaluation of the biopsy by an experienced pathologist is essential for the correct identification of microinvasion with its respective measurement and characterization of the presence or not of invasion of the lymphovascular space. Also, it is of great importance that the pathologist can determine the presence of compromise of the margins and the grade of these lesions. Therefore, for young patients with the intention of preserving fertility, the identification of these parameters can translate to conservative treatment.

4. Treatment

Based on the premise that the neoplastic cell with malignant differentiation has the potential to metastasize through the lymphatic and vascular systems, it should be takrm into consideration that this could occur even at initial stages of invasion of the basement membrane. Meanwhile, various lines of epidemiological evidence indicate stage IA1 as having a low potential for lymph node metastasis and good disease-free survival rates. Lee and et al. found that the lymphovascular space was compromised in 0.9% of cases when invasion was less than 1 mm and in 10.2 % when invasion was between 1 and 3 mm deep. [8] Ostor et al. demonstrated compromise of the space lymphovascular in 3% and 15% when invasion was up to 1 mm and between 1 and 3 mm, respectively.[9]

The requirements in relation to the involvement of the lymphovascular space with tumor cells are still points to ponder; therefore, understanding that doubt is part of the thought process, we propose the following reflections: (1) Why ignore the involvement of the lymphovascular space? (2) Why value the involvement of the lymphovascular space?

Why ignore the involvement of the lymphovascular space?

- Conflicting evidence
- Studies not associating the involvement of the lymphovascular space with lymph node metastasis
- Interpretation of invasion of the lymphovascular space is subjective
- Inflammation and retraction artifacts can cause confusion

Why value the involvement of the lymphovascular space?

- Think of invasive tumor
- Associated with greater probability of lymph node metastasis
- Associated with worse prognosis - more radical treatment
- Increased identification with increased serial sections

The initial idea of Mestwerdt of performing serial histologic sections with detailed examination of the sections is still an interesting prerogative in this aspect. In 1975, a study with serial sections of 30 microinvasive carcinomas of the cervix (invasion between 2 and 5 mm) demonstrated that 30% had compromise of the lymphovascular space - based on the first of the blocks; but this percentage increased to 57% with serial sections. No patient showed lymph node metastasis.[10]

5. Lymph nodes

Although FIGO does not include the lymph node status in its staging system for cervical carcinoma, it is known that for patients treated surgically in initial stages, the presence of ganglion metastasis is the most important risk factor for recurrence and mortality. [11] In addition, an adequate knowledge of lymph node compromise is essential for the indication of adjuvant treatment.

Traditionally, for lymph node evaluation, the technique proposed is bilateral retroperitoneal lymphadenectomy. However, this practice, associated with high rates of short- and long-term morbidity, has been questioned in initial stages, since a small portion of patients show lymphatic compromise. Studies with patients in stages IA1 and IA2 demonstrated an incidence of lymph node metastasis in 7.3% (0%-13.8%) of cases.[12, 13] In the work of Sevin et al. [14], no cases of lymph node invasion were found when analyzing 110 cases of microinvasive carcinoma with stromal invasion less than or equal to 5 mm. What we can reflect on the positivity of the lymph nodes is that as the depth of stromal invasion increases, there is an increase in the percent of lymph nodes compromised with metastatic cells. Thus, some studies demonstrate the following relation between depth of invasion and lymph node metastasis: invasion up to 1 mm, presence of <1 to 1.5% of lymph nodes compromised; between 1 and 3 mm, <1 to 4.2%; between 3 and 5 mm, between 2 and 3.7%. [8,9]

Aimed at reducing the rate of complications of lymphadenectomy, the technique of sentinel lymph node biopsy (SLB), introduced by Cabañas, [15] has been studied in cases of cervical carcinoma. Studies evaluating the accuracy and applicability of sentinel lymph node biopsy in cervical carcinoma have shown promising results (high rates of detection and low false-positive rates), mainly when analyzing cases of lesions less than 2 cm.[16] Other authors have demonstrated a 94% rate of detection of sentinel lymph nodes associated with sensitivity and negative predictive value of 100%, for tumors less than 2 cm. [17] The recent study SENTICOL [18], in which SLB was carried out in a uniform manner by experienced surgeons, combining techniques that utilize blue dye and lymphoscintigraphy with technetium (Tc99), demonstrated a sensitivity of 92% and obtained ideal mapping in 75% of patients. These authors concluded that when utilizing the two techniques combined, a negative result in the sentinel lymph nodes on both sides indicates the absence of metastatic disease, with a negative predictive value of 98.2%.

In accordance with studies in 2011, the use of laparoscopy in the detection and removal of sentinel lymph nodes (SL) is evidence-based and safe with either the use of blue dye or Tc99 lymphoscintigraphy. When these two detection techniques were compared, Tc99 showed a significantly higher rate of identification of sentinel lymph nodes. [19] The identification of LS by SPECT-CT has also been the target of studies. The results to date suggest that this examination can increase the detection and improve the preoperative anatomic localization of LS, when compared to lymphoscintigraphy with Tc99. [20, 21]

In relation to microinvasive disease, there are no studies only with this population, the focus of interest of the present chapter. A significant part of the works with initial cases includes patients between FIGO stages IA1 and IB1. Although current studies have shown encouraging results, SLB cannot yet be considered standard treatment for initial cases of cervical carcinoma. Its clinical impact must be demonstrated in randomized studies that compare outcomes such as disease-free survival and global survival between patients submitted to traditional pelvic lymphadenectomy and to the sentinel lymph node technique.

Certainly, one important question in the context of microinvasive carcinoma is the search for more conservative therapies with the establishment of a certain balance between uterine preservation and disease-free surgical margins. On demonstrating a lower lymph node compromise in microinvasive carcinoma, especially when there is no involvement of the lymphovascular space, this balance becomes more appropriate.

The primary treatment of cancer of the cervix and thereby of the microcarcinoma of the cervix is surgery, save exceptions of cases with clinical contraindications to surgery, where radiotherapy combined with chemotherapy and the possibility of brachytherapy are valid options. Extended radical hysterectomy with lymphadenectomia is the standard treatment for those women who do not want more children, certainly observing the considerations previously indicated, which authorize a more conservative approach. This standard treatment -radical hysterectomy- can be executed by the vaginal route, Schauta-Amreich or Schauta-Stoeckel surgery with videolaparoscopic radical pelvic lymphadenectomy, or by the abdominal route, Wertheim-Meigs surgery.

Dargent surgery, radical trachelectomy with videolaparoscopic pelvic lymphadenectomy, is indicated in young patients who wish to preserve fertility, constituting a more radical alternative than conization. [22]

When the discussion of the treatment of cancer of the cervix includes specificities such as the case of microinvasion, it is also necessary to consider other specificities. In this point, we must focus on the characteristics of the disease, with the peculiarities of the stage (IA1 or IA2), of the histologic type and of the presence of invasion of the lymphovascular spaces, as well as on the characteristics of the patient, with possible clinical restrictions, with questions of preservation of fertility and with the consent of treatment options.

For the cases with stage IA1 where we did not find any evidence of involvement of the lymphovascular space, conservative treatment - by conization of the cervix -can be an acceptable option, especially for those patients who wish to preserve fertility. [23, 24] The participation of the patient in agreement with the approach should always be pointed out; at this moment, concordance with a more radical treatment can be an option - with the choice of simple hysterectomy, for example. Current recommendations from the World Health Organization, without specification of histopathologic type, are simple hysterectomy for women with microinvasive cancer stage IA1.[25] Risk for recurrence after this treatment is 1% and overall 5-year survival is 99%. [27] When faced with compromise by tumor cells in the lymphovascular space, the indication should be major radical treatment - consisting of total hysterectomy with parametrectomy, resection of the upper third of the vagina and pelvic lymphadenectomy.

Those patients with stage IA2 have a greater potential of lymph node metastasis at this stage, which could also involve a more radical treatment. The cases where no invasion of the lymphovascular space is observed, the complete excision of the lesion by extrafascial hysterectomy or, in selected cases and when there is desire for preservation of fertility, by conization with free margins can be an option. When fertility is not an issue, the treatment proposed here should also be considered, with an indication of hysterectomy. Alternatively, trachelectomy or radical hysterectomy can also be applied, without the need for pelvic lymphadenectomy. [26]

As in the previously mentioned cases of involvement of the lymphovascular space, also in the cases of stage IA2, there is an indication of radical hysterectomy with pelvic lymphadenectomy. When the preservation of fertility is desired, vaginal radical trachelectomy with extra-peritoneal or laparoscopic pelvic lymphadenectomy is the option. Risk of recurrence of IA2 tumors treated with radical hysterectomy and bilateral pelvic lymphadenectomy is 3–5% and overall 5-year survival is 96%.[27]

6. Follow-up

After treatment, the patients should have a regular periodic follow-up with clinical gynecologic examinations, oncotic colpocytology and colposcopy. Follow-up protocols after the conclusion of the initial treatment are variable, using a number of tests in a variety of intervals with debatable results. The components that should be considered for an ideal follow-up program are: (i) optimal interval for the follow-up; (ii) available tests for follow-up; (iii) modifications in the course of the follow-up in accordance with the risk of recurrence identified in the primary treatment.

The tests available for the follow-up are the following: anamnesis, physical examination, cervical cytology, ultrasonography, magnetic resonance, computed tomography, positron emission tomography (PET) and tumor markers. Physical examination and vaginal cytology are the most commonly used methods in the follow-up. The physical examination, especially, has led to a considerable number of detections in patients in which cyto-detection was low. To date, there is little definitive evidence of the most suitable strategy for follow-up (for patients clinically free of disease after primary treatment). Therefore, it is important that the patient have some understanding to facilitate the follow-up. Among these, general symptoms such as weight loss, loss of appetite, fatigue, pain, cough, dyspnea, confusion, and edema of legs (mainly unilateral), beside local symptoms such as bleeding and vaginal, vesical or anal secretion, distension or abdominal pain.[28]

The periodicity recommended for the doctor visits is as follows: 3 to 4 months in the first 2 years; every 6 months for the next 3 years; and annually after this period, maintaining a follow-up for 10 years.

7. References

[1] Mestwerdt G. Zentralbl Gynakol 1947; 69:198-202
[2] Creasman W. New gynecologic cancer staging. Gynecol Oncol 1995;58:157–8
[3] FIGO. Int J Gynecol Oncol 2009; 105:103-4.
[4] Choo YC, et al. Br J Obstet Gynecol 1984; 91:1156-60
[5] Figueiredo PG, et al. RBGO 2003; 24:37-43
[6] Hopman EH, et al. Aus N Z J Obstet Gynaecol 1998, 53:97-106

[7] Reich O, Pickel H, Tamussino K, Winter R. Microinvasive carcinoma of the cervix: site of the first focus invasion. Obstet Gynecol 2001; 97:890-2.
[8] Lee KBM, et al. Int J Gynecol Cancer 2006, 16:1184-1187
[9] Ostor AG: Pandora's box or Ariadne's thread? Definition and prognostic significance of microinvasion in the uterine cervix: squamous lesions. Pathology Annual 1995; 103-136
[10] Roche WD & Norris HJ. 1975
[11] Biewenga P, Van der Velden J, Mol BW, et al. Prognostic model for survival in patients with early stage cervical cancer. Cancer 2011;117:768–76.
[12] Matsuura Y, Kawagoe T, Toki N, Tanaka M, Kashimura M. Long-standing complications after treatment for cancer of the uterine cervix—clinical significance of medical examination at 5 years after treatment. Int J Gynecol Cancer 2006;16:294–7.
[13] Rogers, Linda J. MMed, FCOG; Luesley, David M. MA, MD, FRCOG.Stage IA2 Cervical Carcinoma: How Much Treatment Is Enough?. International Journal of Gynecological Cancer. 19(9):1620-1624, December 2009.
[14] Sevin BU, Nadji M, Averette HE, Hilsenbeck S, Smith D, Lampe A. Microinvasive carcinoma of the cervix. Cancer 1992 ;70:2121-8.
[15] Cabanas RM: An approach for the treatment of penile carcinoma. Cancer 39:456-466, 1977
[16] Robison K, Holman LL, Moore RG. Update on sentinel lymph node evaluation in gynecologic malignancies. Curr Opin Obstet Gynecol. 2011 Feb;23(1):8-12.
[17] Darlin L, Persson J, Bossmar T, et al. The sentinel node concept in early cervical cancer performs well in tumors smaller than 2 cm. Gynecol Oncol 2010; 117:266–269
[18] LeCuru F, Mathevet P, Querleu D, et al. Bilateral negative sentinel nodes accurately predict absence of lymph node metastasis in early cervical cancer: results of the SENTICOL study. J Clin Oncol 2011;29:1686–91
[19] Roy M, et al, Value of sentinel node mapping in cancer of the cervix, Gynecol Oncol (2011), doi:10.1016; 2011.04.002
[20] Martinez A, Zerdoud S, Mery E, Bouissou E, Ferro G, Querleu D. Hybrid imaging by SPECT/CT for sentinel lymph node detection in patients with cancer of the uterine cervix. Gynecol Oncol. 2010;119(3):431-5.
[21] Pandit-Taskar N, Gemignani ML, Lyall A, Larson SM, Barakat RR, Abu Rustum NR. Single photon emission computed tomography SPECT-CT improves sentinel node detection and localization in cervical and uterine malignancy. Gynecol Oncol. 2010 Apr;117(1):59-64.
[22] Querleu D, Childers JM, Dargent D. Laparoscopic Surgery in Gynecological Oncology. Oxford: Blackwell Science, 1999.
[23] Stehman FB, Rose PG, Greer BE, Roy M, Plante M, Penalver M et al. Innovations in the treatment of invasive cervical cancer. Cancer 2003;98(9 Suppl):2052-63.
[24] Kesic V. Management of cervical cancer. Eur J Surg Oncol 2006;32(8):832-7.
[25] Comprehensive cervical cancer control: a guide to essential practice. WHO Press. Geneva, Switzerland. 2006. pp179-181.
[26] Creasman WT, Zaino RJ, Major FJ, DiSaia PJ, Hatch KD, Homesley HD. Early invasive carcinoma of the cervix (3 to 5 mm invasion): risk factors and prognosis. A Gynecologic Oncology Group study. Am J Obstet Gynecol 1998;178:62-5.
[27] Benedet JL, Odicino F, Maisonneuve P, et al. Carcinoma of the cervix uteri. Int J Gynaecol Obstst 2003;83(Suppl 1):41-78.
[28] Elit L, Fyles AW, Devries MC, Oliver TK, Fung-Kee-Fung M; Gynecology Cancer Disease Site Group. Follow-up for women after treatment for cervical cancer: a systematic review. Gynecol Oncol. 2009 Sep;114(3):528-35. Epub 2009 Jun 26.

9

The Clinical Outcome of Patients with Microinvasive Cervical Carcinoma

Špela Smrkolj
Department of Gynecology and Obstetrics,
University Medical Centre Ljubljana
Slovenia

1. Introduction

Cervical cancer, the second most common cancer in women, develops through well-defined precursor lesions with potential to progress to invasive disease if not properly detected and eradicated. In cervical carcinogenesis, human papillomavirus (HPV) plays an important causal role. Besides the evidental causal role in cervical carcinogenesis, HPV is an important prognostic factor for disease progression as well (Syrjänen, 2000). Early invasive carcinoma is an intermediate state in the development of invasive carcinoma from a cervical intraepithelial neoplasia. According to clinical experience, the early stage of invasion has much better prognosis when compared to an advanced invasive cancer. This warrants the recognition of microinvasive carcinoma (MIC) as a separate entity among cervical cancer that is not visible at inspection, and therefore only diagnosed by histological examination of a biopsy specimen that contains the complete lesion (Wright et al., 1994).

Mestwerdt was the first to notice that cervical cancers with less than 5 mm of invasion behave less malignant and therefore could be treated by less radical surgery. He named these tumours "Mikrokarcinom". Mestwerdt also introduced tumour depth of 5 mm as a parameter of the management of cervical carcinoma and suggested a less radical surgery for such cases. Subsequent authors proposed different maximal depths as the upper limit of an invasive growth (Mestwerdt, 1947). Following Mestwerdt's publication and before the most recent FIGO definition of stage IA cervical cancer in the 1994, an intense discussion has continued concerning the definition of microinvasion, terminology and treatment modalities as related to disease outcome, e.g. lymph node metastasis, reccurence and cancer death (Creasman, 1995). The latest FIGO definition of stage IA1 cervical cancer is defined as cervical carcinoma confined to the uterus with stromal invasion less than 3.0 mm and stage IA2 cervical cancer with stromal invasion more than 3.0 mm but not more than 5.0 mm, with limited horizontal spread beyond 7.0 mm (World Health Organization, 2006). Because of the effective use of screening, an increasing number of women are being diagnosed with cervical cancer in an early stage of the disease. However, many of these cases occur in younger women, for whom the preservation of fertility is desirable. More conservative methods have emerged as alternative treatment modalities for these women, as they may allow for future fertility, without having a considerable adverse effect on cure rates.

The objective of this review is to discuss the management of patients with microinvasive cervical cancer and present the Ljubljana experience on management of FIGO stage IA (both IA1 and IA2) cervical cancer.

2. Management of stage IA cervical carcinoma

Lesions of the microinvasive type present a paradox in that they breach the basement membrane yet are rarely associated with metastasis. Traditionally the presence of stromal invasion predetermines a belief that metastasis is imminent and radical surgery obligatory. There is now considerable debate on the necessity for obligate radicality by radical hysterectomy and lymphadenectomy or radical irradiation such that conservative management, simple hysterectomy or even therapeutic cone biopsy, are alternatives in most cases. Individualization of treatment to reduce therapy-associated early and late morbidity is the most current trend in cervical cancer surgery. Despite advances over the past 3 decades in decreasing the morbidity of treatment, the cure rate associated with radical surgery (approximately 90%) has not changed appreciably. The limited risk of parametrial and nodes involvement in case of MIC unbalances the morbidity of radical hysterectomy and pelvic node removal.

Figure 1 shows the treatment options for microinvasive carcinoma of the cervix, based on the latest guidelines within the ESGO community and prepared by ESGO Educational Committee (ESGO, 2010).

Conization as definitive therapy should be reserved for patients who desire fertility preservation. The candidates for this procedure would be those patients with FIGO stage IA1 disease (less than or equal to 3 mm stromal invasion). The selection criteria for this conservative approach to definitive therapy should include squamous histology, negative conization margin, and adequate pathologic processing of the tissue specimen. The patient needs to be compliant with a follow-up regimen. In patients with 3 mm or less depth of stromal invasion who do not desire fertility preservation, a simple extrafascial hysterectomy can be performed.

Patients with FIGO stage IA2 cervical carcinoma can be treated with modified radical hysterectomy and pelvic and para-aortic lymph node dissection. Selection of such patients for a modified radical hysterectomy include squamous histology with negative conization margins following adequate pathologic processing of tissue.

Patients with positive cone margins should be treated as if they had frankly invasive disease and undergo a radical hysterectomy with pelvic and para-aortic lymph node dissection.

The patients who are nonsurgical candidates or individuals not opting for surgical management should be treated with primary radiation therapy.

The use of adjuvant radiation therapy in lymph node positive patients has been controversial. A recent studies indicates that postoperative radiotherapy in node positive cervix cancer significantly improves pelvic control, disease-free survival, and overall survival.

Stage IA1, LVSI negative:	
	Conization if preservation of fertility is desired or Simple (extrafascial, type A) hysterectomy with or without salpingoophorectomy
Stage IA1 with extensive LVSI and Stage IA2:	
	Conization or radical trachelectomy if preservation of fertility is desired or Modified radical hysterectomy (type B) and Pelvic lymphadenectomy
Stage IA1 or IA2 nonsurgical candidates:	
	Primary radiation therapy.

Fig. 1. Treatment options for MIC: accurate pathologic evaluation and negative cone margins for 2009 FIGO staging.

Reports describing primary radiotherapy for microinvasive cervical cancer are limited and generally include patients who have medical contraindications to surgery. As opposed to patients with larger volume invasive disease , brachytherapy is often the sole, or major, component of radiation used. Brachytherapy alone is an effective treatment for nonsurgical candidates with microinvasive cervical carcinoma. The incidence of lymph node metastasis and regional relapse following brachytherapy, is very low for small-volume invasive cervical carcinoma, particularly in those with maximal depth of stromal invasion less than 5 mm (Greer et al., 1990).

Recommended follow-up for patients with MIC after completed therapy is every 3 months during the first year, then every 6 months up to 5 years and annually afterwards. Investigations in addition to gynaecological examination, including cytology and colposcopy, should be performed depending on symptoms, local findings and general condition of the patient (ESGO, 2010).

3. The Ljubljana experience on management of stage IA cervical carcinoma and the clinical outcome of our patients

The Ljubljana experience on management of stage IA (both IA1 and IA2) cervical cancer consists of accumulated experience during several observation periods. During the period of 1960-1972, the surgical treatment in our institution followed the principle that cancer is cancer, therefore radical treatment is justified. During that period, 290 cases of stage IA cervical carcinoma were treated, the great majority by vaginal radical hysterectomy and abdominal radical hysterectomy with lymphadenectomy. Positive lymph nodes were found in none of these cases (Kovačič et al., 1989).

Our accumulated experience on the minimal risk of metastatic spread and reccurence, improved understanding of the development of early stages of cervical carcinoma, and the increasing frequency of young women wishing to preserve fertility were the reasons for the increased use of conservative treatment. A conservative surgical approach for MIC, FIGO stage IA was adopted when a scoring system was implemented in 1979, based on the evaluation of morphological criteria and exact estimation of the tumor size (Rainer, 1978). This scoring system has been used since 1979 as the basis for selecting treatment for all patients with stage IA cervical carcinoma. Table 1 shows the Rainer's scoring system.

The present scoring system was established when there was no definitive international consensus on the classification of MIC. The definition was vague and the criteria for identification varied. The applied score enabled uniform estimation of all histological criteria in every case and was effective in making decisions about the treatment modalities in individual cases. To obtain an unbiased estimation of the tumor size and its various histological parameters, 70 cases of MIC were subjected to stereological analysis (Eržen et al., 1995). The results of this analysis were used to define the criteria for the scoring system. The depth of stromal invasion, mitotic activity, pattern of invasion, host defence reaction and lymph-vascular space invasion (LVSI) were evaluated and scored. The patient's age and her wish to preserve fertility were also taken into consideration.

During the first observation period (1960 - 1972), the cases with the depth of infiltration more than 3 mm were classified as stage IB. If the clinical data including the patient›s general condition and the surgeon›s competence were not taken into consideration, the following total scores were used as the criteria of selection for the different treatment modalities.

Between 1989 and 1993 conization was the definitive treatment for patients with a score of 7 points or less, simple vaginal or abdominal hysterectomy was performed in those who scored 8 to 12 points, and radical hysterectomy with lymphadenectomy was suggested in patients with more than 12 points, using the Rainer's scoring system. According to this scoring system which was further modified in 1994 for MIC stage IA2, radical hysterectomy was no longer indicated. Until 1997 lymphadenectomy was performed only in patients with LVSI, and thereafter in all of the patients with MIC IA2.

During the observation period from 1973 to 2009 the rate of conisation with/without pelvic lymphadenectomy as the sole mode of treatment of MIC, FIGO stage IA has increased continuously and was the definitive treatment for almost 75% of all our

Morphological criteria		Points
I. Cellular type	- large cell type	1
	- keratinizing type	2
	- small cell type	2
II. Mitotic activity (per high power field)	- 5 -10 mitoses	1
	- more than 10 mitoses	2
III. Type of invasion	- pushing borders, singular buds	1
	- dropping off type	5
	- reticular or confluent type	7
IV. Defence reaction	- poor	1
V. Capillary-like space invasion	- present	10
VI. Depth of invasion	- less than 3 mm	2
	- 3 to 5 mm	4
	- morc than 5 mm	8

Table 1. Scoring of the morphological criteria of MIC

patients. If resection margins were not disease-free or lateral clearance was not adequate, the suggested treatment was hysterectomy to avoid late recurrence. However the frequency of Wertheim radical hysterectomy and simple hysterectomy have declined accordingly. The Wertheim radical hysterectomy was performed only in 9,0 % of the cases, mostly due to incorrect preoperative diagnosis of invasive carcinoma, based on scanty biopsy material. The pelvic lymphadenectomy was performed in 11,2% of the cases, in these cases LVSI was present and the pelvic nodes were invariably free of cancer. The frequency of lymph node metastases in stage IA2 cervical cancer is reported to range from 0% to 9,7%. LVSI seems to play an important role in the risk of lymph node metastases in stage IA2 cervical cancer. The recent published article from Rogers LJ et al.

suggests that the latest studies adhering to the FIGO definitions showed a 0,5% incidence of lymph node metastases in stage IA2 cervical carcinomas, which is not as high as was previously believed. The very low rate of positive lymph nodes in correctly staged IA2 cases therefore cannot justify the inclusion of lymphadenectomy as part of standardised care for these patients (Eržen et al, 2001).

The first abdominal radical trachelectomy in our Department was performed by Professor Novak in 1954, but it did not become part of the standardized protocol; it was performed only in a few cases. In 2008 radical trachelectomy (abdominal and laparoscopic) was re-introduced and has been a treatment tool in our Department since.

The Rainer's scoring system has been used at the Department since 1979 as the basis for selecting the treatment option for all patients with stage IA cervical carcinoma, but has generally not gained acceptance. When all the unfavorable prognostic factors are discussed and excluded by the tumor board the treatment of patients with IA MIC wishing to preserve fertility is individualized (Smrkolj et al., 2012).

4. Conclusion

We suggest that treatment of MIC IA can be less radical, particularly for young women who want to preserve their fertility and anatomical integrity, especially if LVSI is absent. The treatment of stage IA should be based on the evaluation of prognostic factors in addition to an adequate assessment of the tumour size. Both parameters should be accurately evaluated by examination of numerous or serial step sections of cervical cones. Individualisation of treatment in patients wishing to preserve fertility should be done when all the unfavourable prognostic factors are excluded. Standardisation of the microscopic examination of the cervix is highly recommended. Cone margins should be carefully examined and proven disease-free. Cases with incorrect clinical estimation of the tumour size, associated with histological diagnosis of invasive carcinoma in punch biopsy, may still result in over-treatment when stage IA is found in cervical specimen after radical hysterectomy. Preoperative high resolution magnetic resonance imaging with an endovaginal coil or preoperative 3D-ultrasound perhaps could identify such patients with small tumour volume and might avoid unnecessary radical operation. According to our experience, follow-up of the patients after conization by regular pelvic examination, cytology and colposcopy is mandatory at least every six months for two years, and yearly thereafter.

Correct diagnosis and adequate treatment of early invasive cervical carcinoma, stage IA, should take into account the existing information of the prognostic factors. This is essential to individualise the treatment to avoid unnecessary risks, as well as over- or under-treatment. Such prognostic factors include: adequate estimation of the tumour size, lymphatic vessel invasion, type of confluence of the invasion, mitotic activity, host defence reaction and accurate examination of the surgical margins. Unfortunately, the existing FIGO staging systems disregard some other important prognostic factors in early cervical carcinoma such as capillary-like space invasion, type of invasion and mitotic activity. The most frequently reported factors increasing the risk for lymph node metastasis, reccurence and cancer death are: depth and pattern of stromal invasion, involvement of lymphatic and vascular space, tumour volume and state of the resection margins. In addition to the above listed major prognostic factors, the outcome of early invasive carcinoma of the uterine cervix could also be significantly affected by: subjectivity of microscopical examination and estimation of histological parameters in differential diagnosis, adequate sampling and technical preparation of all cervical biopsy specimen, particularly adequate handling and sampling of the cones and hysterectomy specimens.

Each of these factors should be considered thoroughly when the prognosis of the disease is assessed, not just from the standpoint of eradicating the cancer, but also to avoid unnecessary over-treatment and with respect to the functional integrity of the patients wishing to preserve fertility. In the near future, the diagnostic procedure should also benefit from immunohistochemical and molecular methods used to predict the behaviour of all tumours classified as microinvasive carcinoma that reccur and progress to frankly invasive carcinomas.

5. References

Creasman WT. *Modification of the staging for stage I vulvar and stage Icervical cancer.* Int J Gynecol Obstet 1995; 50: 215-6.

Eržen M, Rainer S, Kališnik M, Kovačič J, Blejec A. *Classification of microinvasive carcinoma of the uterine cervix using quantitative analysis of pathological features and linear discriminant function.* Advances on Gynecological Oncology. CIC Edizioni Internationali, Roma, 1995.

Eržen M, Rakar S. *Prognostic factors in microinvasive cervical carcinoma.* CME J Gynecol Oncol 2001; 6: 307-23.

Kesić V, Cibula D, Kimmig R, Lopez A, Marth C, Reed N, et al. *Algorithms for management of cervical cancer.* ESGO Educational Committee, 2010.

Greer BE et al. *Gynecologic radiotherapy fields defined by intraoperative measurements.* Gynecol Oncol 1990; 38: 421-4.

Kovačič J, Eržen M, Rainer S. *Current surgical controversies in the management of early cancer of the cervix.* 4th round table: Current treatments in cervical and endometrial cancer. Eur J Gynecol Oncol 1989; 10: 216-7.

Mestwerdt G. *Die Frúhdiagnose des Kollumkarzinoms.* Zentralbl Gynákol 1947; 69: 198-202.

Rainer S. *Patohistološka merila pri zdravljenju karcinoma cerviksa stadija Ia /Pathohistologic factors / features in the treatment of cervical cancer stage Ia/.* Jugoslov Ginek Obstet 1978: 18; 149-54.

Syrjänen K. *Early detection of CIN, HPV and prevention of cervical cancer.* In: Syrjänen K, Syrjänen S, eds. Papillomavirus infections in human pathology. Chapter 8. J. Wiley & Sons, New York, 2000: 252-80.

Smrkolj S, Pogačnik RK, Slabe N, Rakar S. *Clinical outcome of patients with FIGO stage IA2 squamous cell carcinoma of the uterine cervix.* Gynecol Oncol 124 (2012): 63-66.

World Health Organization. *Comprehensive cervical cancer control: A guide to essential practice.* Geneva: World Health Organization; 2006. (http://www.who.int/reproductive-heealth/publications/cervical_cancer_gep/text.pdf.).

Wright TC, Ferenczy A, Kurman RJ. et al. *Carcinoma and other tumours of the cervix*. In: Kurman RJ, ed. Blaussteins Pathology of the female genital tract. 4th edn. New York, Springer –Verlag, 1994: 284-7.

10

New Therapeutic Targets

Magali Provansal[1], Maria Cappiello[1],
Frederique Rousseau[1], Anthony Goncalves[1,2] and Patrice Viens[1,2]
[1]*Paoli-Calmettes Institute, Marseille*
[2]*Faculty of Medicine of Marseille*
France

1. Introduction

Cervical cancer occurs in approximately 500,000 women and kills 288,000 women worldwide each year. Prognosis is highly dependent on disease stage at diagnosis. When detected early, cervical cancer is generally curable. Early lesions are treated surgically and locally advanced lesions are managed with concurrent cisplatin chemotherapy and pelvic radiation. Unfortunately, responses to chemoradiation are partial and are of short duration.

Metastatic disease or recurrent lesions not amenable to radical local excision or regional radiation are treated with palliative chemotherapy. Current chemotherapeutic regimens are associated with significant side effects and only limited activity making the identification of active and tolerable novel targeted agents a high priority.

The evidence supporting the biological rational to combine novel non-cytotoxic agents with chemoradiotherapy is strong, and drugs targeting different molecular pathways are currently under clinical development (EGFR inhibitors, COX-2 inhibitors, hypoxia targeted agents, etc). Early pre-clinical and clinical strategies also favor the use of vascular-targeted agents with the aim to normalize the abnormal tumor vasculature, increase tumor oxygenation, and reduce interstitial fluid pressure. The integration of these novel targeted therapies with chemoradiotherapy in clinical trials is discussed, as well as new and promising biomarkers to test drug activity (Herrera, 2008).

2. Overexpression of epidermal growth factor type-1 receptor (EGF-R1) in cervical cancer: A possible therapeutic target for cervical carcinoma

Overexpression of epidermal growth factor type-1 receptor (EGF-R1) has been found in more than 70% of carcinomas of the cervix.

2.1 Cetuximab

Cetuximab, a monoclonal antibody, binds specifically to the epidermal growth factor receptor (EGFR) and competitively inhibits the binding of epidermal growth factor and other ligands. Cetuximab is clinically approved for the treatment of EGFR-expressing metastatic colorectal cancer and advanced head and neck cancer. Cetuximab might be a novel and attractive therapeutic strategy in patients harboring chemotherapy-resistant, recurrent, or metastatic cervical cancer.

As anti-EGFR monoclonal antibodies sensitise tumours, Cetuximab's toxicity plus chemoradiation on cervical cancer cells which express different EGFR levels was investigated. This study showed that Cetuximab combined with chemoradiation, trastuzumab or MAPK inhibitors has useful applications for cervical cancer treatment, independently of EGFR expression (Meira, 2009).

In cervical cancer the expression of EGFR is reported in up to 85% of the tumour cells. Therefore, Cetuximab monotherapy could be a new option in the treatment of patients with advanced cervical cancer.

In a retrospective study, 5 patients with stage IIB to IVB cervical cancer were treated with Cetuximab monotherapy 250 mg/m^2 weekly after an initial loading dose of 400 mg/m^2 as third- to fifth-line therapy. Only one patient (20%) had a stable disease, and the other four a progressive disease. Four out of five patients (80%) developed an acneiform rash. The median survival time was 8.6 months.

This study showed no advantage in the treatment with Cetuximab monotherapy in patients with advanced cervical cancer. Further studies are necessary to evaluate the significance of Cetuximab in the treatment of advanced cervical cancer (Hertlein, 2011).

In a phase II GINECO trial, patients with advanced cervical squamous cell cancer or adenocarcinoma and at least one measurable target received intravenous cisplatin 50 mg/m^2 on day 1 plus topotecan 0.75 mg/m^2/day from days 1 to 3 every 3 weeks combined with cetuximab (initial dose of 400 mg/m^2 followed by subsequent weekly dose of 250 mg/m^2).

Nineteen out of the 44 planned patients were accrued before the study was stopped early due to excessive toxicity. The most frequent adverse event was severe myelosuppression. The main grades 3-4 non-hematologic toxicities were infection (39%) and febrile neutropenia (28%), skin reactions (22%), renal toxicity (11%), and pulmonary embolism (11%). Five (28%) patients died during the treatment including 3 deaths related to treatment toxicity. Six (32%) evaluable patients achieved a partial response. The median times of progression free survival and overall survival were 172 and 220 days, respectively.

In this phase II trial, the combination cisplatin - topotecan - cetuximab induced a high rate of serious adverse and/or fatal events at standard dose and schedule (Kurtz, 2009).

2.2 Erlotinib

A phase I trial was aimed to determine the maximum tolerated dose and related toxicity of erlotinib when administered concurrently with cisplatin and radiotherapy (CRT) for patients with locally advanced cervical squamous cell cancer. There was three cohorts of at least three patients receiving escalating doses of erlotinib combined with cisplatin (40 mg/m^2, weekly, 5 cycles) and radiotherapy (external beam 4,500 cGy in 25 fractions, followed by 4 fractions/600 cGy/weekly of brachytherapy) in squamous cell cervical carcinoma patients, stage IIB to IIIB.

Fifteen patients were enrolled, 3 at dose level (DL) 50 mg, 4 at DL 100 mg, and 8 at DL 150 mg. Patients presented median age 47 (36-59), stage IIB (46.2%) and IIIB (53.8%). Overall, erlotinib+CRT was well-tolerated. Three patients did not complete the planned schedule. One patient at DL 100 mg withdrew informed consent due to grade 2 rash; at DL 150 mg, 1 patient presented Raynaud's Syndrome and had C interrupted, and another patient presented grade 4 hepatotoxicity. The latter was interpreted as dose limiting toxicity and a new cohort of 150 mg was started. No further grade 4 toxicity occurred. Grade 3 toxicity occurred in 6 cases: diarrhea in 3 patients, rash in 2 patients, and leukopenia in 1 patient. Erlotinib +CRT did not lead to limiting in-field toxicity.

This study showed that erlotinib + CRT was feasible to locally advanced squamous cell cervical cancer and was well tolerated. The maximum tolerated dose has been defined as 150 mg (Nogueira-Rodrigues, 2008).

A phase II trial of erlotinib in recurrent squamous cell carcinoma of the cervix was aimed to determine the proportion of patients with tumor response, the proportion who survived progression-free for at least 6 months and the frequency and severity of toxicities of patients with recurrent squamous cell carcinoma of the uterine cervix treated with erlotinib. This multicenter, open-label, single-arm trial evaluated the toxicity and efficacy of oral erlotinib at an initial dosage of 150 mg daily until progressive disease or adverse effects prohibited further therapy.

Twenty-eight patients with squamous cell carcinoma were enrolled and 25 patients were evaluable. There were no objective responses, with 4 (16%) patients achieving stable disease; only 1 patient had a progression-free survival of 6 months (4%) or more. Erlotinib was well tolerated, with the most common drug-related adverse events being gastrointestinal toxicities, fatigue, and rash. This study showed that erlotinib was inactive as monotherapy in patients with recurrent squamous cell carcinoma of the uterine cervix (Schilder, 2009).

2.3 Gefitinib

Evidence suggests the epidermal growth factor receptor (EGFR) is expressed at moderate to high levels in cervical carcinomas. A multicenter, open-label, non-comparative phase II trial (study 1839IL/0075) investigated whether gefitinib (IRESSA), an EGFR tyrosine kinase inhibitor, is a potential second- or third-line treatment option for patients with recurring locoregionally advanced or metastatic cervical cancer. This study evaluated the clinical outcomes of 500 mg/day gefitinib.

Thirty patients with squamous-cell carcinoma or adenocarcinoma were recruited from six centers in France. Of these, 28 patients were evaluable for efficacy. Although there were no objective responses, six (20%) patients experienced stable disease with a median duration of 111.5 days. Median time to progression was 37 days and median overall survival was 107 days. Disease control did not appear to correlate with levels of EGFR expression. Gefitinib was well tolerated, with the most common drug-related adverse events being skin and gastrointestinal toxicities.

This study showed that gefitinib has only minimal monotherapy activity in recurrent disease resistant to standard treatment. However, the observation that 20% of patients treated with gefitinib had stable disease may warrant further investigation (Goncalves, 2008).

3. NF-κB inhibition

Nuclear factor-kappa B (NF-kappaB) is a transcription factor that plays a critical role across many cellular processes including embryonic and neuronal development, cell proliferation, apoptosis, and immune responses to infection and inflammation. Dysregulation of NF-kappaB signaling is associated with inflammatory diseases and certain cancers.

Constitutive activation of NF-kappaB signaling has been found in some types of tumors including breast, colon, prostate, skin and lymphoid, hence therapeutic blockade of NF-kappaB signaling in cancer cells provides an attractive strategy for the development of anticancer drugs.

Miller *and al.* indicated that many currently approved pharmaceuticals have previously unappreciated effects on NF-kappaB signaling, which may contribute to anticancer therapeutic effects. Comprehensive profiling of approved drugs provides insight into their molecular mechanisms, thus providing a basis for drug repurposing (Miller, 2010).

Kima *and al.* suggested that the HPV 16 E5 oncoprotein mediates cervical carcinogenesis at least in part via upregulation of COX-2 expression through NF-kappaB and AP-1, with NF-kappaB playing a larger role (Kim, 2009).

NF-kappaB activation is known to reduce the efficiency of chemotherapy in cancer treatment. Ursolic acid, a minimally toxic compound, has shown the capability to inhibit NF-kappaB activation in living cells. Li *and al.* investigated the effects and mechanisms of NF-kappaB inhibition by ursolic acid on chemotherapy treatment (Taxol or cisplatin) of cancerBy supplementing chemotherapy with minimally toxic ursolic acid, it is possible to improve the efficacy of cancer treatment by significantly reducing the necessary drug dose without sacrificing the treatment results (Li, 2010).

This recent studies suggested that NF-kappaB may contribute to the resistance of human cervical cancer cells to cisplatin and highlight the potential use of combination therapy involving cisplatin and NF-kappaB inhibitors.

4. Cyclooxygenase-2 inhibitor

Evidence from clinical and preclinical studies indicates that COX-2-derived prostaglandins participate in carcinogenesis, inflammation, immune response suppression, apoptosis inhibition, angiogenesis, and tumor cell invasion and metastasis. Clinical trial results have demonstrated that selective inhibition of COX-2 can alter the development and the progression of cancer. In animal models, selective inhibition of COX-2 activity is associated with the enhanced radiation sensitivity of tumors without appreciably increasing the effects of radiation on normal tissue, and preclinical evidence suggests that the principal mechanism of radiation potentiation through selective COX-2 inhibition is the direct increase in cellular radiation sensitivity and the direct inhibition of tumor neovascularization (Choy, 2003).

A phase I-II accrued 31 women with locally advanced cervical cancer to receive celecoxib 400 mg by mouth twice per day for 2 weeks before and during chemoradiotherapy (CRT). Tumor oxygenation (HP(5)) and interstitial fluid pressure (IFP) were measured before and 2 weeks after celecoxib administration alone. The median follow-up time was 2.7 years.

The most common acute G3/4 toxicities were hematologic and gastrointestinal largely attributed to chemotherapy. Late G3/4 toxicity was seen in 4 of 31 patients, including fistulas in 3 patients. Within the first year of follow-up, 25 of 31 patients achieved complete response (CR), of whom 20 remained in CR at last follow-up. After 2 weeks of celecoxib administration before CRT, the median IFP decreased slightly, whereas HP(5) did not change significantly. No significant associations were seen between changes in HP(5) or IFP and response to treatment.

Celecoxib in combination with definitive CRT is associated with acceptable acute toxicity, but higher than expected late complications. Celecoxib is associated with a modest reduction in the angiogenic biomarker IFP, but this does not correspond with tumor response (Herrera, 2007).

A phase II study determined the efficacy, patterns of initial failure and treatment-related acute toxicity rates in patients with locally advanced cancer of the cervix treated by oral celecoxib, intravenous cisplatin and 5-fluorouracil, and concurrent pelvic radiation therapy in patients with locally advanced cancer of the cervix.

Eligible patients included FIGO Stage IIB-IVA or patients with FIGO Stage IB through IIA with biopsy proven pelvic node metastases or tumor size > or =5 cm. Celecoxib was prescribed at a dose of 400 mg twice daily for 1 year beginning on the first day of radiotherapy. Cisplatin (75 mg/m^2) and 5-FU ($1g/m^2$ for 4 days) were administered every 3 weeks times 3. A total of 84 patients were accrued, of whom 78 were eligible and 77 were evaluable for toxicity.

At 2 years, the estimated disease-free survival and overall survival rate for patients with advanced cervical cancer who underwent a combination of chemoradiotherapy and celecoxib treatment was 69% and 83%, respectively. Of the 78 patients, 24 had treatment failure and, of those patients, 18 had a component of locoregional failure as a site of first failure (Gaffney, 2007a). Toxicities were observed in the following areas: blood/bone marrow (16), gastrointestinal (14), pain (7), renal/genitourinary (6), cardiovascular (3), hemorrhage (1), and neurologic (1). For the first 75 evaluable patients, a toxicity failure was identified in 36 patients for a rate of 48% (Gaffney, 2007b).

Thus, locoregional control continues to be problematic after chemoradiotherapy (Gaffney, 2007a). Celecoxib at 400 mg twice daily together with concurrent cisplatin and 5-FU and pelvic radiotherapy has a high incidence of acute toxicities. The most frequent toxicities were hematologic (Gaffney, 2007b).

Previous data demonstrate an association between cyclooxygenase activity and development of cervical cancer. A review investigated the role of cyclooxygenase-2 (COX-2) in the development of cervical cancer and potential therapeutic options targeting this pathway.

Studies in vivo and in vitro confirm the role of COX-2 in the development of cervical cancer. In addition, COX-2 overexpression is associated with an increase in angiogenesis markers. Clinical correlation found that COX-2 overexpression in cervical cancer patients is a poor prognostic marker associated with increased risk for recurrent or metastatic disease. Despite early promise, two phase II trials in use of specific COX-2 inhibitors as radio-sensitizers in locally advanced cervical cancer demonstrated increased toxicity with no change in therapeutic effect. Results of studies using COX-2 inhibitors in pre-invasive cervical disease are encouraging (Young, 2008).

Jung *and al.* evaluated 67 FIGO stage IB2-IVA cervical cancer patients treated with cisplatin-based chemoradiotherapy (CCRT). The study group included patients who received rofecoxib (N=30) and the control group included patients who received CCRT only (N=37).

There were no significant differences in toxicity between the two groups. The most common acute grade 3/4 toxicity was neutropenia. Grade 3/4 late toxicity was observed in 2 patients in the study group and 3 in the control group. There was no treatment-related deaths in either group. Six patients in the study group had treatment failure. In the control group, 6 patients experienced treatment failure. There were no differences in progression-free and overall survival between the 2 groups.

This data indicated that rofecoxib, at a dose of 25 mg twice daily, has acceptable acute toxicity as a radiosensitizer during CCRT. Although rofecoxib was not efficacious as a radiosensitizer in the present study, the benefit of rofecoxib as a radiosensitizer should be further evaluated in a prospective study (Jung, 2009).

5. Anti-angiogenesis agents

Angiogenesis is central to cervical cancer development and progression. The dominant role of angiogenesis in cervical cancer seems to be directly related to HPV inhibition of p53 and stabilization of HIF-1 alpha, both of which increase vascular endothelial growth factor (VEGF).

5.1 Bevacizumab

Bevacizumab binding and subsequent inactivation of VEGF seem to shrink cervical tumors and delay progression without appreciable toxicity, and are therefore being studied in a Gynecologic Oncology Group (GOG) phase III trial. Other intracellular tyrosine kinase inhibitors (TKIs) of angiogenesis such as pazopanib are also encouraging, especially in lieu of their oral administration (Monk, 2010).

The Gynecologic Oncology Group (GOG) conducted a phase II trial to assess the efficacy and tolerability of bevacizumab. Eligible patients had recurrent cervical cancer, measurable disease, and GOG performance status < or = 2. Treatment consisted of bevacizumab 15 mg/kg intravenously every 21 days until disease progression or prohibitive toxicity. Forty-six patients were enrolled. Grade 3 or 4 adverse events at least possibly related to bevacizumab included hypertension, thrombo-embolism, gastro-intestinal, anemia, other cardiovascular, vaginal bleeding, neutropenia, and fistula. One grade 5 infection was observed. Eleven patients (23.9%) survived progression free for at least 6 months, and five patients (10.9%) had partial responses. The median response duration was 6.21 months. The median PFS and overall survival times were 3.40 months and 7.29 months, respectively (Monk, 2009).

A retrospective analysis of women with recurrent cervical cancer treated with bevacizumab combination therapy was performed. Six patients were identified. The patients had a median of 3 prior regimens. All of the patients had multisite, metastatic disease. The combination regimen included IV 5-fluorouracil in 5 (83%) patients and capecitabine in one (17%) subject. Treatment was well tolerated. Grade 4 toxicity occurred in one patient who developed neutropenic sepsis. Clinical benefit (CR, PR, or SD) was noted in 67% of the subjects. This included 1 (17%) complete response, 1 (17%) partial response and two (33%) patients with stable disease. The median time to progression for the four women who demonstrated clinical benefit was 4.3 months (Wright, 2006).

5.2 Pazopanib

Pazopanib is an oral multi-targeted TKI that binds to the vascular endothelial growth factor receptor (VEGFR), platelet-derived growth factor receptor (PDGFR) and c-Kit or epidermal growth factor receptor (EGFR) and human epidermal growth factor receptor 2 (HER2/neu), responsible for angiogenesis, tumor growth and cell survival.

Pazopanib exhibited in vivo and in vitro activity against tumor growth and, in early clinical trials, was well tolerated with the main side effects being hypertension, fatigue and gastrointestinal disorders. Pazopanib showed clinical activity in several tumors including renal cell cancer (RCC), breast cancer, soft tissue sarcoma, thyroid cancer, hepatocellular cancer and cervical cancer (Schutz, 2011).

A phase II open-label study compared pazopanib or lapatinib monotherapy with pazopanib plus lapatinib combination therapy in patients with advanced and recurrent cervical cancer.

Patients with measurable stage IVB persistent/recurrent cervical carcinoma not amenable to curative therapy and at least one prior regimen in the metastatic setting were randomly assigned in a ratio of 1:1:1 to pazopanib at 800 mg once daily, lapatinib at 1,500 mg once daily, or lapatinib plus pazopanib combination therapy (lapatinib at 1,000 mg plus pazopanib at 400 mg once daily or lapatinib at 1,500 mg plus pazopanib at 800 mg once daily).

Of 230 patients enrolled, 152 were randomly assigned to the monotherapy arms: pazopanib (n = 74) or lapatinib (n = 78). Most patients (62%) had recurrent cancer. Pazopanib improved PFS (hazard ratio [HR], 0.66; 90% CI, 0.48 to 0.91; P = .013) and OS (HR, 0.67; 90% CI, 0.46 to 0.99; P = .045). Median OS was 50.7 weeks and 39.1 weeks and RRs were 9% and 5% for pazopanib and lapatinib, respectively. The only grade 3 AE > 10% was diarrhea (11% pazopanib and 13% lapatinib). Grade 4 AEs were 9% (lapatinib) and 12% (pazopanib).

This study confirms the activity of antiangiogenesis agents in advanced and recurrent cervical cancer and demonstrates the benefit of pazopanib based on the prolonged PFS and favorable toxicity profile. Further study of angiogenesis and its inhibition are ongoing (Monk, 2010).

6. References

Choy H, Milas L (2003). Enhancing radiotherapy with cyclooxygenase-2 enzyme inhibitors: a rational advance? *J Natl Cancer Inst.* Vol 1;95(19):1440-52.

Gaffney DK, Winter K, Dicker AP, Miller B, Eifel PJ, Ryu J, Avizonis V, Fromm M, Small W, Greven K (2007). Efficacy and patterns of failure for locally advanced cancer of the cervix treated with celebrex (celecoxib) and chemoradiotherapy in RTOG 0128. *Int J Radiat Oncol Biol Phys.* Vol 1;69(1):111-7.

Gaffney DK, Winter K, Dicker AP, Miller B, Eifel PJ, Ryu J, Avizonis V, Fromm M, Greven K (2007). A Phase II study of acute toxicity for Celebrex (celecoxib) and chemoradiation in patients with locally advanced cervical cancer: primary endpoint analysis of RTOG 0128. *Int J Radiat Oncol Biol Phys.* Vol 1;67(1):104-9.

Goncalves A, Fabbro M, Lhommé C, Gladieff L, Extra JM, Floquet A, Chaigneau L, Carrasco AT, Viens P (2008). A phase II trial to evaluate gefitinib as second- or third-line treatment in patients with recurring locoregionally advanced or metastatic cervical cancer. *Gynecol Oncol.* Vol 108(1):42-6.

Herrera FG, Chan P, Doll C, Milosevic M, Oza A, Syed A, Pintilie M, Levin W, Manchul L, Fyles A (2007). A prospective phase I-II trial of the cyclooxygenase-2 inhibitor celecoxib in patients with carcinoma of the cervix with biomarker assessment of the tumor microenvironment. *Int J Radiat Oncol Biol Phys.* Vol 1;67(1):97-103.

Herrera FG, Vidal L, Oza A, Milosevic M, Fyles A (2008). Molecular targeted agents combined with chemo-radiation in the treatment of locally advanced cervix cancer. *Rev Recent Clin Trials.* Vol 3(2):111-20.

Hertlein L, Lenhard M, Kirschenhofer A, Kahlert S, Mayr D, Burges A, Friese K (2011). In a retrospective study, Cetuximab monotherapy was applied in advanced cervical cancer. *Arch Gynecol Obstet.* Vol 283(1):109-13.

Jung YW, Lee SH, Paek JH, Nam EJ, Kim SW, Kim JH, Kim JW, Kim YT (2009). Acute toxicity of cyclooxygenase-2 inhibitor rofecoxib as a radiosensitizer for concurrent chemoradiation in the treatment of uterine cervical cancer. *J Gynecol Oncol.* Vol 20(3):151-7.

Kim SH, Oh JM, No JH, Bang YJ, Juhnn YS, Song YS (2009). Involvement of NF-kappaB and AP-1 in COX-2 upregulation by human papillomavirus 16 E5 oncoprotein. *Carcinogenesis.* Vol 30(5):753-7.

Kurtz JE, Hardy-Bessard AC, Deslandres M, Lavau-Denes S, Largillier R, Roemer-Becuwe C, Weber B, Guillemet C, Paraiso D, Pujade-Lauraine E (2009). Cetuximab, topotecan and cisplatin for the treatment of advanced cervical cancer: A phase II GINECO trial. *Gynecol Oncol.* Vol 113(1):16-20.

Li Y, Xing D, Chen Q, Chen WR (2010). Enhancement of chemotherapeutic agent-induced apoptosis by inhibition of NF-kappaB using ursolic acid. *Int J Cancer.* Vol 15;127(2):462-73.

Meira DD, de Almeida VH, Mororó JS, Nóbrega I, Bardella L, Silva RL, Albano RM, Ferreira CG (2009). Combination of cetuximab with chemoradiation, trastuzumab or MAPK inhibitors: mechanisms of sensitisation of cervical cancer cells. *Br J Cancer.* Vol 1;101(5):782-91.

Miller SC, Huang R, Sakamuru S, Shukla SJ, Attene-Ramos MS, Shinn P, Van Leer D, Leister W, Austin CP, Xia M (2010). Identification of known drugs that act as inhibitors of NF-kappaB signaling and their mechanism of action. *Biochem Pharmacol.* Vol 1;79(9):1272-80.

Monk BJ, Sill MW, Burger RA, Gray HJ, Buekers TE, Roman LD (2009). Phase II trial of bevacizumab in the treatment of persistent or recurrent squamous cell carcinoma of the cervix: a gynecologic oncology group study. *J Clin Oncol.* Vol 1;27(7):1069-74.

Monk BJ, Mas Lopez L, Zarba JJ, Oaknin A, Tarpin C, Termrungruanglert W, Alber JA, Ding J, Stutts MW, Pandite LN (2010). Phase II, open-label study of pazopanib or lapatinib monotherapy compared with pazopanib plus lapatinib combination therapy in patients with advanced and recurrent cervical cancer. *J Clin Oncol.* Vol 1;28(22):3562-9.

Monk BJ, Willmott LJ, Sumner DA (2010). Anti-angiogenesis agents in metastatic or recurrent cervical cancer. *Gynecol Oncol.* Vol 116(2):181-6.

Nogueira-Rodrigues A, do Carmo CC, Viegas C, Erlich F, Camisão C, Fontão K, Lima R, Herchenhorn D, Martins RG, Moralez GM, Small IA, Ferreira CG (2008). Phase I trial of erlotinib combined with cisplatin and radiotherapy for patients with locally advanced cervical squamous cell cancer. *Clin Cancer Res.* Vol 1;14(19):6324-9.

Schilder RJ, Sill MW, Lee YC, Mannel R (2009). A phase II trial of erlotinib in recurrent squamous cell carcinoma of the cervix: a Gynecologic Oncology Group Study. *Int J Gynecol Cancer.* Vol 19(5):929-33.

Schutz FA, Choueiri TK, Sternberg CN (2011). Pazopanib: Clinical development of a potent anti-angiogenic drug. *Crit Rev Oncol Hematol.* Vol 77(3):163-71.

Wright JD, Viviano D, Powell MA, Gibb RK, Mutch DG, Grigsby PW, Rader JS (2006). Bevacizumab combination therapy in heavily pretreated, recurrent cervical cancer. *Gynecol Oncol.* Vol 103(2):489-93.

Young JL, Jazaeri AA, Darus CJ, Modesitt SC (2008). Cyclooxygenase-2 in cervical neoplasia: a review. *Gynecol Oncol.* Vol 109(1):140-5.

11

A Transcriptome- and Marker-Based Systemic Analysis of Cervical Cancer

Carlos G. Acevedo-Rocha[1,2], José A. Munguía-Moreno[3], Rodolfo Ocádiz-Delgado[3] and Patricio Gariglio[3]
[1]*Max-Planck-Institut für Kohlenforschung, Organische Chemie*
[2]*Philipps-Universität-Marburg, Fakultät für Chemie*
[3]*Departamento de Genética y Biología Molecular, CINVESTAV-IPN*
[1,2]*Germany*
[3]*Mexico*

1. Introduction

The 20th century witnessed a great development of genetics and molecular biology, laying the foundations for a new era in medicine. The elucidation of the mechanism of heredity, for example, helped us understanding the connection between cells, chromosomes, DNA and the genetic code, an historical journey to the center of biology (Lander & Weinberg, 2000). This process strongly consolidated when "the central dogma of molecular biology" (Crick, 1970) was proposed long time ago, whereby the genetic information flows from DNA to RNA to protein. Since then, however, our understanding in the molecular and cellular organization, as well as physiology of living systems has radically changed, partially challenging the validity of the central 'dogma'- by the way, dogma strictly means a belief that people are expected to accept without any doubts, a word to be expectedly seen outside the scientific method lexicon - of molecular biology (Shapiro, 2009). The main paradigm is that cells are able to make decisions based on actively sensing their environment; hence, information processing in living systems can be regarded at least bidirectional. In any case, the recent sequencing of the human genome is a great milestone (Human Genome Sequencing, 2004), whereby the language of the "common thread of humanity" in this new medicine era is just "the end of the beginning" (Stein, 2004).

Genomics studies the total DNA sequence of an organism. Of the approximately 3,000 million base pairs that comprise the human genome, only 1% was firstly estimated to correspond to as low as 25,000 proteins (Southan, 2004), a number that has been changing since the initial sequence drafts of the Human Genome Project (HGP). One motivation behind genome-sequencing projects is the assumption that the nucleotide sequence of an organism provides a description of the genes, its products and interaction networks that orchestrate programs like those sustaining the metabolic activity of a cell or deploying a body plan. However, new discoveries in transcriptome functions significantly expand—and even challenge—the classical concept of the gene and how post-transcriptional molecular events are becoming key to understand gene regulation in higher eukaryotes.

The success of the HGP has provided a blueprint of genes encoding the entire human protein set potentially expressed in any of the approximately 230 cell types comprising the human proteome. Considering that both the current and sometimes limited knowledge of only two-thirds of the 20,300 protein-coding human genes mapped through the HGP is at hand (Legrain *et al.*, 2011), the recently launched Human Proteome Project (HPP) aims to provide for the remaining one-third of proteins experimental evidence related to abundance, distribution, subcellular localization, functions, and interactions (Bustamante *et al.*, 2011).

In the current "post-genomic era" scientists aim not only to build a catalog of all genes, but also to translate the knowledge obtained into benefits for humanity (Collins *et al.*, 2003). By examining tumors at the genomic, transcriptomic, and proteomic levels, for instance, it is possible to better understand cancer biology and improve patient care, diagnosis, prognosis, and therapy (Lin & Li, 2008). Importantly, one key development that has emerged between the interface of the HGP and the HPP is the area of functional genomics or transcriptomics, which aims to assign a function to all transcripts. But this is not a trivial task because talking about transcriptomes involves considering these as entities as diverse as the cell types, developmental stages, environmental conditions and pathological states that an organism harbors or faces. Therefore, we must include a global vision for the process of transcription, i.e. the process by which information contained in DNA is converted (or transcribed) into RNA and how this process is regulated by protein(s) (Fig. 1).

Importantly, it should bear on mind that 57% - a scalable number up to 90% (Costa, 2010) - of the genome is transcribed into RNA but does not code for proteins (Frith *et al.*, 2005). Moreover, very recently non-coding RNAs (microRNAs, small RNAs, small interfering RNAs or siRNAs as well as medium and large RNAs) have emerged as key elements in carcinogenesis. The amazing complexity of the transcriptome and its expansion (Mendes Soares & Valcarcel, 2006), has led to scientists eager to hunt transcriptomes. Fortunately, there are tools to examine the expression of genes at many levels, allowing us to globally understand complex diseases like cancer.

The current manuscript introduces the most common techniques to study the transcription of the 1% protein-coding genes encoded in the human genome, followed by a review of microarray studies that had provided invaluable information of the carcinogenesis of cervical cancer (CC), the most and second most common cancer disease in women from the developing and developed world, respectively. The integration of all this information is very important to not only understand CC from a global perspective, but also to identify key tumor markers that could help for CC diagnosis, prognosis and/or therapy, as discussed in the last part of the manuscript. As for cancer progression involving noncoding RNAs – importantly considered the "masters of regulation" (Costa, 2010), the reader is encouraged to read an excellent recent review (Gibb *et al.*, 2011).

Importantly, CC is largely associated to Human Papillomavirus (HPV) infection, from which there are over hundred types but of these 40 infecting the genital tract and 15 of high-risk related to the development of CC. Thus, HPV is a common sexually transmitted agent after a woman starts her first sexual relationship and responsible of *ca.* 30% of the global cancer burden associated to infective agents (20% of the total) (zur Hausen, 2009).

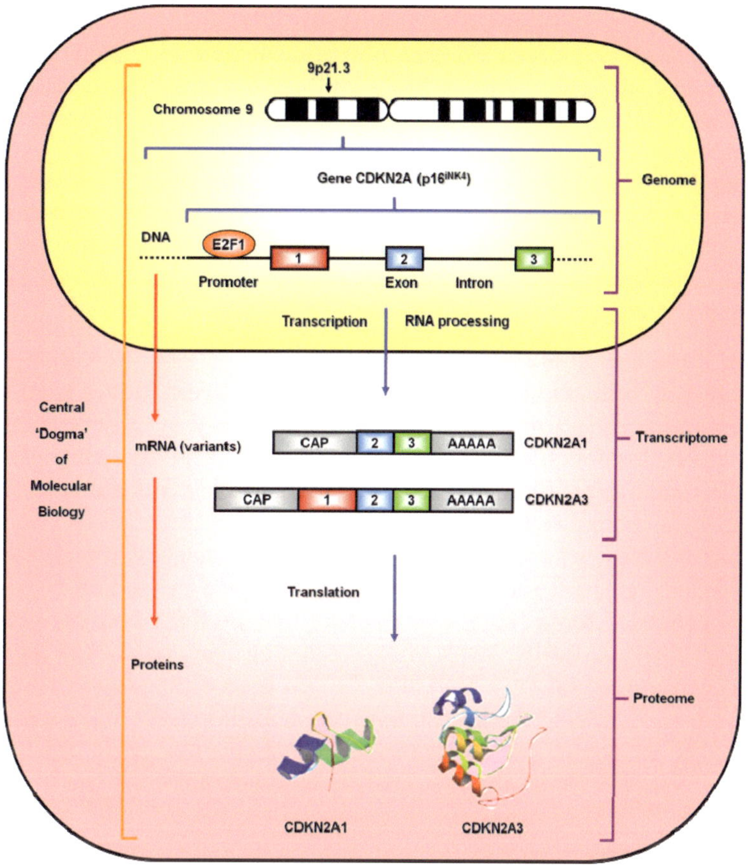

Fig. 1. Role of transcription in the central 'dogma' of molecular biology. According to this 'dogma', the genetic information flows from DNA to messenger RNA (mRNA) to proteins. The gene CDKN2A/p16INK4a, for example, is located at position "21.3" of the short arm of the human chromosome 9, which resides inside the nucleus. Upon activation by the transcription factor (E2F1), its mRNA is transcribed and the corresponding proteins are translated in the cytoplasm (CDKN2A encodes three but only two variants are displayed). The interplay between the genome, transcriptome and proteome is oversimplified.

2. Probing the transcriptome

The relationship between a particular molecule and cellular phenotype has allowed us to better understand the molecular mechanisms of complex diseases such as cancer. In the course of molecular biology many useful techniques to analyze DNA, RNA and proteins were developed. For about half century, reasonably, the practice of molecular biology was comfortable with its reductionism; however, in the coming era of genomics, the tendency to probe in a single experiment hundreds or thousands of biomolecules allows us talking of two mechanisms: (i) The "reductionist mechanism" employs tools to analyze one or few different molecules in a single experiment; it is a slow but comprehensive conclusions can be reliably obtained; (ii) The "holistic mechanism" allows the assessment of thousands of different molecules in a single experiment; it is a fast mechanism but the obtained hypotheses remained to be tested (Coulton, 2004). While single gene analyses gradually shifted towards large mutational screens and complete genome mapping, whole genome sequencing moved towards bioinformatics with exhaustive functional genomics and proteomics data. Systems biology aims to understand this complexity. Ironically, the holism in systems biology has re-emerged out of the traditional molecular biology, carrying with it the *reductionism-holism* debate since the past years (Gatherer, 2010). Interestingly, it has been boldly argued that traditional molecular biology represents a greedy reductionist approach (to some authors a naively reductionist one) that requires either extensive complementation from, or even replacement by systems biology. However, as we discuss along the text, it is more meaningful to combine both approaches.

The study of transcription is important because the levels of mRNA transcripts in a cell correlate frequently with the expression levels of the corresponding proteins. There are several techniques used in transcriptomics, which are based on gene amplification by the polymerase chain reaction (PCR), hybridization and sequencing. All these tools permit analyzing differential expression, and determine what transcripts are mainly expressed in cancerous tissue in comparison with normal tissue and *vice versa*. This is important because knowing what and how genes are differentially expressed suggests that these may play an important role in carcinogenesis. This scenario can be found in the case of proto-oncogenes and anti-oncogenes (or tumor suppressor genes) that promote and prevent cell growth, respectively. In other words, the levels of expression of many oncogenes (normally known as proto-oncogenes) may be very high and the levels of expression of tumor suppressor genes may be low. Following the reductionist and holistic classification, the most common techniques used in transcriptomics can be classified into high, medium, and low performance, with respect to its ability to analyze different molecules in a single experiment.

2.1 Low-throughput techniques

One of the first developed methods to detect a mRNA transcript was *in situ* hybridization (ISH) (Harrison *et al.*, 1973). ISH requires labelling either fluorescently or radioactively a RNA or complementary DNA (cDNA) corresponding to the transcript of interest. Through the formation of hybrid cDNA:RNA or RNA:RNA duplexes, the amount of the specific transcript can be determined as well as its cellular position can be localized. Thereafter, the popular technique Northern Blot (NB) was developed. NB uses a labeled probe that recognizes the transcript of interest in a similar manner to the ISH, but the hybridization is performed on cellulose, because the RNA of a tissue is previously separated by electrophoresis and transferred to a special paper surface. If the transcript of interest forms a hybrid with the radioactively labeled probe, it will reveal the presence of a band in a autoradiography upon exposure (Alwine *et al.*, 1977). Because of its sensitivity, this technique is commonly used in molecular biology. Another similar technique, called ribonuclease protection assay (RPA), is based on hybrid formation between the mRNA of the gene in question and a labeled probe (RNA or cDNA), being the non-hybridized single-strand RNA part degraded by a RNAse enzyme (Berk & Sharp, 1977). This way, the hybrids can be detected because the RNA chain is radiolabelled; this method is 50 times more sensitive than NB (Bartlett, 2002).

Another old technique is subtractive hybridization (SH), which employs single-strand RNA or cDNA labeled probes. Using SH one can remove commonly expressed genes between two samples (e.g. cancerous and normal tissue) by hybrid formation between cDNA:RNA and identified those differentially expressed genes in a particular tissue (Zimmermann *et al.*, 1980). The tumor-suppresor gene p21WAF1/CIP1, also known as CDKN1A, involved in the negative regulation of the cell cycle as well as the induction of apoptosis, was identified using SH (el-Deiry et al, 1993). Finally, the Retro-Transcription coupled to PCR (RT-PCR) allows the amplification of a cDNA synthesized from a specific mRNA using a reverse transcriptase (Rappolee *et al.*, 1988). RT-PCR can also be applied to tissues (*in situ* RT-PCR) similarly to the ISH but the sensitivity differs: While ISH can detect from 20 to 200 copies of transcript per cell, *in situ* RT-PCR can detect one transcript per cell (Bartlett, 2002). The enormous sensitivity of RT-PCR has allowed the development of a technique to quantify quickly and accurately the amount of transcripts in a given biological sample. It is called quantitative RT-PCR or Real-Time PCR (qRT-PCR) (Bustin, 2000). All these methods mainly based on hybridization and PCR can generally characterize one transcript per experiment.

2.2 Medium-throughput techniques

When a mRNA is converted to cDNA, the fragments obtained can be cloned or inserted into a vector (plasmid), which can be introduced into bacteria to obtain many copies of the transcript. At the end, the fragment of interest must be sequenced. In this way, various types of sequences can be generated: A EST (Expressed Sequence Tags) corresponds to an arbitrary portion of a cDNA sequence, i.e. a random sequence that allows identification of a transcript (Adams *et al.*, 1991), whereas "ORESTES" (Open Reading Frame Expressed Sequence Tags) contain an open reading frame, which generally corresponds to a central portion of the cDNA sequence (Dias Neto *et al.*, 2000); it is also possible to alternatively clone the entire sequence of cDNA without tag (Strausberg *et al.*, 2002). Importantly, all these partial or complete cDNA sequences had enabled the characterization of large numbers of transcripts and their differential expression depending on their frequency and tissue of origin.

Similarly, the techniques of Differential Display (DD) and Representational Differential Analysis (RDA) permit the identification of differentially expressed transcripts e.g. coming from different sources or coming from the same source but subjected to different conditions. DD is essentially based on a series of RT-PCR amplifications where the transcripts of two samples are fluorescently or radioactively labeled, compared by electrophoresis, selected and finally sequenced (Liang & Pardee, 1992). The RDA technique is based on SH and RT-PCR, so that common transcripts between two samples are removed after the formation of hybrid cDNA:cDNA and genes only expressed in a tissue are amplified in a sensitive and accurate way (Hubank & Schatz, 1994). Since both techniques are of easy accessibility and use, their use has allowed the identification of many genes altered in cancer (Liang & Pardee, 2003; Hollestelle & Schutte, 2005). For example, while the Cyclin G was identified using the DD technique (Okamoto & Beach, 1994) the anti-oncogene PTEN was characterized through RDA (Li *et al.*, 1997). The medium-throughput methods basically depend on sequencing and differ from those of low-performance because many transcripts can be characterized at a single experiment, but not as many as when using high-performance ones.

2.3 High-throughput techniques

In general, these methods are based on sequencing and hybridization. Sequencing includes Serial Analysis of Gene Expression (SAGE) and Massively Parallel Signature Sequencing

(MPSS) and, in the case of hybridization, the best example is DNA microarrays. SAGE is similar to the sequencing of ESTs or cDNA clones, but the performance is much higher because in a single vector a lot of small tags corresponding to different mRNAs can be inserted. After sequencing, the abundance of these tags can be measured doing a bioinformatics analysis, whereby the fold expression change of a gene in different tissues/conditions can be estimated (Velculescu *et al.*, 1995). MPSS is similar to SAGE but the main difference is that in the former small tags are attached to microbead arrays, increasing the capacity of the system (Brenner *et al.*, 2000). Although MPSS is similar to SAGE, the later method has been widely used, uncovering many genes with a potential role in cancer (Yamashita *et al.*, 2008), and allowing the identification of known oncogenes such as ERBB2 and EGFR (Polyak & Riggins, 2001; Forrest *et al.*, 2006).

The DNA microarrays are a set of gene sequences (which may correspond to transcripts) arranged on a flat surface. There are two types of DNA microarrays: cDNA microarrays, in which transcripts of interest are amplified by PCR and deposited on sites identified in a paper or small glass slide (Schena *et al.*, 1995) and oligonucleotide microarrays, in which small sequences corresponding to a gene are synthesized and arranged on a particular area of a slide (Lockhart *et al.*, 1996; Singh-Gasson *et al.*, 1999; Hughes *et al.*, 2001). While the former arrays are normally produced in-house by researchers, the latter one are usually obtained from companies, being the most known "Affymetrix". During the experiment, the mRNA of a tissue of interest is firstly converted into cDNA and labeled either radioactively or fluorescently. Then, through the formation of hybrids between the labeled cDNA and the unlabelled cDNA or oligonucleotides attached to the surface, differentially expressed genes between two samples can be identified. Finally, the ratios of frequency can be estimated using different bioinformatics methods. Both cDNA and oligonucleotide microarrays have been widely used, the difference lies in the number of genes per square centimeter: On paper there may be hundreds of genes, whereas in a glass slide it is possible to bear sequences representing up to 10,000 and 25,000 genes in the case of cDNA and oligonucleotide microarrays, respectively. This allows the simultaneous quantification of thousands of gene transcripts in two samples when they are tagged with different fluorophores, for example, if the transcripts from tumor cells are stained with red (e.g. Cy5) and those from normal cells with green (e.g. Cy3), upon locating spots on a cDNA microarray, while the red and green ones would respectively correspond to genes differentially expressed in the tumor and normal tissue, the yellow (and alike degrees of color) would correspond to genes similarly expressed in both tissues. This is usually done on cDNA microarrays because the spots can be compared directly in one experiment, but in the case of oligonucleotide microarrays, the spots are compared indirectly in separate experiments because the detection and analysis methods differ. In either case, the different spot intensities can be transformed into transcript levels present in each sample. The numerical data are analyzed with a computer and mathematical algorithms, allowing various genes to display a characteristic pattern or "Gene Expression Profile" (GEP) related to the phenotype of the different samples. Depending on the intensity in which the various genes from the GEP are expressed, the sample acquires a particular "expression signature".

The transcriptome should study not only the expression of transcripts, but also the DNA sites where transcription factors bind as well as chromatin modifications that regulate gene expression. Chromatin Immunoprecipitation (ChIP) is a old technique to identify genes that can be activated by a protein *in vivo* (Orlando, 2000), but can be of high-throughput when it is coupled with: i) DNA microarrays (Ren *et al.*, 2000), also known as "ChIP-on-Chip", for instance, many genes that can be activated by the transcription factors E2F have been identified (Bracken *et al.*, 2004); or 2) Sequencing-based techniques like Paired-end di-tags (PET) that is equivalent to SAGE but in contrast to a tag, two gene extremes are joined (Ng *et al.*, 2005). Using ChIP-PET, several TP53-regulated genes have been identified (Wei *et al.*, 2006). TP53 and E2F are the most important transcription factors known in cancer development, activating or deactivating genes involved in cell cycle and apoptosis.

Last but not least, another successful tool combined with microarrays is Laser Capture Microdissection (LCM), which uses a laser beam targeted to specific tissue sections under microscopic control to isolate cell clusters, allowing the molecular comparison of cell populations that are histologically or pathologically distinct but topographically contiguous (Kalantari *et al.*, 2009). The main limitation of this technique, however, is that it requires trained personnel to visually select cell populations of interest. One approach to increase dissection performance is to utilize molecular probes to facilitate the process. Expression microdissection (xMD) is such an example, where an antibody is used for cell targeting in place of an investigator (Tangrea *et al.*, 2004; Hanson *et al.*, 2011). In fact, large numbers of cells can be greatly analyzed by using the recently described SIVQ feature matching algorithm, making possible the development of a high-throughput cell procurement instrument. This approach permits histologically constrained morphologies (e.g. automated selection of only the malignant epithelium of solid tissue tumours) to be acquired in a semi-autonomous fashion, allowing the generation of large, preparative quantities of DNA, RNA, or protein for subsequent high-throughput analysis. In fact, SIVQ–LCM holds unique potential as a discovery tool for molecular pathology, since individual cells with particular computer-defined morphologic features can be microdissected and profiled, thus generation new integrated and composite morphological data types (e.g. morpho-genomics or -proteomics) (Hipp *et al.*, 2011). Importantly, there is increasing evidence demonstrating the necessity of upfront malignant cell enrichment techniques for specific molecular profiles, being especially desirable for clinical trials that require accurate, disease cell-specific molecular measurements (Harrell *et al.*, 2008; Klee *et al.*, 2009; Silvestri *et al.*, 2010). This technique has opened new and promising avenues to molecularly enquire histology and pathology in many fields of cancer research (Fuller *et al.*, 2003; Domazet *et al.*, 2008).

All the techniques mentioned above (Fig. 2) have favorable characteristics, while the high-throughput methods have a great capacity for data management; the low-throughput ones confer higher specificity, sensitivity, and reproducibility. Due to this, high- and medium-performance techniques are complementary, but they must be validated with those of low-performance. These tools have generated much information that should be integrated to extract biological meaning, allowing the complete characterization of the transcriptome of a cell. Indeed, a complete integrative analysis of the cancer transcriptome cannot only be obtained by analyzing the genome, transcriptional networks and the interactome, (Rhodes & Chinnaiyan, 2005), but also by delineating the subtypes of cancer obtained from DNA microarrays with relation to a particular phenotype.

3. A brief overview on microarrays and cancer

Microarrays are one of the most versatile tools used in transcriptomics, whereby many benefits for oncogenomics have been found. For example, thanks to the determination of

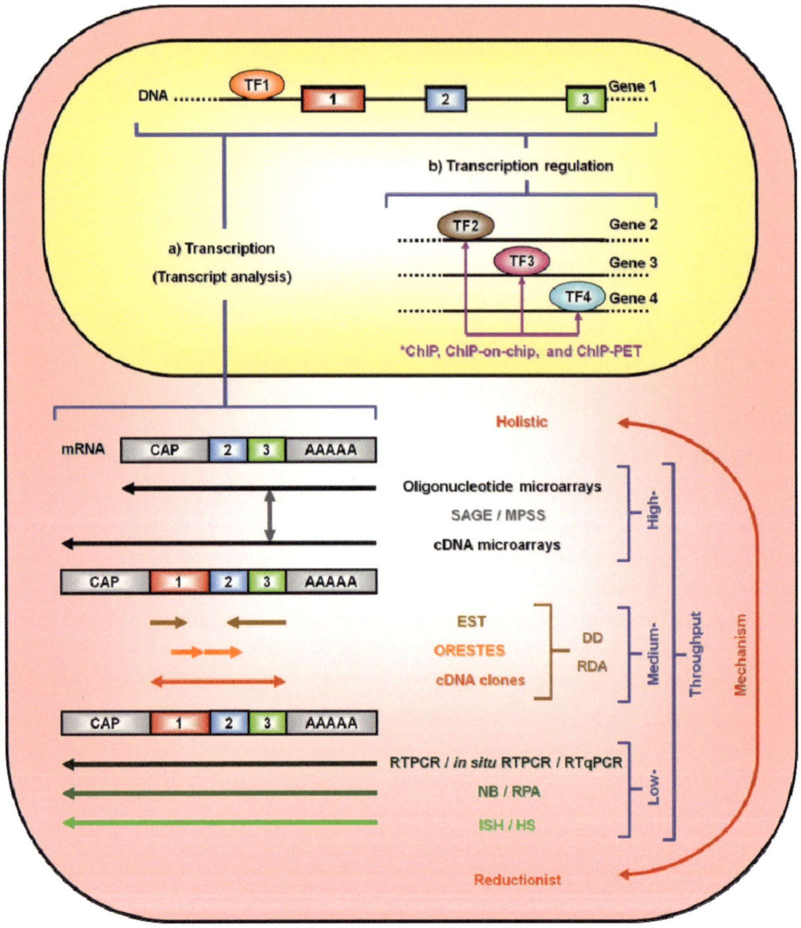

Fig. 2. Probing the transcriptome at different performances. a) Upon DNA transcription, messenger RNA (mRNA) molecules can be analyzed in a single experiment: i) For one or few transcripts, low-throughput methods include *in situ* hybridization (ISH), subtractive hybridization (SH), "Northern Blot" (NB), Ribonuclease-Protection Assay (RPA), Reverse-Transcriptase Polymerase Chain Reaction (RT-PCR), *in situ* RT-PCR and quantitative or real time RT-PCR (qRT-PCR). ii) For various transcripts there are medium-throughput tools based on cDNA clones, Expressed Sequence Tags (ESTs), Open Reading Frame ESTs (ORESTES), Differential Display (DD) and Representative Differential Analysis (RDA). iii) For thousands of transcripts, Serial Analysis of Gene Expression (SAGE), Massive-Parallel Signature Sequencing as well as DNA and oligonucleotide microarrays are high-throughput approaches. b) Transcription regulation: To identify Transcription Factors (TF) that bind specifically to DNA sites, one can use Chromatin Immunoprecipitation in a low- (ChIP) or high-throughput manner when it is coupled to microarrays (ChIP-to-Chip) or Pair-End di-Tags (ChIP-PET). These methods are classified according to the holism-reductionism approach.

Gene Expression Profiles (GEPs) using DNA microarrays, a new molecular classification and subclassification, as well as clinical prediction and diagnosis of many cancer (sub)types have been developed (Macoska, 2002; Ciro *et al.*, 2003; Wadlow & Ramaswamy, 2005). Likewise, new potential markers for therapy have been identified and there is a better understanding of the molecular mechanisms of cancer (Clarke *et al.*, 2004). There are classic studies that have demonstrated the potentials of microarray technology, for instance, one of the first reports was the molecular classification of human acute leukemias using an oligonucleotide microarray (Affymetrix) representing 6817 genes (Golub *et al.*, 1999). In this study, 50 genes were found aid to distinguish between acute myeloid leukemia and acute lymphoblastic leukemia. To validate the gene set, 34 samples were analyzed without knowledge of its type (unsupervised analysis) and classified in their respective type with a high accuracy. This was a very important achievement because the right diagnosis of this cancer is often difficult but essential to discern because an effective treatment relies on an accurate identification of the cancer subtype.

Another classical study was applied on the Diffuse Large-B-Cell Lymphoma since it is known that patients exhibit different prognoses and variable responses to therapy. Using a microarray containing over 18,000 cDNA clones, a GEP with little more than 100 genes and 96 different samples was established (Alizadeh *et al.*, 2000). This pattern allowed the classification of this cancer into two subtypes regarding the status of differentiation of B cells: one similar to germ B cells and other similar to activated B cells *in vitro*. Interestingly, the two subtypes showed a strong correlation with clinical prognosis, which was the best for the subtype bearing germinal B cells. These patients are usually treated with a combination of chemotherapy based on anthracyclines, but if they don´t have a good prognosis then a bone marrow transplantation is rather recommended. Therefore, the GEP of about hundred genes can help to determine what kind of treatment and prognosis a patient should have. Thereafter, this work was validated by using 240 samples that allowed the identification of only 17 genes capable to correlate disease with prognosis (Rosenwald *et al.*, 2002). Similarly, another laboratory studied the prognosis of the same cancer type but whose patients received different treatments, allowing the identification of two groups of patients with different life expectancy for 5 years (72% good versus 12% bad prognosis) using only a predictor of 13 out of 6,817 genes included in a "Genechip" from Affymetrix (Shipp *et al.*, 2002). It is noteworthy that 3 tumor markers were detected in both the 17 and 13 gene predictors developed independently by those laboratories.

The best example of GEPs, nonetheless, has been demonstrated in the prognosis of breast cancer. Using an oligonucleotide microarray of 25,000 and 78 samples of primary breast tumors obtained from patients with negative lymph node status for metastasis, a 70-gene "poor-prognosis" molecular signature was identified (van 't Veer *et al.*, 2002). This signature corresponds to a high probability of developing metastasis in the short term and most likely die. What is interesting about this study is that tumors are not "good" nor "bad" when the disease progresses as was proposed not so long time ago with the clonal model of development (Couzin, 2003); rather, the malignant cell is destined to metastasize very early. Through this genetic signature, experts can decide what patients should receive adjuvant therapy consisting of Tamoxifen (an antagonist of the estrogen receptor in breast tissue via its active metabolite, hydroxytamoxifen). Shortly after, this study was clinically validated using 217 new samples, which reconfirmed that the signature of 70 genes is the best criterion for deciding whether a patient requires adjuvant therapy or not (van de Vijver *et al.*, 2002).

Since the first two studies were developed using samples from young patients with relatively early tumours from the same institution, it was not clear whether the 70-gene could also be applied to other patients. Interestingly, the TRANSBIG consortium, a network of 28 institutions promoting international collaboration in translational research across 11 countries, independently validated the 70-gene signature using 302 samples from patients from different age groups (up to 61 years) and from 5 different European hospitals (Buyse *et al.*, 2006). Despite its achievements, the same group questioned whether this 70-gene signature could be used as a standard high-throughput diagnostic test, so, using the samples from the first two mentioned reports, they validated a customized mini-array containing a reduced set of 1,900 probes known as the "MammaPrint" (Glas *et al.*, 2006). The "MammaPrint" prognostic assay is currently being validated under the clinical MINDACT (Microarray in Node-Negative Disease May Avoid Chemotherapy) randomized trial that includes 6,000 patient samples from various centers, even though the 70-gene signature has been validated several times in patients with negative (Bueno-de-Mesquita *et al.*, 2009) or positive (Mook *et al.*, 2009) lymph-node status as well as from other populations, including Japanese (Ishitobi *et al.*, 2010). Remarkably, the MammaPrint 70-gene signature, whose genes reflect the hallmarks of cancer (Tian *et al.*, 2010), can be considered as a milestone in the personalized care for breast cancer patients (Slodkowska & Ross, 2009).

4. Microarrays and cervical cancer

The origin of cervical cancer (CC) is linked to the infection of High-Risk Human Papilloma Virus (HR-HPV) mainly type 16 and 18. The genome of these viruses contain 8 viral oncogenes, 2 of which code for the early-expressed oncoproteins E6 and E7 that inhibit the activity of the anti-oncoproteins p53 and pRb, respectively. This way, the oncoproteins deregulate the necessary balance between proliferation and apoptosis, promoting the development of cancer. These imbalances have been studied at the transcriptional level and in a comprehensive manner using microarrays in both clinical samples and cell lines derived from CC with and without therapy. Although there are much fewer reports of microarrays compared to other tissues e.g. for every CC microarray paper, there are 7 for breast cancer (Acevedo Rocha *et al.*, 2007); these few studies have provided invaluable information on the molecular mechanisms of CC.

4.1 Studying carcinogenesis using *in vitro* HPV models

A key event in the development of CC is the infection by HR-HPVs. Using microarray technology, gene expression profiles in cell lines as well as keratinocytes containing HR-HPVs have been assessed (Chang & Laimins, 2000; Nees *et al.*, 2000; Nees *et al.*, 2001; Duffy *et al.*, 2003; Garner-Hamrick *et al.*, 2004; Lee *et al.*, 2004; Toussaint-Smith *et al.*, 2004). Similarly, the overall effect upon infection of cultured human keratinocytes with low-risk HPVs (LR-HPVs) has been described (Thomas *et al.*, 2001). Interestingly, in contrast to HR-HPVs, LR-HPVs induce the overexpression of a larger number of genes from the family TGF-β (Tumor Growth Factor) and apparently, LR-HPVs do not suppress interferon-inducible genes (Thomas *et al.*, 2001). This is very interesting as members of the TGF-β family play a role as tumor suppressor genes (at least at the early development of CC) and interferons are key molecules that counteract viral infections mediated by the immune system. These findings help to explain why the LR-HPVs episomes, conversely to those of HR-HPVs, are easily eliminated in many cases.

Another important event in the carcinogenesis of CC is the integration of viral genomes into the cellular genome. It is known that upon viral DNA integration into the host genome, the E2 protein expression is usually lost. Since E2 normally represses both E6 and E7, its absence deregulates the latter oncoproteins. Using microarrays, the overall effect upon viral genome integration of HR-HPV type 16, 18, and 33 into cell lines and keratinocytes has been determined (Alazawi *et al.*, 2002; Ruutu *et al.*, 2002; Pett *et al.*, 2006). Notably, these studies found that the integration of the viral genome into the host genome is a critical step because, besides the high chromosomal instability of the infected cells, interferon-inducible genes are accordingly activated, thus eliminating the cells containing mainly viral episomes but promoting the selection of the more unstable cells.

In addition, the overall effect of expressing E2 in some cervical carcinoma cell lines has been also determined (Thierry *et al.*, 2004), inducing in some cases cellular senescence or exit to the G0 cell cycle phase (Wells *et al.*, 2003). Last but not least, the general effect of eliminating the gene E6AP, an important gene involved in the E6-mediated TP53 protein degradation, has been also assessed in multiple CC-derived (HPV+) cell lines (Kelley *et al.*, 2005). All the studies mentioned in this section have identified significant changes in the expression patterns of hundreds of genes including cyclins, kinases, oncogenes, and anti-oncogenes; some known to be involved in CC but other previously unknown, so all these gathered information is essential to systematically study the HPV-mediated CC carcinogenesis.

4.2 Studying carcinogenesis using patient samples

To identify key genes in the development of CC several strategies have been followed. Some of them had focused on the progress of the lesions while others had compared their origin, i.e. squamous and/or glandular lesions vs normal tissue. In any case, these studies had allowed the identification of gene expression profiles useful for the molecular classification and subclassification of CC.

In the first attempts to classify CC, an expression profile of only 18 differentially expressed genes involved in apoptosis, cell adhesion, and transcription regulation was found between cervical squamous cell carcinoma (SCC) and normal cervical tissue using a microarray of 588 genes (Shim *et al.*, 1998). In another interesting study, employing a 10,000-gene microarray, 40 genes allowed the classification of 34 samples of patients into a normal and a tumoral group (Wong *et al.*, 2003). Moreover, from the 34 samples, 16 could be sub-classified as patients with grade IB and IIB tumors, from which four genes displayed key expression levels in both the previous classification and subclassification, suggesting their role as possible tumor markers (Wong *et al.*, 2003). In a similar analysis but using only 1,276 genes together with 10 samples of SCC and 20 of cervical intraepithelial neoplasia grade 3 (CIN3), a gene expression profile showed that, from all the samples corresponding to CIN3, some correlated with the progression to cancer while others did not, implying the existence of a new subdivision of precancerous lesions histologically indistinguishable (Sopov *et al.*, 2004).

The selection and characterization of tumor samples is critical as this has permitted the establishment of significant gene expression differences between samples from squamous and glandular origin in both normal and pathological conditions (Contag *et al.*, 2004). Obviously, these differences arise by the transcriptional activity of genes particularly expressed in the histological subtypes of CC, but other strategies had also compared the expression profiles between normal and squamous (Cheng *et al.*, 2002b; Chen *et al.*, 2003; Wong *et al.*, 2006) or glandular (Chen *et al.*, 2003; Fujimoto *et al.*, 2004; Chao *et al.*, 2006) tumor samples. Importantly, with a correct histological characterization of the samples, other factors can also be correlated, for example, using more than 40 samples derived from invasive CC (HPV+), it was found that a high burden of viral DNA correlates with high levels of E6 and E7 transcripts, poor prognosis, genomic instability and overexpression of more than 100 genes related to the cell cycle, from which many were identified as oncogenes and at least 50 target genes for the relevant E2F transcription factor family (Rosty *et al.*, 2005). Although the sample description in other studies has remained considerably poor (Ahn *et al.*, 2004a; Guelaguetza Vázquez-Ortíz, 2005; Santin *et al.*, 2005; Vazquez-Ortiz *et al.*, 2005a; Vazquez-Ortiz *et al.*, 2005b), these also had generated long lists of genes possibly important for the molecular study of CC.

Lastly, there are two more examples displaying the great power of microarray technology as these have enriched samples from cytological screening (Papanicolaou). For instance, by obtaining normal and cancerous cells from a cytobrush and from simple exfoliated cells, it was possible to identify known and potential tumor markers in epithelial cells (Hudelist *et al.*, 2005) and CIN3 lesions (Steinau *et al.*, 2005), respectively.

4.3 Treatment

In the CC treatment, besides surgery there is radiotherapy and chemotherapy. However, it's not possible to predict the individual response of patients. The ability of tumor cells to evade treatments suggests that there are different resistance-induced mechanisms. It is believed that by monitoring the genes involved in the resistance against therapy, will help not only to understand the molecular mechanisms of CC, but also to improve its treatment. Accordingly, depending on the gene expression profiles of tumor samples that indicate sensitivity to radiation or chemotherapy, it could be possible to classify patients, allowing a customized CC treatment (Chin *et al.*, 2005).

4.3.1 Radiation

The survival of patients diagnosed with cervical cancer has been improved by combining radiotherapy and chemotherapy. However, it has been estimated that about 65% of patients can be cured with radiation alone (Usmani *et al.*, 2005) but such patients have not been identified so far and therefore they suffer the unnecessary and lethal chemotherapy effects. The long-term goal of the first report using microarrays in combination with radiotherapy against CC, was to find a GEP that would help deciding whether a patient would benefit or not with this treatment, avoiding in this way chemotherapy (Achary *et al.*, 2000). Using a microarray of 5,776 genes, 70 identified genes allowed the differentiation of two cell lines derived from a single carcinoma, which had been previously characterized as radiosensitive and radiotolerant. Interestingly, some genes were previously associated with a cellular response against radiation, suggesting a key role in therapy resistance (Achary *et al.*, 2000). Likewise, it was possible to classify 19 samples with 100% accuracy in two groups: sensitive and tolerant to ionizing radiation (IR) by using 62 out of 23.000 (Kitahara *et al.*, 2002). Moreover, from the genes identified in the previous study, it was found that low levels of the gene XRCC5, and its corresponding protein Ku80, correlated with a good prognosis in CC patients (Harima *et al.*, 2003). Thereafter, but using instead 35 genes, the same group classified samples from patients treated with radiation and hyperthermia in two groups: sensitive and tolerant (Harima *et al.*, 2004). Importantly, not only the combined treatment offered a better prognosis than radiotherapy alone, but a long list of genes with a possible role in the molecular mechanisms associated with therapy was obtained.

There are other studies where samples of patients with CC were classified in radiotolerant or radiosensitive (Wong *et al.*, 2003), as well as in different radiosensitivity degrees (Tewari *et al.*, 2005). In addition, *in vitro* studies using human keratinocytes (Chen *et al.*, 2002), cervical carcinoma cell lines lacking HPV (Liu *et al.*, 2003) and harboring HPV type either 16 (Liu *et al.*, 2003; Chung *et al.*, 2005) or 18 (Crawford & Piwnica-Worms, 2001; Chaudhry *et al.*, 2003) have been also useful to improve the understanding of the molecular mechanisms that occur when tumor cells are treated with IR. Moreover, high levels of cyclin D1 mRNA (a molecule that promotes the progression of cell cycle) and low mRNA levels of the "Insulin-like Growth Factor-Binding Protein 2" or IGFBP2 (protein that can inhibit or promote tumor growth in many cancers) (Hoeflich *et al.*, 2001) correlate with a radioresistant phenotype in immortalized human keratinocytes and CC cell lines (Chen *et al.*, 2002; Liu *et al.*, 2003; Chung *et al.*, 2005). Other up-regulated genes, primarily involved in the cell cycle, that were detected in patients and radio-resistant cell lines include GAPDH (Kitahara *et al.*, 2002; Harima *et al.*, 2004), E2F3 (Chaudhry *et al.*, 2003; Liu *et al.*, 2003), DDB1 (Chaudhry *et al.*, 2003; Wong *et al.*, 2003) and ICAM5 (Achary *et al.*, 2000; Chung *et al.*, 2005). However, cyclin B1 and D1 have been determined to be overexpressed in immortalized human keratinocytes and several CC-derived radio-resistant cell lines (Chen *et al.*, 2002; Liu *et al.*, 2003), but suppressed in radiosensitive cell lines (Crawford & Piwnica-Worms, 2001; Chaudhry *et al.*, 2003).

Unfortunately, is difficult to find a clear correlation of differentially expressed genes between different microarray studies related to radiation therapy because the response is not only different in every patient, but it also depends on the dose, type, time, etc. In spite of this, other radiation-related tumor markers (Haffty & Glazer, 2003) have also been detected including cyclin D1 (CCND1), the factor vascular endothelial growth factor (VEGF) and the proliferating cell nuclear antigen (PCNA), though in isolated studies (Chen *et al.*, 2002; Chaudhry *et al.*, 2003; Liu *et al.*, 2003).

4.3.2 Chemotherapy

Similar to radiation, there are several studies but using instead chemical agents. For example, using cell lines derived from CC with and without HPV infection, the effect of anticancer substances that stop cell cycle like lovastatin has been study in a comprehensive manner (Dimitroulakos *et al.*, 2002). Other chemicals have been used like the apoptosis-inducing di-indol-methane (Carter *et al.*, 2002), catechin EGCG (found in green tea) (Ahn *et al.*, 2003), arsenic-derived (As_2O_3 and As_4O_6) (Ahn *et al.*, 2004b), and platinum-derived compounds (Gatti *et al.*, 2004) as well as the antibiotic zeocin (Hwang *et al.*, 2005). In addition, several effects exerted by chemicals that inhibit the epidermal growth factor receptor (EGFR) oncogene (Woodworth *et al.*, 2005) and phosphatidylinositol kinase (PIK3CA) (Lee *et al.*, 2006) signaling pathways had been also assessed. However, since these compounds are highly toxic, with broad action spectra, similar to those of radiotherapy, only very slight correlations of activated or deactivated genes across all these studies can be observed. For example, the expression of pro-metastatic factor JAG2 is suppressed when CC cell lines were treated with platinum-containing compounds (Gatti *et al.*, 2004) or di-indolymethane (Carter *et al.*, 2002). Di-indolymethane (Carter *et al.*, 2002) or arsenic compounds (Ahn *et al.*, 2004b), on the other hand, suppressed the transcripts of the proliferation marker PCNA.

It has been likewise reported that the transcription factor E2F4 can be suppressed by the competitive inhibition (in the ATP binding-site) of the EGFR (Woodworth *et al.*, 2005) or simply using zeocin (Hwang *et al.*, 2005). Another gene involved in cell proliferation is CHEK1, which can be suppressed by zeocin (Hwang *et al.*, 2005) and derivatives of arsenic (Ahn *et al.*, 2004b). Lastly, the membrane marker CD83 (antigen involved in immunologic response) has also been down-regulated using arsenic compounds (Ahn *et al.*, 2004b) and EGCG (Ahn *et al.*, 2003). Despite efforts to improve the prognosis of patients through the use of diverse chemotherapy regimens, radiation and their combinations, the quality of life, generally speaking, has not been yet improved significantly (Duenas-Gonzalez *et al.*, 2003). Owed to this, the search for new tumor markers and the development of drugs specifically targeted against these molecules is an important step to control CC.

5. A systematic view on cervical cancer

Systems biology (SB) seeks to explain biological phenomena through the study of networks that emerge because of the interactions of the cellular and biochemical components of a cell or organism (Kitano, 2002). This can be achieved with the aid of bioinformatics, as it allows the integration of large amounts of information that are generated every day as well as the construction of biology-oriented mathematical models. In fact, not only transcriptional network models for the understanding of cancer have been simulated, but also the integration of microarray-derived data has been a useful tool for identifying gene modules involved in different cancer-altered pathways (Segal *et al.*, 2005). Furthermore, it has been shown that cancer alterations can be better correlated when these are compared to different organisms, suggesting that combining data obtained from both cell lines and various techniques can provide more compelling ideas to understand biological phenomena.

5.1 Systems biology and cervical cancer

All available information from the cancer transcriptome could be easily correlated if the respective studies would share a universal language e.g. MIAME (Minimal Information About a Microarray Experiment) (Quackenbush, 2004).

Most microarray reports and in particular those in CC, however, contain no standardized data. Using a database and different computational tools (Kent, 2002; Wain *et al.*, 2004; Wheeler *et al.*, 2008) to assign all genes the same nomenclature, it is nonetheless possible to assess their expression levels and correlate them in different scenarios. For example, from all the aforementioned CC microarray studies, when assessing only "on"/"off" expression, we observed genes commonly found between some studies (Table 1).

Many of the genes in Table 1 have been implicated before in CC. Nevertheless, these genes can be related to other high performance techniques, such as the identification of tumor suppressor genes among a big set of genes that increase their expression during loss of tumorigenicity in HeLa cells (Mikheev *et al.*, 2004) or the quantification of transcripts present in samples of CC (Frigessi *et al.*, 2005) or normal cervix (Perez-Plasencia *et al.*, 2005).

Up-regulated genes in cervical cancer		Down-regulated genes in cervical cancer	
Gene	*References*	*Gene*	*References*
TOP2A	(Nees *et al.*, 2000), (Nees *et al.*, 2001), (Garner-Hamrick *et al.*, 2004), (Thierry *et al.*, 2004), (Sopov *et al.*, 2004), (Chen *et al.*, 2003), (Rosty *et al.*, 2005), (Santin *et al.*, 2005)	CDKN1A	(Chang & Laimins, 2000), (Nees *et al.*, 2000), (Nees *et al.*, 2001), (Duffy *et al.*, 2003), (Thierry *et al.*, 2004), (Wells *et al.*, 2003), (Kelley *et al.*, 2005)
CCNA2	(Nees *et al.*, 2000), (Nees *et al.*, 2001), (Garner-Hamrick *et al.*, 2004), (Thierry *et al.*, 2004), (Sopov *et al.*, 2004), (Rosty *et al.*, 2005), (Santin *et al.*, 2005)	FN1	(Nees *et al.*, 2000), (Nees *et al.*, 2001), (Toussaint-Smith *et al.*, 2004), (Kelley *et al.*, 2005), (Santin *et al.*, 2005), (Hudelist *et al.*, 2005)
CCNB1	(Nees *et al.*, 2000), (Nees *et al.*, 2001), (Garner-Hamrick *et al.*, 2004), (Rosty *et al.*, 2005), (Santin *et al.*, 2005), (Vazquez-Ortiz *et al.*, 2005a), (Liu *et al.*, 2003)	TRIM22	(Chang & Laimins, 2000), (Nees *et al.*, 2001), (Duffy *et al.*, 2003), (Pett *et al.*, 2006), (Kelley *et al.*, 2005), (Santin *et al.*, 2005)
CDKN2A	(Nees *et al.*, 2001), (Garner-Hamrick *et al.*, 2004), (Wong *et al.*, 2006), (Rosty *et al.*, 2005), (Santin *et al.*, 2005) , (Hudelist *et al.*, 2005)	IL1RN	(Chang & Laimins, 2000), (Duffy *et al.*, 2003), (Ruutu *et al.*, 2002), (Wong *et al.*, 2006), (Santin *et al.*, 2005)
PLK1	(Nees *et al.*, 2000), (Nees *et al.*, 2001), (Pett *et al.*, 2006), (Wells *et al.*, 2003), (Rosty *et al.*, 2005), (Santin *et al.*, 2005)	SPRR1A	(Chang & Laimins, 2000), (Duffy *et al.*, 2003), (Alazawi *et al.*, 2002), (Wong *et al.*, 2006), (Santin *et al.*, 2005)
BIRC5	(Nees *et al.*, 2000), (Nees *et al.*, 2001), (Garner-Hamrick *et al.*, 2004), (Rosty *et al.*, 2005), (Santin *et al.*, 2005)	TNC	(Duffy *et al.*, 2003), (Garner-Hamrick *et al.*, 2004), (Pett *et al.*, 2006), (Kelley *et al.*, 2005), (Santin *et al.*, 2005)
MCM2	(Garner-Hamrick *et al.*, 2004), (Wells *et al.*, 2003), (Wong *et al.*, 2006), (Rosty *et al.*, 2005), (Santin *et al.*, 2005)	IGFBP6	(Garner-Hamrick *et al.*, 2004), (Wong *et al.*, 2006), (Hudelist *et al.*, 2005), (Liu *et al.*, 2003)
NEK2	(Nees *et al.*, 2001), (Garner-Hamrick *et al.*, 2004), (Thierry *et al.*, 2004), (Rosty *et al.*, 2005), (Santin *et al.*, 2005)	LCN2	(Chang & Laimins, 2000), (Nees *et al.*, 2001), (Duffy *et al.*, 2003), (Santin *et al.*, 2005)
BUB1	(Nees *et al.*, 2001), (Garner-Hamrick *et al.*, 2004), (Wells *et al.*, 2003), (Rosty *et al.*, 2005)	ABCA1	(Garner-Hamrick *et al.*, 2004), (Kelley *et al.*, 2005), (Santin *et al.*, 2005)
CCNB2	(Garner-Hamrick *et al.*, 2004), (Thierry *et al.*, 2004), (Rosty *et al.*, 2005), (Santin *et al.*, 2005)	BNIP2	(Nees *et al.*, 2001), (Thierry *et al.*, 2004), (Wong *et al.*, 2006)
CDC2	(Nees *et al.*, 2001), (Garner-Hamrick *et al.*, 2004), (Wells *et al.*, 2003), (Rosty *et al.*, 2005)	CSPG2	(Duffy *et al.*, 2003), (Ruutu *et al.*, 2002), (Santin *et al.*, 2005)
CDC20	(Nees *et al.*, 2001), (Wells *et al.*, 2003), (Rosty *et al.*, 2005), (Santin *et al.*, 2005)	DDB2	(Duffy *et al.*, 2003), (Thierry *et al.*, 2004), (Kelley *et al.*, 2005)
CKS1B	(Nees *et al.*, 2001), (Thierry *et al.*, 2004), (Rosty *et al.*, 2005), (Santin *et al.*, 2005)	GSN	(Garner-Hamrick *et al.*, 2004), (Thierry *et al.*, 2004), (Kelley *et al.*, 2005)
E2F1	(Wells *et al.*, 2003), (Rosty *et al.*, 2005), (Santin *et al.*, 2005), (Hudelist *et al.*, 2005)	INPP5D	(Nees *et al.*, 2001), (Duffy *et al.*, 2003), (Wells *et al.*, 2003)
FOXM1	(Garner-Hamrick *et al.*, 2004), (Thierry *et al.*, 2004), (Rosty *et al.*, 2005), (Santin *et al.*, 2005)	IVL	(Duffy *et al.*, 2003), (Garner-Hamrick *et al.*, 2004), (Wong *et al.*, 2006)
KRT18	(Garner-Hamrick *et al.*, 2004), (Thierry *et al.*, 2004), (Sopov *et al.*, 2004), (Rosty *et al.*, 2005)	KLK7	(Chang & Laimins, 2000), (Duffy *et al.*, 2003), (Wong *et al.*, 2006)
MEST	(Duffy *et al.*, 2003), (Chen *et al.*, 2003), (Rosty *et al.*, 2005), (Santin *et al.*, 2005)	KRT4	(Duffy *et al.*, 2003), (Ruutu *et al.*, 2002), (Wong *et al.*, 2006)
MKI67	(Garner-Hamrick *et al.*, 2004), (Thierry *et al.*, 2004), (Rosty *et al.*, 2005), (Vazquez-Ortiz et al, 2005b)	KRT16	(Alazawi *et al.*, 2002), (Ruutu *et al.*, 2002), (Wong *et al.*, 2006)
MSH6	(Garner-Hamrick *et al.*, 2004), (Sopov *et al.*, 2004), (Rosty *et al.*, 2005), (Santin *et al.*, 2005)	LAMA3	(Chang & Laimins, 2000), (Kelley *et al.*, 2005), (Santin *et al.*, 2005)

Up-regulated genes in cervical cancer		Down-regulated genes in cervical cancer	
Gene	*References*	*Gene*	*References*
MYBL2	(Thierry *et al.*, 2004), (Chen *et al.*, 2003), (Rosty *et al.*, 2005), (Santin *et al.*, 2005)	SMPG	(Garner-Hamrick *et al.*, 2004), (Wong *et al.*, 2006), (Santin *et al.*, 2005)
PRIM1	(Nees *et al.*, 2001), (Garner-Hamrick *et al.*, 2004), (Rosty *et al.*, 2005), (Santin *et al.*, 2005)	PI3	(Duffy *et al.*, 2003), (Alazawi *et al.*, 2002), (Santin *et al.*, 2005)
RRM2	(Nees *et al.*, 2001), (Thierry *et al.*, 2004), (Wong *et al.*, 2006), (Rosty *et al.*, 2005)	PPP2R5B	(Garner-Hamrick *et al.*, 2004), (Ruutu *et al.*, 2002), (Santin *et al.*, 2005)
SPARC	(Nees *et al.*, 2001), (Duffy *et al.*, 2003), (Chen *et al.*, 2003), (Ahn *et al.*, 2004a)	SERPINB2	(Chang & Laimins, 2000), (Ruutu *et al.*, 2002), (Santin *et al.*, 2005)
TTK	(Garner-Hamrick *et al.*, 2004), (Wells *et al.*, 2003), (Rosty *et al.*, 2005), (Santin *et al.*, 2005)	SPRR2B	(Duffy *et al.*, 2003), (Wong *et al.*, 2006), (Santin *et al.*, 2005)
VEGF	(Garner-Hamrick *et al.*, 2004), (Toussaint-Smith *et al.*, 2004), (Wong *et al.*, 2006), (Vazquez-Ortiz *et al.*, 2005a)	SULT2B1	(Chang & Laimins, 2000), (Duffy *et al.*, 2003), (Wong *et al.*, 2006)

Table 1. Genes primarily found to be up- or down-regulated in cervical cancer across different DNA microarray platforms comparing non-pathogenic vs tumor samples and cell lines. The internationally accepted nomenclature for each gene can be found in: http://www.genenames.org/ or http://cgap.nci.nih.gov/Genes/GeneFinder.

Moreover, it is even possible to combine all this information with that derived of techniques of medium- (Nees *et al.*, 1998; Cheng *et al.*, 2002a; Brentani *et al.*, 2003; Ahn *et al.*, 2005; Ranamukhaarachchi *et al.*, 2005; Seo *et al.*, 2005; Sgarlato *et al.*, 2005) and low- (Helliwell, 2001; Keating *et al.*, 2001; Follen *et al.*, 2003; Gray & Herrington, 2004) performance in CC.

In addition, the to-be-integrated information can be further correlated with genes that have been (a) implied as potential markers in several metastatic solid tumors, including some of uterine origin (Ramaswamy *et al.*, 2003); (b) associated with cervical cancer and other kind of cancers whose somatic or germline mutations frequently favor the development of neoplasia (Forbes *et al.*, 2006); or (c) proposed as common tumor proliferation markers overexpressed across microarray reports in very diverse tumor tissues (Whitfield *et al.*, 2006). Last but not least, a more comprehensive systematic analysis of CC can be done by correlating gene up-regulation mediated via the transcription factors E2F (Bracken *et al.*, 2004) and TP53 (Wei *et al.*, 2006), being this integration crucial for a general understanding of the transcriptional regulation during CC development because the functions E2F and TP53 are respectively altered by the oncoproteins E7 and E6. The idea of integrating all these additional supporting studies from many sources poses great potential in the diagnosis, prevention, and treatment of cancer as has been shown in liver carcinoma (Thorgeirsson *et al.*, 2006).

5.2 Systematic model of HPV-mediated cervical carcinogenesis

The invaluable information provided by all the aforementioned microarray-based CC reports can be related to those additional supporting studies through an integrative disease model as the HPV-mediated cervix carcinogenesis develops in a complex multiple-step process (Sherman & Kurman, 1998; Klaes *et al.*, 1999; zur Hausen, 2002; Sherman, 2003; Ahn *et al.*, 2004a; Frazer, 2004; Pett *et al.*, 2006; Snijders *et al.*, 2006). It starts with the HR-HPV infection and episomes formation thereof, followed by the production of virions and/or the integration of the viral genome into the host one that can lead to precancerous and cancerous lesions of squamous and/or glandular origin and ultimately to death. In other words, with this model (Fig. 3) it is not only possible to correlate the up/down regulation of

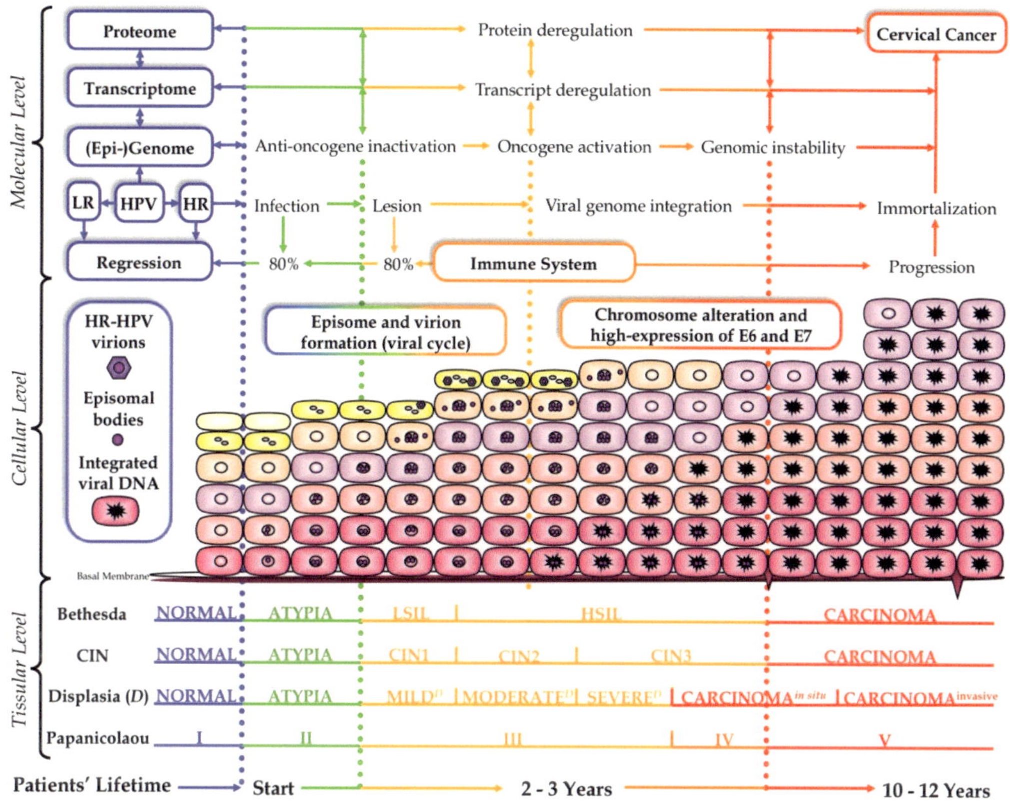

Fig. 3. Cervix carcinogenesis systematic model. The various nomenclatures employed in the histopathology of cervical cancer are aligned by dashed lines and extended to key cellular and molecular events that occur during the transformation of the epithelium. The solid lines indicate a direct relationship between key events. A key event is the infection of cells in the basal membrane by HR-HPVs. These can turn into episomal bodies, which will be in charge of, on one hand, producing infective virions and, on the other, integrating into the genome of epithelial cells. Upon infection, an average of 2-3 years are necessary to develop cervical intraepithelial neoplasia of low- (CIN1/2) and/or high-grade (CIN3), often characterized by the integration of the viral genome, another key event for the disease progression as this often triggers the deregulation of the oncogenes E6 and E7, mayor chromosomal alterations and cellular immortalization. The immune system plays a key role during carcinogenesis since the majority of HR-HPV infections (80%) as well as most low-grade lesions (80%) regress. Due to this and the long periods of time between viral infection and the progression to invasive disease, the infection by HR-HPVs is necessary but not sufficient for the development of cervical cancer; in addition, the inactivation of anti-oncogenes (besides pRb and p53) and activation of oncogenes are necessary to consequently provoke changes at the (epi-)genomic, transcriptomic and protemic level. *D* = Displasia; L- or HSIL = Low- or High-grade squamous intraepithelial lesion.

specific genes upon presence/absence of HR-HPVs episomes or genome integration as well as that of the oncoproteins E6 and/or E7, but also to identify specific carcinogenesis targets.

Depending on the study, however, the gene correlation has to be carefully done, for example, the processes of cell differentiation and senescence (Nees *et al.*, 2000; Wells *et al.*, 2003; Ranamukhaarachchi *et al.*, 2005) have been considered as anti-cell proliferation molecular events (Gandarillas, 2000). Similarly, an indirect correlation could be observed for gene activation mediated by LR-HPVs (Thomas *et al.*, 2001) but not HR-HPVs or E6 and E7 oncogene suppression (Wells *et al.*, 2003; Thierry *et al.*, 2004; Kelley *et al.*, 2005) by E2 (Dowhanick *et al.*, 1995) or RNA interference (Novina & Sharp, 2004). More importantly, nonetheless, as will be discussed in the coming subsections, this model allows the comparison of candidate tumor markers to data obtained from other CC studies at the genomic (Lazo, 1999; Wilting *et al.*, 2006), transcriptomic (Martin *et al.*, 2006), proteomic (Bae *et al.*, 2005; Choi *et al.*, 2005; Yim & Park, 2006) and epigenomic (Duenas-Gonzalez *et al.*, 2005; Sova *et al.*, 2006) level.

5.3 Up-regulated candidate tumor markers

Although many genes frequently activated in CC have been reported using microarrays, other techniques and analyses strongly suggest that these are tumor markers. This can be illustrated with the inhibitor of cyclin-dependent kinases (CDKs) $p16^{INK4a}$ or *CDKN2A*, which is involved in cell cycle and has been categorized as a tumor marker in the development of CC (Keating *et al.*, 2001). Overexpression of $p16^{INK4a}$ at both the transcript and protein level can be detected in samples of cervical dysplasia, squamous and glandular HR-HPV positive and negative lesions when compared with normal cervix by low-throughput techniques (Martin *et al.*, 2006). As summarized in Table 2, $p16^{INK4a}$ up-regulation has been also found using medium- (Brentani *et al.*, 2003) and high-performance methods when the oncoprotein E7 is expressed in cell lines *in vitro* (Nees *et al.*, 2001; Garner-Hamrick *et al.*, 2004), in patient samples *in vivo* (Rosty *et al.*, 2005) and when comparing tumors vs normal tissue (Hudelist *et al.*, 2005; Rosty *et al.*, 2005; Santin *et al.*, 2005; Wong *et al.*, 2006).

Interestingly, $p16^{INK4a}$ is one of the genes that can display somatic mutations in CC; an abnormal status that has been linked to the development of cervical squamous cell cancer (SCC) (Forbes *et al.*, 2006). Dozens of references in the literature demonstrate that the overexpression of $p16^{INK4a}$ is useful as a CC tumor marker; however, using patient samples, others have determined transcript inactivation due to strong hypermethylation on its promoter region (Duenas-Gonzalez *et al.*, 2005). Although these findings are contradictory at first glance, some subpopulations of dysplastic cervical cells can also display epigenetic silencing of $p16^{INK4a}$ and associated low protein levels (Nuovo *et al.*, 1999). This suggests that the expression of $p16^{INK4a}$ is inhibited in some cells within the tumor, whereas its overexpression can be abundant in other cells, most probably expressing the oncoprotein E7. In spite of this, the detection of $p16^{INK4a}$ is very useful in the cytological diagnosis of CC and, furthermore, recent evidence suggests that the determination of the $p16^{INK4a}$ protein may be even more useful than the already-established HR-HPVs detection in the cytological diagnosis (Nieh *et al.*, 2005).

Another important up-regulated gene is "survivin" or *BIRC5* (Table 2). Although surviving expression is undetectable in normal adult tissues, its expression can be detected normally

Biological Process	Gene (Locus)[A]	References: Throughput[B] High-	Medium-	Low-	Marker[C] Metastasis	Cancer	Proliferation	TF[D] E2F	TP53	Analysis[E] Genome	Transcriptome	Proteome	Epigenome
Cell Cycle	MKI67 (Ag Ki-67) (10q25-ter)	(Garner-Hamrick *et al.*, 2004), (Thierry *et al.*, 2004), (Rosty *et al.*, 2005), (Vazquez-Ortiz *et al.*, 2005b)	(Brentani *et al.*, 2003)	(Follen *et al.*, 2003)	-	-	(Whitfield *et al.*, 2006)	(Bracken *et al.*, 2004)	-	-	-	-	-
	CDKN2A (p16[INK4a]) (9p21)	(Nees *et al.*, 2001), (Garner-Hamrick *et al.*, 2004), (Wong *et al.*, 2006), (Rosty *et al.*, 2005), (Santin *et al.*, 2005), (Hudelist *et al.*, 2005)	(Brentani *et al.*, 2003)	(Keating *et al.*, 2001)	-	(Forbes *et al.*, 2006)	-	-	-	-	(Martin *et al.*, 2006)	-	Gonzalez *et*
	CCNB1 (5q12)	(Nees *et al.*, 2000), (Nees *et al.*, 2001), (Garner-Hamrick *et al.*, 2004), (Rosty *et al.*, 2005), (Santin *et al.*, 2005), (Vazquez-Ortiz *et al.*, 2005a), (Liu *et al.*, 2003)	(Brentani *et al.*, 2003) (Sgarlato *et al.*, 2005) (Cheng *et al.*, 2002a)	-	-	-	(Whitfield *et al.*, 2006)	-	-	(Wilting *et al.*, 2006)	-	-	-
	PLK1 (16p12.1)	(Nees *et al.*, 2000), (Nees *et al.*, 2001), (Pett *et al.*, 2006), (Wells *et al.*, 2003), (Rosty *et al.*, 2005), (Santin *et al.*, 2005)	(Brentani *et al.*, 2003)	-	-	-			-	-	-	-	-
	CCNA2 (4q25-31)	(Nees *et al.*, 2000), (Nees *et al.*, 2001), (Garner-Hamrick *et al.*, 2004), (Thierry *et al.*, 2004), (Sopov *et al.*, 2004), (Rosty *et al.*, 2005), (Santin *et al.*, 2005)	(Brentani *et al.*, 2003)	-	-	-			-	-	-	-	-
	MSH6 (2p16)	(Garner-Hamrick *et al.*, 2004), (Sopov *et al.*, 2004), (Rosty *et al.*, 2005), (Santin *et al.*, 2005)	(Ranamukhaarachchi *et al.*, 2005)	-	-	(Forbes *et al.*, 2006)	-	(Bracken *et al.*, 2004)	*al.*,	-	-	-	-
	MAD2L1 (4q27)	(Nees *et al.*, 2001), (Thierry *et al.*, 2004), (Wells *et al.*, 2003), (Rosty *et al.*, 2005)	(Brentani *et al.*, 2003)	-	-	-	(Whitfield *et al.*, 2006)		-	-	-	-	-
	CKS1B (1q21.2)	(Nees *et al.*, 2001), (Thierry *et al.*, 2004), (Rosty *et al.*, 2005), (Santin *et al.*, 2005)	-	-	-	-	-		-	(Wilting *et al.*, 2006)	-	-	-
	SMC4L1 (3q26.1)	(Rosty *et al.*, 2005), (Santin *et al.*, 2005)	(Brentani *et al.*, 2003) (Ranamukhaarachchi *et al.*, 2005)	-	-	-	-		-		-	-	-
	ZWINT (10q21-22)	(Thierry *et al.*, 2004), (Rosty *et al.*, 2005), (Santin *et al.*, 2005)	(Brentani *et al.*, 2003) (Sgarlato *et al.*, 2005)	-	-	-	-	-	-	-	-	-	-
Apoptosis	BIRC5 (17q25)	(Nees *et al.*, 2000), (Nees *et al.*, 2001), (Garner-Hamrick *et al.*, 2004), (Rosty *et al.*, 2005), (Santin *et al.*, 2005)	(Brentani *et al.*, 2003)	-	-	-	(Whitfield *et al.*, 2006)	-	-	-	-	-	-

	MYBL2 (20q13.1)	(Thierry *et al.*, 2004), (Chen *et al.*, 2003), (Rosty *et al.*, 2005), (Santin *et al.*, 2005)	(Brentani *et al.*, 2003) (Sgarlato *et al.*, 2005)	-	-	-		(Bracken *et al.*, 2004)	-	(Wilting *et al.*, 2006)	(Martin *et al.*, 2006)	-	-
	LMNB1 (5q23.3-31)	(Garner-Hamrick *et al.*, 2004), (Rosty *et al.*, 2005), (Santin *et al.*, 2005)	-	-	(Ramaswamy *et al.*, 2003)	-	-	-	-	-	-	-	-
DNA replication	TOP2A (17q21-22)	(Nees *et al.*, 2000), (Nees *et al.*, 2001), (Garner-Hamrick *et al.*, 2004), (Thierry *et al.*, 2004), (Sopov *et al.*, 2004), (Chen *et al.*, 2003), (Rosty *et al.*, 2005), (Santin *et al.*, 2005)	(Brentani *et al.*, 2003)	-	-	-	(Whitfield *et al.*, 2006)	(Bracken *et al.*, 2004)	-	-	(Martin *et al.*, 2006)	-	-
	MCM2 (3q21)	(Garner-Hamrick *et al.*, 2004), (Wells *et al.*, 2003), (Wong *et al.*, 2006), (Rosty *et al.*, 2005), (Santin *et al.*, 2005)	(Brentani *et al.*, 2003) (Sgarlato *et al.*, 2005)	-	-	-	-		-	(Wilting *et al.*, 2006)		-	-
	MCM4 (8q11.2)	(Ruutu *et al.*, 2002), (Chen *et al.*, 2003), (Rosty *et al.*, 2005), (Santin *et al.*, 2005)	-	-	-	-	(Whitfield *et al.*, 2006)		-			-	-
Morphogenesis	KRT19 (17q21-23)	(Garner-Hamrick *et al.*, 2004), (Alazawi *et al.*, 2002), (Wong *et al.*, 2006), 113	(Brentani *et al.*, 2003)	-	-	-	-	-	-	-	-	[illegible] *al.*, [illegible]	-
	KRT18 (12q13)	(Garner-Hamrick *et al.*, 2004), (Thierry *et al.*, 2004), (Sopov *et al.*, 2004), (Rosty *et al.*, 2005)	(Brentani *et al.*, 2003)	-	-	-	-	-	-	-	-	-	-
Angiogenesis	VEGF (6p21-12)	(Garner-Hamrick *et al.*, 2004), (Toussaint-Smith *et al.*, 2004), (Wong *et al.*, 2006), (Vazquez-Ortiz *et al.*, 2005a)	-	(Helliwell, 2001)	-	-	-	-	-	-	(Martin *et al.*, 2006)	-	-
	VEGFC (4q33-34)	(Nees *et al.*, 2001), (Duffy *et al.*, 2003), (Pett *et al.*, 2006)	-	-	-	-	-	-	-	-	-	-	-

Table 2. Genes frequently reported as up-regulated in cervical cancer (CC). A) For each biological process, genes are listed in descending order by the mayor number of reports related to CC e.g. the gene MKI67 has been reported at least 190 times in CC. Genes in bold have been used as therapeutic targets in cancer, whereas genes in italics are not so known in CC. The chromosomal localization of the gene is shown in brackets. B) Techniques of high-throughput are DNA microarrays; medium- DD, RDA and ESTs; and low- are tumor markers previously defined in CC. C) Genes proposed as metastasis markers (in solid tumors), tumoral cancer markers (due to frequent mutations) and proliferation markers (large number of cancers). D) Transcription factor (TF) that might regulate the corresponding gene. E) The analysis of the genome refers to the most common chromosomal gains in CC (1q, 3q, 5p, 8q, 20q and Xq); transcriptome to the importance of genes in CC; proteome to overexpressed proteins in CC and; epigenome to genes whose promoter has been found methylated in samples derived from CC. For gene nomenclature see Table 1.

in embryogenesis and abnormally in cancer (mainly inhibiting apoptosis). Due to this, survivin has been generally proposed as a proliferation tumor marker in cancer (Whitfield *et al.*, 2006) and particularly in CC (Branca *et al.*, 2005), opening promising therapeutic strategies (Altieri, 2006). Other emergent useful target genes are the members 2 and 4 from the "minichromosome maintenance deficient" complex or *MCM* found, genes primary involved in DNA replication that have been considered useful for cancer diagnosis and therapy (Rosty et al., 2005; Santin et al., 2005). Similarly, other up-regulated genes that could be specifically targeted are the 2α topoisomerase or *TOP2A* (Whitfield *et al.*, 2006), cyclin B1 or *CCNB1* (Yuan *et al.*, 2004), the kinase 1 polo type or *PLK1* (Strebhardt & Ullrich, 2006) and keratin 19 or *KRT19* (Chang *et al.*, 2005). The transcripts of the latter gene have been abundantly estimated not only in CC-derived samples (Frigessi *et al.*, 2005), but also determined as overexpressed at both the messenger (Alazawi *et al.*, 2002; Brentani *et al.*, 2003; Garner-Hamrick *et al.*, 2004; Wong *et al.*, 2006), and protein (Bae *et al.*, 2005) level in cervical neoplasia compared to normal tissue. As *KRT19*, a protein part of the intermediate filaments of epithelial cells, *KRT18* (Table 2) could likewise play an important role in the molecular diagnosis of cancer.

It should be noted that several genes reported in Table 2 only have been linked to CC using high and average performance techniques, such as the gene involved in the structural maintenance of chromosomes "*SMC4L1*". As far as we known, a single report correlated the expression levels of this gene to esophageal squamous cancer (Yen *et al.*, 2005), but a genomic analysis showed that chromosomal gains in the region 3q12.1- 28 (where *SMC4L1* lies) are most common in SCC (Wilting *et al.*, 2006). This gene might be activated by E2F (Bracken *et al.*, 2004), but it is desirable to check the expression levels of SMC4L1 with low-yield techniques to determine its relevance in CC as well as for potential metastatic markers like LMNB1 or proliferation ones like MAD2L1 gene (Table 2).

5.4 Down-regulated candidate tumor markers

Using microarrays and other techniques it has been possible to find genes frequently down-regulated in CC, suggesting that these may play a role as tumor markers e.g. the tumor suppressor gene $p21^{WAF1/CIP1}$ or *CDKN1A*, which regulates the cell cycle via CDKs inhibition, senescence as well as TP53-dependent and -independent apoptosis (Table 3). Upon degradation or inactivation of the nuclear phosphoprotein TP53 by E6 or PLK1, respectively, the transcription of $p21^{WAF1/CIP1}$ is reduced as observed in several types of cancer (Gartel & Radhakrishnan, 2005) and particularly in CC samples using DNA microarrays (Chang & Laimins, 2000; Nees *et al.*, 2000; Nees *et al.*, 2001; Duffy *et al.*, 2003; Wells *et al.*, 2003; Thierry *et al.*, 2004; Kelley *et al.*, 2005). In addition, it has been suggested that low $p21^{WAF1/CIP1}$ expression correlates with poor prognosis in cervical adenocarcinoma (AC) (Lu *et al.*, 1998). Moreover, in samples derived from CC it has been observed a decrease in cell growth and induction of $p21^{WAF1/CIP1}$ by platinum-based chemotherapy (Gatti *et al.*, 2004) as well as radioimmunotherapy directed against KRT19 (Chang *et al.*, 2005).

Other down-regulated genes in CC include the gene desmoglein 1 or *DSG1*, which encodes a protein involved in the homeostasis of cell-cell epithelial junctions and belongs to the family of "cadherins", proteins whose expression decreases as it progresses in many kinds of cancers, such as cervical cancer (de Boer *et al.*, 1999). It has been determined that the expression of *DSG1* increases in presence of LR-HPVs episomal bodies in human keratinocytes, but its expression levels highly decrease when HR-HPV episomes are present in cell lines and SCC samples. Moreover, DSG1 importantly lies in an area that often presents chromosomal losses during CC (Table 3) and has been assigned as a pro-apoptotic factor mediated by the caspase 3 in keratinocytes (Dusek *et al.*, 2006).

Biological Process	Gene (Locus)[A]	References						
		Throughput[B]			Marker[C]		TF[D]	Analysis[E]
		High-	*Medium-*	*Low-*	*Metastasis*	*Cancer*	*TP53*	*Genome*
Cell Cycle	CDKN1A (p21[WAF1/CIP1]) (6p21.1)	(Chang & Laimins, 2000), (Nees *et al.*, 2000), (Nees *et al.*, 2001), (Duffy *et al.*, 2003), (Thierry *et al.*, 2004), (Wells *et al.*, 2003), (Kelley *et al.*, 2005)	-	-	-	-	(Nees *et al.*, 2000)	-
Cell Adhesion	FN1 (2q34-36)	(Nees *et al.*, 2000), (Nees *et al.*, 2001), (Toussaint-Smith *et al.*, 2004), (Kelley *et al.*, 2005), (Santin *et al.*, 2005), (Hudelist *et al.*, 2005)	-	-	-	-	-	(Wilting *et al.*, 2006)
	DSG1 (18q12.1)	(Chang & Laimins, 2000), (Thomas *et al.*, 2001), (Wong *et al.*, 2006)	-	-	-	-	-	(Wilting *et al.*, 2006)
	CSPG2 (5q12-14)	(Duffy *et al.*, 2003), (Ruutu *et al.*, 2002), (Santin *et al.*, 2005)	(Brentani *et al.*, 2003)	-	-	-	-	(Wilting *et al.*, 2006)
Apoptosis	SERPINB2 (18q21.3)	(Chang & Laimins, 2000), (Ruutu *et al.*, 2002), (Santin *et al.*, 2005)	(Brentani *et al.*, 2003)	-	-	-	-	(Lazo, 1999)
	BNIP2 (10q26.3)	(Nees *et al.*, 2001), (Thierry *et al.*, 2004), (Wong *et al.*, 2006)	-	-	-	-	-	-
Immune Response	IL1RN (2q14.2)	(Chang & Laimins, 2000), (Duffy *et al.*, 2003), (Ruutu *et al.*, 2002), (Wong *et al.*, 2006), (Santin *et al.*, 2005)	-	-	-	-	-	(Wilting *et al.*, 2006)
	TRIM22 (11p15)	(Chang & Laimins, 2000), (Nees *et al.*, 2001), (Duffy *et al.*, 2003), (Pett *et al.*, 2006), (Kelley *et al.*, 2005), (Santin *et al.*, 2005)	-		-	-	(Nees *et al.*, 2000)	-
Epidermal Development	KLK7 (19q13.41)	(Chang & Laimins, 2000), (Duffy *et al.*, 2003), (Wong *et al.*, 2006)	-	-	-	-	-	(Lazo, 1999)
	KRT4 (12p12-11)	(Duffy *et al.*, 2003), (Ruutu *et al.*, 2002), (Wong *et al.*, 2006)	(Brentani *et al.*, 2003)	(Contag *et al.*, 2004)	-	-	-	-
	KRT16 (17q12-21)	(Alazawi *et al.*, 2002), (Ruutu *et al.*, 2002), (Wong *et al.*, 2006)	(Brentani *et al.*, 2003)	-	-	-	-	-
	LAMA3 (18q11.2)	(Chang & Laimins, 2000), (Kelley *et al.*, 2005), (Santin *et al.*, 2005)	-	-	-	-	-	(Wilting *et al.*, 2006)
	SPRR3 (1q21-22)	(Wong *et al.*, 2006), (Santin *et al.*, 2005), (Perez-Plasencia *et al.*, 2005)	-	-	-	-	-	-

	SPRR1A (1q21-22)	(Chang & Laimins, 2000), (Duffy *et al.*, 2003), (Alazawi *et al.*, 2002), (Wong *et al.*, 2006), (Santin *et al.*, 2005)	-	-	-	-	-	-
Signal Transduction	*INPP5D* (2q36-37)	(Nees *et al.*, 2001), (Duffy *et al.*, 2003), (Wells *et al.*, 2003)	-	-	-	-	-	(Wilting *et al.*, 2006)
Signal Transduction	*IGFBP6* (12q13)	(Garner-Hamrick *et al.*, 2004), (Wong *et al.*, 2006), (Hudelist *et al.*, 2005), (Liu *et al.*, 2003)	-	-	-	-	-	-
Signal Transduction	*PPP2R5B* (11q12)	(Garner-Hamrick *et al.*, 2004), (Ruutu *et al.*, 2002), (Santin *et al.*, 2005)	-	-	-	-	-	(Wilting *et al.*, 2006)
DNA Repair	MPG (16p13.3)	(Garner-Hamrick *et al.*, 2004), (Wong *et al.*, 2006), (Santin *et al.*, 2005)	(Seo *et al.*, 2005)	-	-	-	-	-
DNA Repair	*DDB2* (11p12-11)	(Duffy *et al.*, 2003), (Thierry *et al.*, 2004), (Kelley *et al.*, 2005)	-	-	-	(Forbes *et al.*, 2006)	(Nees *et al.*, 2000)	-
DNA Transcription	*RUNX1* (21q22.3)	(Garner-Hamrick *et al.*, 2004), (Wong *et al.*, 2006)	-	-	(Ramaswamy *et al.*, 2003)	(Forbes *et al.*, 2006)	-	-
Cellular Transport	*LCN2* (9q34)	(Chang & Laimins, 2000), (Nees *et al.*, 2001), (Duffy *et al.*, 2003), (Santin *et al.*, 2005)	(Brentani *et al.*, 2003)	-	-	-	-	-

Table 3. Genes frequently reported as down-regulated in cervical cancer (CC). A) For each biological process, genes are listed in descending order by the mayor number of reports related to CC e.g. the gene *CDKN1A* has been reported at least 70 times in CC. Genes in bold represent increased expression levels upon different schemes of radio and/or chemotherapy, whereas genes in *italics* are not so known in CC. The chromosomal localization of the gene is shown in brackets. B) Techniques of high-throughput are mainly DNA microarrays; medium- DD, and ESTs; and low- are tumor markers previously defined in CC. C) Genes proposed as metastasis markers (in solid tumors) and tumoral cancer markers (due to frequent mutations). D) Transcription factor (TF) that might regulate the corresponding gene. E) The analysis of the genome refers to the most common chromosomal alterations in CC (2q, 3p, 4p, 5p, 5q, 6p, 6q, 11q, 13q, 18q and 19q). For gene nomenclature see Table 1.

Another gene that could be of interest in CC is *SERPINB2*. The gene product is an inhibitor of the serine-type proteases like the plasminogen activator (also known as *PLAU*). On one hand, *SERPINB2* suppression has been determined using both microarrays as well as genomic studies in CC (Table 3); but on the other, its expression in HeLa cells can stabilize the expression levels of the Rb protein and suppress the oncoproteins E6 and E7 of HPV18 (Darnell *et al.*, 2005). This suggests that low levels of *SERPINB2* promote CC development, being this a potentially good molecular marker.

Of genes not known in CC there are several examples, being the gene *TRIM22* or "tripartite motif-containing 22", which has been found down-regulated in at least 6 microarray studies (Table 3). *TRIM22* belongs to a conserved family of antiviral proteins, where the member 22 has been implicated in inhibiting the replication of the human immunodeficiency virus 1 (HIV1) (Nisole *et al.*, 2005). This suggests that TRIM22 may be relevant in the immune response HR-HPVs and that these viruses may be responsible for its inhibition.

Table 3 also lists genes from the epidermal differentiation complex (EDC, located in the band 21 of the long arm of chromosome 1), for instance, using SAGE, abundant transcripts of *SPRR3* have been found in normal cervical tissue, but a low *SPRR3* expression has been determined in tumor tissue using microarrays (Table 3). This suggests that *SPRR3* and perhaps *SPRR1A,* which also belongs to the EDC, may be useful tumor markers in CC. Last, other suppressed genes in CC are *IGFBP6* and *RUNX1* (Table 3). While the first one is responsible for inactivating a potent growth factor similar to insulin (IGF2), a gene in turn required by IGFBP6 to reduce metastatic characteristics in tumors from different origin (Bach, 2005), the second gene belongs to a family of transcription factors that can inhibit angiogenesis (Sakakura *et al.*, 2005).

5.5 Candidate tumor markers in cervical cancer subtypes

Although HPV-16-infections are more frequently detected than HPV-18 ones in squamous cell carcinoma (SCC), the latter ones are more often associated to adenocarcinoma of the cervix (AC), whose incidence is growing at the same time as SCC incidence. Interestingly, several genes with a clinically usefulness for the molecular differentiation between the two major histological subtypes of CC have been found using DNA microarrays (Table 4). The genes *TACSTD1* and *CEACAM5,* which encode transmembrane proteins that transmit signals for development, motility and cell growth, for example, were found to be upregulated in AC compared to SCC (Chao *et al.*, 2006).

Up-regulated genes in squamous cell carcinoma		Up-regulated genes in adenocarcinoma	
Gene	*Reference*	*Gene*	*Reference*
CRABP2	(Chao *et al.*, 2006)	BIRC3	(Fujimoto *et al.*, 2004)
NDRG1	(Chao *et al.*, 2006)	CEACAM1	(Fujimoto *et al.*, 2004)
CDH13	(Fujimoto *et al.*, 2004)	CEACAM5-7	(Chao *et al.*, 2006)
KRT13	(Chao *et al.*, 2006)	FOLR1	(Fujimoto *et al.*, 2004)
KRT15	(Chao *et al.*, 2006)	MSLN	(Chao *et al.*, 2006)
PTHLH	(Fujimoto *et al.*, 2004)	S100P	(Chao *et al.*, 2006)
S100A9	(Chao *et al.*, 2006)	TACSTD1	(Chao *et al.*, 2006)
SPRR1B	(Chao *et al.*, 2006)	TSPAN3	(Chao *et al.*, 2006)

Table 4. Genes with a possible clinical utility for the molecular differentiation between squamous cell carcinoma (SCC) and adenocarcinoma (AC) in cervical cancer. The internationally accepted nomenclature for each gene can be found in: http://www.genenames.org/ or http://cgap.nci.nih.gov/Genes/GeneFinder.

Furthermore, high levels of the corresponding proteins served by themselves as poor prognostic factors in patients with AC compared with SCC (Chao *et al.*, 2006). Other genes for potential use as markers in CC that have been found with microarrays are:

1. *CRABP2* (belongs to the EDC and encodes the retinoic acid binding protein 2) has been identified as up-regulated in SSC compared to normal tissue (Shim *et al.*, 1998; Seo *et al.*, 2005) and AC (Chao *et al.*, 2006).
2. *NDRG1* (N-myc Downstream Regulated Gene 1) is involved in cell growth and differentiation and was found overexpressed in SCC compared to AC (Chao *et al.*, 2006) and normal cervical tissue (Sgarlato *et al.*, 2005).
3. Other members of the "Carcinoembryonic antigen-related cell adhesion molecule" family such as the *CEACAM-1, -5, -6,* and *-7,* are shown as up-regulated in AC compared to SCC (Fujimoto *et al.*, 2004; Chao *et al.*, 2006).
4. *MSLN* or mesothelin encodes a membrane glycoprotein involved in cell adhesion whose transcripts are detectable in normal tissue but abundant in tumors of glandular origin or HeLa cells. In CC, *MSLN* is overexpressed in AC compared to SCC (Chao *et al.*, 2006) and in HPV-18-derived samples of SCC/AC compared to normal tissue (Rosty *et al.*, 2005). It is worth noting that *MSLN* is a therapeutic target in various malignancies (Hassan *et al.*, 2004).
5. Finally, high expression levels of *FOLR1* (folate receptor) have been associated with an AC phenotype (Fujimoto *et al.*, 2004) and tumorigenicity in cell lines derived from AC (Mikheev *et al.*, 2004). However, further studies are required to demonstrate the relevance of this receptor in both AC and SCC because it is known that via FOLR1 and folic acid, its ligand, some drugs can be bound and directed into over-expressing high levels of *FOLR1,* as suggested in several types of cancer (Kelemen, 2006).

The aforementioned "tumoral markers" could be potentially important for the diagnosis, prevention, and treatment of CC because these were identified using cell lines from various sources as well as samples of SCC and/or AC for comparative studies with normal tissues. Last but not least, a recent and interesting CC review not only proposed a similar systematic model of HPV infection highlighting the current debate on the viral status as hallmark of disease progression (episomal vs integrated forms where HPV-18 genome integration seems to prevail in women with advance disease in contrast to HPV-16), but also provided overlapping and additional tumor markers at some of those analyzed herein (Woodman *et al.*, 2007). Along these lines, it would be worth saying that cancer, including its hundred subtypes, is such a complex phenomenon (Vogelstein & Kinzler, 2004), which should be rather seen as an average of key molecular events displaying often specific hallmarks (Hanahan & Weinberg, 2000) of disease progression.

6. Conclusions

Thanks to the comparison of the cervix in normal and abnormal conditions via transcriptomics in general and particularly using DNA microarrays, it is possible to identify known and unknown clinically relevant genes for the disease progression. The next goal is to identify and validate specific tumor markers for profiling histo- and pathological subtypes. This will allow not only a molecular subclassification and more understanding of CC, but also choosing the right treatment for each patient according to its gene expression signature if there is prior knowledge about the most likely response she would have. This is the only way to fully understand more about this complex disease.

The intention of this manuscript is to provide the reader a broad view of the transcriptome, an area that is developing rapidly, especially in cancer. It is worthwhile reemphasize that the transcriptome also consists of non-coding RNAs regulating the transcription of many genes and likewise acting as oncogenes or tumor suppressor genes. With such complexity, the best tackling to cancer will rely on predictive hypothesis, so it is important to take into account systems biology, which will allow us to better understand transcriptional networks and identify specific therapy targets for a tailored therapy.

Although there are improved programs for the early diagnosis of CC as well as very effective prophylactic vaccines against HR-HPVs, the high mortality rates triggered by CC will not diminish soon, not even in the medium-term after optimizing CC monitoring programs and broadly executing vaccination schemes. An alternative for CC patients is therefore to look at those tumor markers that could aid in the stratification of the disease and therapy. Unfortunately, genomics and all its derivatives are exacerbating global inequalities in terms of scientific research and health between developed and developing countries since the first cause of death of women in the former countries is breast cancer whereas in the latter ones CC kills every 2 hours, on average, a Mexican woman in productive age.

7. Acknowledgments

We thank the library at the MPI of Coal Research for financial support.

8. References

Acevedo Rocha CG, Alvarez E, Zafra de la Rosa G, Alvarez Navarro M & Gariglio P (2007) [Cervical cancer and DNA microarrays: tumour marker identification]. *Ginecologia y Obstetricia de Mexico* 75, 205-213.

Achary MP, Jaggernauth W, Gross E, Alfieri A, Klinger HP & Vikram B (2000) Cell lines from the same cervical carcinoma but with different radiosensitivities exhibit different cDNA microarray patterns of gene expression. *Cytogenetics and cell genetics* 91, 39-43.

Adams MD, Kelley JM, Gocayne JD, Dubnick M, Polymeropoulos MH, Xiao H, Merril CR, Wu A, Olde B, Moreno RF & et al. (1991) Complementary DNA sequencing: expressed sequence tags and human genome project. *Science* 252, 1651-1656.

Ahn WS, Bae SM, Lee JM, Namkoong SE, Han SJ, Cho YL, Nam GH, Seo JS, Kim CK & Kim YW (2004a) Searching for pathogenic gene functions to cervical cancer. *Gynecologic oncology* 93, 41-48.

Ahn WS, Bae SM, Lee KH, Kim YW, Lee JM, Namkoong SE, Lee IP, Kim CK, Seo JS & Sin JI (2004b) Comparison of effects of As2O3 and As4O6 on cell growth inhibition and gene expression profiles by cDNA microarray analysis in SiHa cells. *Oncology reports* 12, 573-580.

Ahn WS, Huh SW, Bae SM, Lee IP, Lee JM, Namkoong SE, Kim CK & Sin JI (2003) A major constituent of green tea, EGCG, inhibits the growth of a human cervical cancer cell line, CaSki cells, through apoptosis, G(1) arrest, and regulation of gene expression. *DNA and cell biology* 22, 217-224.

Ahn WS, Seo MJ, Bae SM, Lee JM, Namkoong SE, Kim CK & Kim YW (2005) Cellular process classification of human papillomavirus-16-positive SiHa cervical carcinoma cell using Gene Ontology. *International journal of gynecological cancer: official journal of the International Gynecological Cancer Society* 15, 94-106.

Alazawi W, Pett M, Arch B, Scott L, Freeman T, Stanley MA & Coleman N (2002) Changes in cervical keratinocyte gene expression associated with integration of human papillomavirus 16. *Cancer research* 62, 6959-6965.

Alizadeh AA, Eisen MB, Davis RE, Ma C, Lossos IS, Rosenwald A, Boldrick JC, Sabet H, Tran T, Yu X, Powell JI, Yang L, Marti GE, Moore T, Hudson J, Jr., Lu L, Lewis DB, Tibshirani R, Sherlock G, Chan WC, Greiner TC, Weisenburger DD, Armitage JO, Warnke R, Levy R, Wilson W, Grever MR, Byrd JC, Botstein D, Brown PO & Staudt LM (2000) Distinct types of diffuse large B-cell lymphoma identified by gene expression profiling. *Nature* 403, 503-511.

Altieri DC (2006) Targeted therapy by disabling crossroad signaling networks: the survivin paradigm. *Molecular cancer therapeutics* 5, 478-482.

Alwine JC, Kemp DJ & Stark GR (1977) Method for detection of specific RNAs in agarose gels by transfer to diazobenzyloxymethyl-paper and hybridization with DNA probes. *Proceedings of the National Academy of Sciences of the United States of America* 74, 5350-5354.

Bach LA (2005) IGFBP-6 five years on; not so 'forgotten'? *Growth hormone & IGF research* 15, 185-192.

Bae SM, Lee CH, Cho YL, Nam KH, Kim YW, Kim CK, Han BD, Lee YJ, Chun HJ & Ahn WS (2005) Two-dimensional gel analysis of protein expression profile in squamous cervical cancer patients. *Gynecologic oncology* 99, 26-35.

Bartlett JM (2002) Approaches to the analysis of gene expression using mRNA: a technical overview. *Molecular biotechnology* 21, 149-160.

Berk AJ & Sharp PA (1977) Sizing and mapping of early adenovirus mRNAs by gel electrophoresis of S1 endonuclease-digested hybrids. *Cell* 12, 721-732.

Bracken AP, Ciro M, Cocito A & Helin K (2004) E2F target genes: unraveling the biology. *Trends in Biochemical Sciences* 29, 409-417.

Branca M, Giorgi C, Santini D, Di Bonito L, Ciotti M, Costa S, Benedetto A, Casolati EA, Favalli C, Paba P, Di Bonito P, Mariani L, Syrjanen S, Bonifacio D, Accardi L, Zanconati F & Syrjanen K (2005) Survivin as a marker of cervical intraepithelial neoplasia and high-risk human papillomavirus and a predictor of virus clearance and prognosis in cervical cancer. *American journal of clinical pathology* 124, 113-121.

Brenner S, Johnson M, Bridgham J, Golda G, Lloyd DH, Johnson D, Luo SJ, McCurdy S, Foy M, Ewan M, Roth R, George D, Eletr S, Albrecht G, Vermaas E, Williams SR, Moon K, Burcham T, Pallas M, DuBridge RB, Kirchner J, Fearon K, Mao J & Corcoran K (2000) Gene expression analysis by massively parallel signature sequencing (MPSS) on microbead arrays. *Nature Biotechnology* 18, 630-634.

Brentani H, Caballero OL, Camargo AA, da Silva AM, da Silva WA, Jr., Dias Neto E, Grivet M, Gruber A, Guimaraes PE, Hide W, Iseli C, Jongeneel CV, Kelso J, Nagai MA, Ojopi EP, Osorio EC, Reis EM, Riggins GJ, Simpson AJ, de Souza S, Stevenson BJ, Strausberg RL, Tajara EH, Verjovski-Almeida S, Acencio ML, Bengtson MH,

Bettoni F, Bodmer WF, Briones MR, Camargo LP, Cavenee W, Cerutti JM, Coelho Andrade LE, Costa dos Santos PC, Ramos Costa MC, da Silva IT, Estecio MR, Sa Ferreira K, Furnari FB, Faria M, Jr., Galante PA, Guimaraes GS, Holanda AJ, Kimura ET, Leerkes MR, Lu X, Maciel RM, Martins EA, Massirer KB, Melo AS, Mestriner CA, Miracca EC, Miranda LL, Nobrega FG, Oliveira PS, Paquola AC, Pandolfi JR, Campos Pardini MI, Passetti F, Quackenbush J, Schnabel B, Sogayar MC, Souza JE, Valentini SR, Zaiats AC, Amaral EJ, Arnaldi LA, de Araujo AG, de Bessa SA, Bicknell DC, Ribeiro de Camaro ME, Carraro DM, Carrer H, Carvalho AF, Colin C, Costa F, Curcio C, Guerreiro da Silva ID, Pereira da Silva N, Dellamano M, El-Dorry H, Espreafico EM, Scattone Ferreira AJ, Ayres Ferreira C, Fortes MA, Gama AH, Giannella-Neto D, Giannella ML, Giorgi RR, Goldman GH, Goldman MH, Hackel C, Ho PL, Kimura EM, Kowalski LP, Krieger JE, Leite LC, Lopes A, Luna AM, Mackay A, Mari SK, Marques AA, Martins WK, Montagnini A, Mourao Neto M, Nascimento AL, Neville AM, Nobrega MP, O'Hare MJ, Otsuka AY, Ruas de Melo AI, Paco-Larson ML, Guimaraes Pereira G, Pesquero JB, Pessoa JG, Rahal P, Rainho CA, Rodrigues V, Rogatto SR, Romano CM, Romeiro JG, Rossi BM, Rusticci M, Guerra de Sa R, Sant' Anna SC, Sarmazo ML, Silva TC, Soares FA, Sonati Mde F, de Freitas Sousa J, Queiroz D, Valente V, Vettore AL, Villanova FE, Zago MA & Zalcberg H (2003) The generation and utilization of a cancer-oriented representation of the human transcriptome by using expressed sequence tags. *Proceedings of the National Academy of Sciences of the United States of America* 100, 13418-13423.

Bueno-de-Mesquita JM, Linn SC, Keijzer R, Wesseling J, Nuyten DS, van Krimpen C, Meijers C, de Graaf PW, Bos MM, Hart AA, Rutgers EJ, Peterse JL, Halfwerk H, de Groot R, Pronk A, Floore AN, Glas AM, Van't Veer LJ & van de Vijver MJ (2009) Validation of 70-gene prognosis signature in node-negative breast cancer. *Breast cancer research and treatment* 117, 483-495.

Bustamante C, Cheng W & Mejia YX (2011) Revisiting the central dogma one molecule at a time. *Cell* 144, 480-497.

Bustin SA (2000) Absolute quantification of mRNA using real-time reverse transcription polymerase chain reaction assays. *Journal of molecular endocrinology* 25, 169-193.

Buyse M, Loi S, van't Veer L, Viale G, Delorenzi M, Glas AM, d'Assignies MS, Bergh J, Lidereau R, Ellis P, Harris A, Bogaerts J, Therasse P, Floore A, Amakrane M, Piette F, Rutgers E, Sotiriou C, Cardoso F & Piccart MJ (2006) Validation and clinical utility of a 70-gene prognostic signature for women with node-negative breast cancer. *Journal of the National Cancer Institute* 98, 1183-1192.

Carter TH, Liu K, Ralph W, Jr., Chen D, Qi M, Fan S, Yuan F, Rosen EM & Auborn KJ (2002) Diindolylmethane alters gene expression in human keratinocytes in vitro. *The Journal of nutrition* 132, 3314-3324.

Chang CH, Tsai LC, Chen ST, Yuan CC, Hung MW, Hsieh BT, Chao PL, Tsai TH & Lee TW (2005) Radioimmunotherapy and apoptotic induction on CK19-overexpressing human cervical carcinoma cells with Re-188-mAbCx-99. *Anticancer research* 25, 2719-2728.

Chang YE & Laimins LA (2000) Microarray analysis identifies interferon-inducible genes and Stat-1 as major transcriptional targets of human papillomavirus type 31. *Journal of virology* 74, 4174-4182.

Chao A, Wang TH, Lee YS, Hsueh S, Chao AS, Chang TC, Kung WH, Huang SL, Chao FY, Wei ML & Lai CH (2006) Molecular characterization of adenocarcinoma and squamous carcinoma of the uterine cervix using microarray analysis of gene expression. *International journal of cancer* 119, 91-98.

Chaudhry MA, Chodosh LA, McKenna WG & Muschel RJ (2003) Gene expression profile of human cells irradiated in G1 and G2 phases of cell cycle. *Cancer letters* 195, 221-233.

Chen X, Shen B, Xia L, Khaletzkiy A, Chu D, Wong JY & Li JJ (2002) Activation of nuclear factor kappaB in radioresistance of TP53-inactive human keratinocytes. *Cancer research* 62, 1213-1221.

Chen Y, Miller C, Mosher R, Zhao X, Deeds J, Morrissey M, Bryant B, Yang D, Meyer R, Cronin F, Gostout BS, Smith-McCune K & Schlegel R (2003) Identification of cervical cancer markers by cDNA and tissue microarrays. *Cancer research* 63, 1927-1935.

Cheng Q, Lau WM, Chew SH, Ho TH, Tay SK & Hui KM (2002a) Identification of molecular markers for the early detection of human squamous cell carcinoma of the uterine cervix. *British journal of cancer* 86, 274-281.

Cheng Q, Lau WM, Tay SK, Chew SH, Ho TH & Hui KM (2002b) Identification and characterization of genes involved in the carcinogenesis of human squamous cell cervical carcinoma. *International journal of cancer* 98, 419-426.

Chin KV, Alabanza L, Fujii K, Kudoh K, Kita T, Kikuchi Y, Selvanayagam ZE, Wong YF, Lin Y & Shih WC (2005) Application of expression genomics for predicting treatment response in cancer. *Annals of the New York Academy of Sciences* 1058, 186-195.

Choi YP, Kang S, Hong S, Xie X & Cho NH (2005) Proteomic analysis of progressive factors in uterine cervical cancer. *Proteomics* 5, 1481-1493.

Chung YM, Kim BG, Park CS, Huh SJ, Kim J, Park JK, Cho SM, Kim BS, Kim JS, Yoo YD & Bae DS (2005) Increased expression of ICAM-3 is associated with radiation resistance in cervical cancer. *International journal of cancer* 117, 194-201.

Ciro M, Bracken AP & Helin K (2003) Profiling cancer. *Current opinion in cell biology* 15, 213-220.

Clarke PA, te Poele R & Workman P (2004) Gene expression microarray technologies in the development of new therapeutic agents. *European journal of cancer* 40, 2560-2591.

Collins FS, Green ED, Guttmacher AE & Guyer MS (2003) A vision for the future of genomics research. *Nature* 422, 835-847.

Contag SA, Gostout BS, Clayton AC, Dixon MH, McGovern RM & Calhoun ES (2004) Comparison of gene expression in squamous cell carcinoma and adenocarcinoma of the uterine cervix. *Gynecologic oncology* 95, 610-617.

Costa FF (2010) Non-coding RNAs: Meet thy masters. *Bioessays* 32, 599-608.

Coulton G (2004) Are histochemistry and cytochemistry 'Omics'? *Journal of molecular histology* 35, 603-613.

Couzin J (2003) Medicine. Tracing the steps of metastasis, cancer's menacing ballet. *Science* 299, 1002-1006.

Crawford DF & Piwnica-Worms H (2001) The G(2) DNA damage checkpoint delays expression of genes encoding mitotic regulators. *The Journal of biological chemistry* 276, 37166-37177.

Crick F (1970) Central dogma of molecular biology. *Nature* 227, 561-563.

Darnell GA, Antalis TM, Rose BR & Suhrbier A (2005) Silencing of integrated human papillomavirus type 18 oncogene transcription in cells expressing SerpinB2. *Journal of virology* 79, 4246-4256.

de Boer CJ, van Dorst E, van Krieken H, Jansen-van Rhijn CM, Warnaar SO, Fleuren GJ & Litvinov SV (1999) Changing roles of cadherins and catenins during progression of squamous intraepithelial lesions in the uterine cervix. *The American journal of pathology* 155, 505-515.

Dias Neto E, Correa RG, Verjovski-Almeida S, Briones MR, Nagai MA, da Silva W, Jr., Zago MA, Bordin S, Costa FF, Goldman GH, Carvalho AF, Matsukuma A, Baia GS, Simpson DH, Brunstein A, de Oliveira PS, Bucher P, Jongeneel CV, O'Hare MJ, Soares F, Brentani RR, Reis LF, de Souza SJ & Simpson AJ (2000) Shotgun sequencing of the human transcriptome with ORF expressed sequence tags. *Proceedings of the National Academy of Sciences of the United States of America* 97, 3491-3496.

Dimitroulakos J, Marhin WH, Tokunaga J, Irish J, Gullane P, Penn LZ & Kamel-Reid S (2002) Microarray and biochemical analysis of lovastatin-induced apoptosis of squamous cell carcinomas. *Neoplasia* 4, 337-346.

Domazet B, Maclennan GT, Lopez-Beltran A, Montironi R & Cheng L (2008) Laser capture microdissection in the genomic and proteomic era: targeting the genetic basis of cancer. *International journal of clinical and experimental pathology* 1, 475-488.

Dowhanick JJ, McBride AA & Howley PM (1995) Suppression of cellular proliferation by the papillomavirus E2 protein. *Journal of virology* 69, 7791-7799.

Duenas-Gonzalez A, Cetina L, Mariscal I & de la Garza J (2003) Modern management of locally advanced cervical carcinoma. *Cancer treatment reviews* 29, 389-399.

Duenas-Gonzalez A, Lizano M, Candelaria M, Cetina L, Arce C & Cervera E (2005) Epigenetics of cervical cancer. An overview and therapeutic perspectives. *Molecular cancer* 4, 38.

Duffy CL, Phillips SL & Klingelhutz AJ (2003) Microarray analysis identifies differentiation-associated genes regulated by human papillomavirus type 16 E6. *Virology* 314, 196-205.

Dusek RL, Getsios S, Chen F, Park JK, Amargo EV, Cryns VL & Green KJ (2006) The differentiation-dependent desmosomal cadherin desmoglein 1 is a novel caspase-3 target that regulates apoptosis in keratinocytes. *The Journal of biological chemistry* 281, 3614-3624.

Follen M, Meyskens FL, Jr., Alvarez RD, Walker JL, Bell MC, Storthz KA, Sastry J, Roy K, Richards-Kortum R & Cornelison TL (2003) Cervical cancer chemoprevention, vaccines, and surrogate endpoint biomarkers. *Cancer* 98, 2044-2051.

Forbes S, Clements J, Dawson E, Bamford S, Webb T, Dogan A, Flanagan A, Teague J, Wooster R, Futreal PA & Stratton MR (2006) Cosmic 2005. *British journal of cancer* 94, 318-322.

Forrest ARR, Taylor DF, Crowe ML, Chalk AM, Waddell NJ, Kolle G, Faulkner GJ, Rimantas K, Katayama S, Wells C, Kai C, Kawai J, Carninci P, Hayashizaki Y & Grimmond SM (2006) Genome-wide review of transcriptional complexity in mouse protein kinases and phosphatases. *Genome Biology* 7, R5.

Frazer IH (2004) Prevention of cervical cancer through papillomavirus vaccination. *Nature Reviews Immunology* 4, 46-54.

Frigessi A, van de Wiel MA, Holden M, Svendsrud DH, Glad IK & Lyng H (2005) Genome-wide estimation of transcript concentrations from spotted cDNA microarray data. *Nucleic Acids Research* 33, e143.

Frith MC, Pheasant M & Mattick JS (2005) The amazing complexity of the human transcriptome. *European journal of human genetics : EJHG* 13, 894-897.

Fujimoto T, Nishikawa A, Iwasaki M, Akutagawa N, Teramoto M & Kudo R (2004) Gene expression profiling in two morphologically different uterine cervical carcinoma cell lines derived from a single donor using a human cancer cDNA array. *Gynecologic oncology* 93, 446-453.

Fuller AP, Palmer-Toy D, Erlander MG & Sgroi DC (2003) Laser capture microdissection and advanced molecular analysis of human breast cancer. *Journal of mammary gland biology and neoplasia* 8, 335-345.

Gandarillas A (2000) Epidermal differentiation, apoptosis, and senescence: common pathways? *Experimental gerontology* 35, 53-62.

Garner-Hamrick PA, Fostel JM, Chien WM, Banerjee NS, Chow LT, Broker TR & Fisher C (2004) Global effects of human papillomavirus type 18 E6/E7 in an organotypic keratinocyte culture system. *Journal of virology* 78, 9041-9050.

Gartel AL & Radhakrishnan SK (2005) Lost in transcription: p21 repression, mechanisms, and consequences. *Cancer research* 65, 3980-3985.

Gatherer D (2010) So what do we really mean when we say that systems biology is holistic? *BMC systems biology* 4, 22.

Gatti L, Beretta GL, Carenini N, Corna E, Zunino F & Perego P (2004) Gene expression profiles in the cellular response to a multinuclear platinum complex. *Cell Mol Life Sci* 61, 973-981.

Gibb EA, Brown CJ & Lam WL (2011) The functional role of long non-coding RNA in human carcinomas. *Mol Cancer* 10, 38.

Glas AM, Floore A, Delahaye LJ, Witteveen AT, Pover RC, Bakx N, Lahti-Domenici JS, Bruinsma TJ, Warmoes MO, Bernards R, Wessels LF & Van't Veer LJ (2006) Converting a breast cancer microarray signature into a high-throughput diagnostic test. *BMC Genomics* 7, 278.

Golub TR, Slonim DK, Tamayo P, Huard C, Gaasenbeek M, Mesirov JP, Coller H, Loh ML, Downing JR, Caligiuri MA, Bloomfield CD & Lander ES (1999) Molecular classification of cancer: class discovery and class prediction by gene expression monitoring. *Science* 286, 531-537.

Gray LJ & Herrington CS (2004) Molecular markers for the prediction of progression of CIN lesions. *International journal of gynecological pathology* 23, 95-96.

Guelaguetza Vázquez-Ortíz ea (2005) Análisis de expresión global del cáncer cérvico uterino: rutas metabólicas y genes alterados. *Revista de Investigaciones Clinicas* 57 434-441.

Haffty BG & Glazer PM (2003) Molecular markers in clinical radiation oncology. *Oncogene* 22, 5915-5925.

Hanahan D & Weinberg RA (2000) The hallmarks of cancer. *Cell* 100, 57-70.

Hanson JC, Tangrea MA, Kim S, Armani MD, Pohida TJ, Bonner RF, Rodriguez-Canales J & Emmert-Buck MR (2011) Expression microdissection adapted to commercial laser dissection instruments. *Nature protocols* 6, 457-467.

Harima Y, Sawada S, Miyazaki Y, Kin K, Ishihara H, Imamura M, Sougawa M, Shikata N & Ohnishi T (2003) Expression of Ku80 in cervical cancer correlates with response to radiotherapy and survival. *American journal of clinical oncology* 26, e80-85.

Harima Y, Togashi A, Horikoshi K, Imamura M, Sougawa M, Sawada S, Tsunoda T, Nakamura Y & Katagiri T (2004) Prediction of outcome of advanced cervical cancer to thermoradiotherapy according to expression profiles of 35 genes selected by cDNA microarray analysis. *International journal of radiation oncology, biology, physics* 60, 237-248.

Harrell JC, Dye WW, Harvell DM, Sartorius CA & Horwitz KB (2008) Contaminating cells alter gene signatures in whole organ versus laser capture microdissected tumors: a comparison of experimental breast cancers and their lymph node metastases. *Clinical & experimental metastasis* 25, 81-88.

Harrison PR, Conkie D, Paul J & Jones K (1973) Localisation of cellular globin messenger RNA by in situ hybridisation to complementary DNA. *FEBS letters* 32, 109-112.

Hassan R, Bera T & Pastan I (2004) Mesothelin: a new target for immunotherapy. *Clinical cancer research* 10, 3937-3942.

Helliwell TR (2001) Molecular markers of metastasis in squamous carcinomas. *The Journal of pathology* 194, 289-293.

Hipp J, Cheng J, Hanson JC, Yan W, Taylor P, Hu N, Rodriguez-Canales J, Tangrea MA, Emmert-Buck MR & Balis U (2011) SIVQ-aided laser capture microdissection: A tool for high-throughput expression profiling. *Journal of pathology informatics* 2, 19.

Hoeflich A, Reisinger R, Lahm H, Kiess W, Blum WF, Kolb HJ, Weber MM & Wolf E (2001) Insulin-like growth factor-binding protein 2 in tumorigenesis: protector or promoter? *Cancer research* 61, 8601-8610.

Hollestelle A & Schutte M (2005) Representational difference analysis as a tool in the search for new tumor suppressor genes. *Methods in molecular medicine* 103, 143-159.

Hubank M & Schatz DG (1994) Identifying differences in mRNA expression by representational difference analysis of cDNA. *Nucleic Acids Research* 22, 5640-5648.

Hudelist G, Czerwenka K, Singer C, Pischinger K, Kubista E & Manavi M (2005) cDNA array analysis of cytobrush-collected normal and malignant cervical epithelial cells: a feasibility study. *Cancer genetics and cytogenetics* 158, 35-42.

Hughes TR, Mao M, Jones AR, Burchard J, Marton MJ, Shannon KW, Lefkowitz SM, Ziman M, Schelter JM, Meyer MR, Kobayashi S, Davis C, Dai HY, He YDD, Stephaniants SB, Cavet G, Walker WL, West A, Coffey E, Shoemaker DD, Stoughton R, Blanchard AP, Friend SH & Linsley PS (2001) Expression profiling using microarrays fabricated by an ink-jet oligonucleotide synthesizer. *Nature Biotechnology* 19, 342-347.

Human Genome Sequencing C (2004) Finishing the euchromatic sequence of the human genome. *Nature* 431, 931-945.

Hwang J, Kim YY, Huh S, Shim J, Park C, Kimm K, Choi DK, Park TK & Kim S (2005) The time-dependent serial gene response to Zeocin treatment involves caspase-dependent apoptosis in HeLa cells. *Microbiology and immunology* 49, 331-342.

Ishitobi M, Goranova TE, Komoike Y, Motomura K, Koyama H, Glas AM, van Lienen E, Inaji H, Van't Veer LJ & Kato K (2010) Clinical utility of the 70-gene MammaPrint profile in a Japanese population. *Japanese journal of clinical oncology* 40, 508-512.

Kalantari M, Garcia-Carranca A, Morales-Vazquez CD, Zuna R, Montiel DP, Calleja-Macias IE, Johansson B, Andersson S & Bernard HU (2009) Laser capture microdissection of cervical human papillomavirus infections: copy number of the virus in cancerous and normal tissue and heterogeneous DNA methylation. *Virology* 390, 261-267.

Keating JT, Ince T & Crum CP (2001) Surrogate biomarkers of HPV infection in cervical neoplasia screening and diagnosis. *Advances in anatomic pathology* 8, 83-92.

Kelemen LE (2006) The role of folate receptor alpha in cancer development, progression and treatment: cause, consequence or innocent bystander? *International journal of cancer* 119, 243-250.

Kelley ML, Keiger KE, Lee CJ & Huibregtse JM (2005) The global transcriptional effects of the human papillomavirus E6 protein in cervical carcinoma cell lines are mediated by the E6AP ubiquitin ligase. *Journal of virology* 79, 3737-3747.

Kent WJ (2002) BLAT--the BLAST-like alignment tool. *Genome research* 12, 656-664.

Kitahara O, Katagiri T, Tsunoda T, Harima Y & Nakamura Y (2002) Classification of sensitivity or resistance of cervical cancers to ionizing radiation according to expression profiles of 62 genes selected by cDNA microarray analysis. *Neoplasia* 4, 295-303.

Kitano H (2002) Systems biology: a brief overview. *Science* 295, 1662-1664.

Klaes R, Woerner SM, Ridder R, Wentzensen N, Duerst M, Schneider A, Lotz B, Melsheimer P & von Knebel Doeberitz M (1999) Detection of high-risk cervical intraepithelial neoplasia and cervical cancer by amplification of transcripts derived from integrated papillomavirus oncogenes. *Cancer research* 59, 6132-6136.

Klee EW, Erdogan S, Tillmans L, Kosari F, Sun Z, Wigle DA, Yang P, Aubry MC & Vasmatzis G (2009) Impact of sample acquisition and linear amplification on gene expression profiling of lung adenocarcinoma: laser capture micro-dissection cell-sampling versus bulk tissue-sampling. *BMC medical genomics* 2, 13.

Lander ES & Weinberg RA (2000) Genomics: journey to the center of biology. *Science* 287, 1777-1782.

Lazo PA (1999) The molecular genetics of cervical carcinoma. *British journal of cancer* 80, 2008-2018.

Lee CM, Fuhrman CB, Planelles V, Peltier MR, Gaffney DK, Soisson AP, Dodson MK, Tolley HD, Green CL & Zempolich KA (2006) Phosphatidylinositol 3-kinase inhibition by LY294002 radiosensitizes human cervical cancer cell lines. *Clinical cancer research* 12, 250-256.

Lee KA, Shim JH, Kho CW, Park SG, Park BC, Kim JW, Lim JS, Choe YK, Paik SG & Yoon DY (2004) Protein profiling and identification of modulators regulated by the E7 oncogene in the C33A cell line by proteomics and genomics. *Proteomics* 4, 839-848.

Legrain P, Aebersold R, Archakov A, Bairoch A, Bala K, Beretta L, Bergeron J, Borchers C, Corthals GL, Costello CE, Deutsch EW, Domon B, Hancock W, He F, Hochstrasser D, Marko-Varga G, Salekdeh GH, Sechi S, Snyder M, Srivastava S, Uhlen M, Hu CH, Yamamoto T, Paik YK & Omenn GS (2011) The human proteome project: Current state and future direction. *Molecular & cellular proteomics*.

Li J, Yen C, Liaw D, Podsypanina K, Bose S, Wang SI, Puc J, Miliaresis C, Rodgers L, McCombie R, Bigner SH, Giovanella BC, Ittmann M, Tycko B, Hibshoosh H, Wigler MH & Parsons R (1997) PTEN, a putative protein tyrosine phosphatase gene mutated in human brain, breast, and prostate cancer. *Science* 275, 1943-1947.

Liang P & Pardee AB (1992) Differential display of eukaryotic messenger RNA by means of the polymerase chain reaction. *Science* 257, 967-971.

Liang P & Pardee AB (2003) Analysing differential gene expression in cancer. *Nature Reviews Cancer* 3, 869-876.

Lin J & Li M (2008) Molecular profiling in the age of cancer genomics. *Expert review of molecular diagnostics* 8, 263-276.

Liu SS, Cheung AN & Ngan HY (2003) Differential gene expression in cervical cancer cell lines before and after ionizing radiation. *International journal of oncology* 22, 1091-1099.

Lockhart DJ, Dong HL, Byrne MC, Follettie MT, Gallo MV, Chee MS, Mittmann M, Wang CW, Kobayashi M, Horton H & Brown EL (1996) Expression monitoring by hybridization to high-density oligonucleotide arrays. *Nature Biotechnology* 14, 1675-1680.

Lu X, Toki T, Konishi I, Nikaido T & Fujii S (1998) Expression of p21WAF1/CIP1 in adenocarcinoma of the uterine cervix: a possible immunohistochemical marker of a favorable prognosis. *Cancer* 82, 2409-2417.

Macoska JA (2002) The progressing clinical utility of DNA microarrays. *CA Cancer J Clin* 52, 50-59.

Martin CM, Astbury K & O'Leary JJ (2006) Molecular profiling of cervical neoplasia. *Expert review of molecular diagnostics* 6, 217-229.

Mendes Soares LM & Valcarcel J (2006) The expanding transcriptome: the genome as the 'Book of Sand'. *The EMBO Journal* 25, 923-931.

Mikheev AM, Mikheeva SA, Liu B, Cohen P & Zarbl H (2004) A functional genomics approach for the identification of putative tumor suppressor genes: Dickkopf-1 as suppressor of HeLa cell transformation. *Carcinogenesis* 25, 47-59.

Mook S, Schmidt MK, Viale G, Pruneri G, Eekhout I, Floore A, Glas AM, Bogaerts J, Cardoso F, Piccart-Gebhart MJ, Rutgers ET & Van't Veer LJ (2009) The 70-gene prognosis-signature predicts disease outcome in breast cancer patients with 1-3 positive lymph nodes in an independent validation study. *Breast cancer research and treatment* 116, 295-302.

Nees M, Geoghegan JM, Hyman T, Frank S, Miller L & Woodworth CD (2001) Papillomavirus type 16 oncogenes downregulate expression of interferon-responsive genes and upregulate proliferation-associated and NF-kappaB-responsive genes in cervical keratinocytes. *Journal of virology* 75, 4283-4296.

Nees M, Geoghegan JM, Munson P, Prabhu V, Liu Y, Androphy E & Woodworth CD (2000) Human papillomavirus type 16 E6 and E7 proteins inhibit differentiation-dependent expression of transforming growth factor-beta2 in cervical keratinocytes. *Cancer research* 60, 4289-4298.

Nees M, van Wijngaarden E, Bakos E, Schneider A & Durst M (1998) Identification of novel molecular markers which correlate with HPV-induced tumor progression. *Oncogene* 16, 2447-2458.

Ng P, Wei CL, Sung WK, Chiu KP, Lipovich L, Ang CC, Gupta S, Shahab A, Ridwan A, Wong CH, Liu ET & Ruan Y (2005) Gene identification signature (GIS) analysis for transcriptome characterization and genome annotation. *Nature Methods* 2, 105-111.

Nieh S, Chen SF, Chu TY, Lai HC, Lin YS, Fu E & Gau CH (2005) Is p16(INK4A) expression more useful than human papillomavirus test to determine the outcome of atypical squamous cells of undetermined significance-categorized Pap smear? A comparative analysis using abnormal cervical smears with follow-up biopsies. *Gynecologic oncology* 97, 35-40.

Nisole S, Stoye JP & Saib A (2005) TRIM family proteins: retroviral restriction and antiviral defence. *Nature Reviews Microbiology* 3, 799-808.

Novina CD & Sharp PA (2004) The RNAi revolution. *Nature* 430, 161-164.

Nuovo GJ, Plaia TW, Belinsky SA, Baylin SB & Herman JG (1999) In situ detection of the hypermethylation-induced inactivation of the p16 gene as an early event in oncogenesis. *Proceedings of the National Academy of Sciences of the United States of America* 96, 12754-12759.

Okamoto K & Beach D (1994) Cyclin-G Is a Transcriptional Target of the P53 Tumor-Suppressor Protein. *The EMBO Journal* 13, 4816-4822.

Orlando V (2000) Mapping chromosomal proteins in vivo by formaldehyde-crosslinked-chromatin immunoprecipitation. *Trends in Biochemical Sciences* 25, 99-104.

Perez-Plasencia C, Riggins G, Vazquez-Ortiz G, Moreno J, Arreola H, Hidalgo A, Pina-Sanchez P & Salcedo M (2005) Characterization of the global profile of genes expressed in cervical epithelium by Serial Analysis of Gene Expression (SAGE). *BMC Genomics* 6, 130.

Pett MR, Herdman MT, Palmer RD, Yeo GS, Shivji MK, Stanley MA & Coleman N (2006) Selection of cervical keratinocytes containing integrated HPV16 associates with episome loss and an endogenous antiviral response. *Proceedings of the National Academy of Sciences of the United States of America* 103, 3822-3827.

Polyak K & Riggins GJ (2001) Gene discovery using the serial analysis of gene expression technique: Implications for cancer research. *Journal of Clinical Oncology* 19, 2948-2958.

Quackenbush J (2004) Data standards for 'omic' science. *Nature Biotechnology* 22, 613-614.

Ramaswamy S, Ross KN, Lander ES & Golub TR (2003) A molecular signature of metastasis in primary solid tumors. *Nature Genetics* 33, 49-54.

Ranamukhaarachchi DG, Unger ER, Vernon SD, Lee D & Rajeevan MS (2005) Gene expression profiling of dysplastic differentiation in cervical epithelial cells harboring human papillomavirus 16. *Genomics* 85, 727-738.

Rappolee DA, Mark D, Banda MJ & Werb Z (1988) Wound macrophages express TGF-alpha and other growth factors in vivo: analysis by mRNA phenotyping. *Science* 241, 708-712.

Ren B, Robert F, Wyrick JJ, Aparicio O, Jennings EG, Simon I, Zeitlinger J, Schreiber J, Hannett N, Kanin E, Volkert TL, Wilson CJ, Bell SP & Young RA (2000) Genome-wide location and function of DNA binding proteins. *Science* 290, 2306-+.

Rhodes DR & Chinnaiyan AM (2005) Integrative analysis of the cancer transcriptome. *Nature Genetics* 37, S31-S37.

Rosenwald A, Wright G, Chan WC, Connors JM, Campo E, Fisher RI, Gascoyne RD, Muller-Hermelink HK, Smeland EB, Giltnane JM, Hurt EM, Zhao H, Averett L, Yang L, Wilson WH, Jaffe ES, Simon R, Klausner RD, Powell J, Duffey PL, Longo DL, Greiner TC, Weisenburger DD, Sanger WG, Dave BJ, Lynch JC, Vose J, Armitage JO, Montserrat E, Lopez-Guillermo A, Grogan TM, Miller TP, LeBlanc M, Ott G, Kvaloy S, Delabie J, Holte H, Krajci P, Stokke T & Staudt LM (2002) The use of molecular profiling to predict survival after chemotherapy for diffuse large-B-cell lymphoma. *The New England journal of medicine* 346, 1937-1947.

Rosty C, Sheffer M, Tsafrir D, Stransky N, Tsafrir I, Peter M, de Cremoux P, de La Rochefordiere A, Salmon R, Dorval T, Thiery JP, Couturier J, Radvanyi F, Domany E & Sastre-Garau X (2005) Identification of a proliferation gene cluster associated with HPV E6/E7 expression level and viral DNA load in invasive cervical carcinoma. *Oncogene* 24, 7094-7104.

Ruutu M, Peitsaro P, Johansson B & Syrjanen S (2002) Transcriptional profiling of a human papillomavirus 33-positive squamous epithelial cell line which acquired a selective growth advantage after viral integration. *International journal of cancer* 100, 318-326.

Sakakura C, Hagiwara A, Miyagawa K, Nakashima S, Yoshikawa T, Kin S, Nakase Y, Ito K, Yamagishi H, Yazumi S, Chiba T & Ito Y (2005) Frequent downregulation of the runt domain transcription factors RUNX1, RUNX3 and their cofactor CBFB in gastric cancer. *International journal of cancer* 113, 221-228.

Santin AD, Zhan F, Bignotti E, Siegel ER, Cane S, Bellone S, Palmieri M, Anfossi S, Thomas M, Burnett A, Kay HH, Roman JJ, O'Brien TJ, Tian E, Cannon MJ, Shaughnessy J, Jr. & Pecorelli S (2005) Gene expression profiles of primary HPV16- and HPV18-infected early stage cervical cancers and normal cervical epithelium: identification of novel candidate molecular markers for cervical cancer diagnosis and therapy. *Virology* 331, 269-291.

Schena M, Shalon D, Davis RW & Brown PO (1995) Quantitative Monitoring of Gene-Expression Patterns with a Complementary-DNA Microarray. *Science* 270, 467-470.

Segal E, Friedman N, Kaminski N, Regev A & Koller D (2005) From signatures to models: understanding cancer using microarrays. *Nature Genetics* 37 Suppl, S38-45.

Seo MJ, Bae SM, Kim YW, Hur SY, Ro DY, Lee JM, Namkoong SE, Kim CK & Ahn WS (2005) New approaches to pathogenic gene function discovery with human squamous cell cervical carcinoma by gene ontology. *Gynecologic oncology* 96, 621-629.

Sgarlato GD, Eastman CL & Sussman HH (2005) Panel of genes transcriptionally up-regulated in squamous cell carcinoma of the cervix identified by representational difference analysis, confirmed by macroarray, and validated by real-time quantitative reverse transcription-PCR. *Clinical chemistry* 51, 27-34.

Shapiro JA (2009) Revisiting the central dogma in the 21st century. *Annals of the New York Academy of Sciences* 1178, 6-28.

Sherman ME (2003) Chapter 11: Future directions in cervical pathology. *Journal of the National Cancer Institute. Monographs*, 72-79.

Sherman ME & Kurman RJ (1998) Intraepithelial carcinoma of the cervix: reflections on half a century of progress. *Cancer* 83, 2243-2246.

Shim C, Zhang W, Rhee CH & Lee JH (1998) Profiling of differentially expressed genes in human primary cervical cancer by complementary DNA expression array. *Clinical cancer research* 4, 3045-3050.

Shipp MA, Ross KN, Tamayo P, Weng AP, Kutok JL, Aguiar RC, Gaasenbeek M, Angelo M, Reich M, Pinkus GS, Ray TS, Koval MA, Last KW, Norton A, Lister TA, Mesirov J, Neuberg DS, Lander ES, Aster JC & Golub TR (2002) Diffuse large B-cell lymphoma outcome prediction by gene-expression profiling and supervised machine learning. *Nature medicine* 8, 68-74.

Silvestri A, Colombatti A, Calvert VS, Deng J, Mammano E, Belluco C, De Marchi F, Nitti D, Liotta LA, Petricoin EF & Pierobon M (2010) Protein pathway biomarker analysis of human cancer reveals requirement for upfront cellular-enrichment processing. *Laboratory investigation; a journal of technical methods and pathology* 90, 787-796.

Singh-Gasson S, Green RD, Yue Y, Nelson C, Blattner F, Sussman MR & Cerrina F (1999) Maskless fabrication of light-directed oligonucleotide microarrays using a digital micromirror array. *Nature Biotechnology* 17, 974-978.

Slodkowska EA & Ross JS (2009) MammaPrint 70-gene signature: another milestone in personalized medical care for breast cancer patients. *Expert review of molecular diagnostics* 9, 417-422.

Snijders PJ, Steenbergen RD, Heideman DA & Meijer CJ (2006) HPV-mediated cervical carcinogenesis: concepts and clinical implications. *The Journal of pathology* 208, 152-164.

Sopov I, Sorensen T, Magbagbeolu M, Jansen L, Beer K, Kuhne-Heid R, Kirchmayr R, Schneider A & Durst M (2004) Detection of cancer-related gene expression profiles in severe cervical neoplasia. *International journal of cancer* 112, 33-43.

Southan C (2004) Has the yo-yo stopped? An assessment of human protein-coding gene number. *Proteomics* 4, 1712-1726.

Sova P, Feng Q, Geiss G, Wood T, Strauss R, Rudolf V, Lieber A & Kiviat N (2006) Discovery of novel methylation biomarkers in cervical carcinoma by global demethylation and microarray analysis. *Cancer epidemiology, biomarkers & prevention* 15, 114-123.

Stein LD (2004) Human genome: end of the beginning. *Nature* 431, 915-916.

Steinau M, Lee DR, Rajeevan MS, Vernon SD, Ruffin MT & Unger ER (2005) Gene expression profile of cervical tissue compared to exfoliated cells: impact on biomarker discovery. *BMC Genomics* 6, 64.

Strausberg RL, Feingold EA, Grouse LH, Derge JG, Klausner RD, Collins FS, Wagner L, Shenmen CM, Schuler GD, Altschul SF, Zeeberg B, Buetow KH, Schaefer CF, Bhat NK, Hopkins RF, Jordan H, Moore T, Max SI, Wang J, Hsieh F, Diatchenko L, Marusina K, Farmer AA, Rubin GM, Hong L, Stapleton M, Soares MB, Bonaldo MF, Casavant TL, Scheetz TE, Brownstein MJ, Usdin TB, Toshiyuki S, Carninci P, Prange C, Raha SS, Loquellano NA, Peters GJ, Abramson RD, Mullahy SJ, Bosak SA, McEwan PJ, McKernan KJ, Malek JA, Gunaratne PH, Richards S, Worley KC, Hale S, Garcia AM, Gay LJ, Hulyk SW, Villalon DK, Muzny DM, Sodergren EJ, Lu X, Gibbs RA, Fahey J, Helton E, Ketteman M, Madan A, Rodrigues S, Sanchez A, Whiting M, Young AC, Shevchenko Y, Bouffard GG, Blakesley RW, Touchman JW, Green ED, Dickson MC, Rodriguez AC, Grimwood J, Schmutz J, Myers RM, Butterfield YS, Krzywinski MI, Skalska U, Smailus DE, Schnerch A, Schein JE, Jones SJ & Marra MA (2002) Generation and initial analysis of more than 15,000 full-length human and mouse cDNA sequences. *Proceedings of the National Academy of Sciences of the United States of America* 99, 16899-16903.

Strebhardt K & Ullrich A (2006) Targeting polo-like kinase 1 for cancer therapy. *Nature Reviews Cancer* 6, 321-330.

Tangrea MA, Chuaqui RF, Gillespie JW, Ahram M, Gannot G, Wallis BS, Best CJ, Linehan WM, Liotta LA, Pohida TJ, Bonner RF & Emmert-Buck MR (2004) Expression microdissection: operator-independent retrieval of cells for molecular profiling. *Diagnostic molecular pathology* 13, 207-212.

Tewari D, Monk BJ, Al-Ghazi MS, Parker R, Heck JD, Burger RA & Fruehauf JP (2005) Gene expression profiling of in vitro radiation resistance in cervical carcinoma: a feasibility study. *Gynecologic oncology* 99, 84-91.

Thierry F, Benotmane MA, Demeret C, Mori M, Teissier S & Desaintes C (2004) A genomic approach reveals a novel mitotic pathway in papillomavirus carcinogenesis. *Cancer research* 64, 895-903.

Thomas JT, Oh ST, Terhune SS & Laimins LA (2001) Cellular changes induced by low-risk human papillomavirus type 11 in keratinocytes that stably maintain viral episomes. *Journal of virology* 75, 7564-7571.

Thorgeirsson SS, Lee JS & Grisham JW (2006) Functional genomics of hepatocellular carcinoma. *Hepatology* 43, S145-150.

Tian S, Roepman P, Van't Veer LJ, Bernards R, de Snoo F & Glas AM (2010) Biological functions of the genes in the mammaprint breast cancer profile reflect the hallmarks of cancer. *Biomark Insights* 5, 129-138.

Toussaint-Smith E, Donner DB & Roman A (2004) Expression of human papillomavirus type 16 E6 and E7 oncoproteins in primary foreskin keratinocytes is sufficient to alter the expression of angiogenic factors. *Oncogene* 23, 2988-2995.

Usmani N, Foroudi F, Du J, Zakos C, Campbell H, Bryson P & Mackillop WJ (2005) An evidence-based estimate of the appropriate rate of utilization of radiotherapy for cancer of the cervix. *International journal of radiation oncology, biology, physics* 63, 812-827.

van 't Veer LJ, Dai H, van de Vijver MJ, He YD, Hart AA, Mao M, Peterse HL, van der Kooy K, Marton MJ, Witteveen AT, Schreiber GJ, Kerkhoven RM, Roberts C, Linsley PS, Bernards R & Friend SH (2002) Gene expression profiling predicts clinical outcome of breast cancer. *Nature* 415, 530-536.

van de Vijver MJ, He YD, van't Veer LJ, Dai H, Hart AA, Voskuil DW, Schreiber GJ, Peterse JL, Roberts C, Marton MJ, Parrish M, Atsma D, Witteveen A, Glas A, Delahaye L, van der Velde T, Bartelink H, Rodenhuis S, Rutgers ET, Friend SH & Bernards R (2002) A gene-expression signature as a predictor of survival in breast cancer. *The New England journal of medicine* 347, 1999-2009.

Vazquez-Ortiz G, Ciudad CJ, Pina P, Vazquez K, Hidalgo A, Alatorre B, Garcia JA, Salamanca F, Peralta-Rodriguez R, Rangel A & Salcedo M (2005a) Gene identification by cDNA arrays in HPV-positive cervical cancer. *Archives of medical research* 36, 448-458.

Vazquez-Ortiz G, Pina-Sanchez P, Vazquez K, Duenas A, Taja L, Mendoza P, Garcia JA & Salcedo M (2005b) Overexpression of cathepsin F, matrix metalloproteinases 11 and 12 in cervical cancer. *BMC Cancer* 5, 68.

Velculescu VE, Zhang L, Vogelstein B & Kinzler KW (1995) Serial Analysis of Gene-Expression. *Science* 270, 484-487.

Vogelstein B & Kinzler KW (2004) Cancer genes and the pathways they control. *Nature medicine* 10, 789-799.

Wadlow R & Ramaswamy S (2005) DNA microarrays in clinical cancer research. *Current molecular medicine* 5, 111-120.

Wain HM, Lush MJ, Ducluzeau F, Khodiyar VK & Povey S (2004) Genew: the Human Gene Nomenclature Database, 2004 updates. *Nucleic Acids Research* 32, D255-257.

Wei CL, Wu Q, Vega VB, Chiu KP, Ng P, Zhang T, Shahab A, Yong HC, Fu YT, Weng ZP, Liu JJ, Zhao XD, Chew JL, Lee YL, Kuznetsov VA, Sung WK, Miller LD, Lim B, Liu ET, Yu Q, Ng HH & Ruan YJ (2006) A global map of p53 transcription-factor binding sites in the human genome. *Cell* 124, 207-219.

Wells SI, Aronow BJ, Wise TM, Williams SS, Couget JA & Howley PM (2003) Transcriptome signature of irreversible senescence in human papillomavirus-positive cervical cancer cells. *Proceedings of the National Academy of Sciences of the United States of America* 100, 7093-7098.

Wheeler DL, Barrett T, Benson DA, Bryant SH, Canese K, Chetvernin V, Church DM, Dicuccio M, Edgar R, Federhen S, Feolo M, Geer LY, Helmberg W, Kapustin Y, Khovayko O, Landsman D, Lipman DJ, Madden TL, Maglott DR, Miller V, Ostell J, Pruitt KD, Schuler GD, Shumway M, Sequeira E, Sherry ST, Sirotkin K, Souvorov A, Starchenko G, Tatusov RL, Tatusova TA, Wagner L & Yaschenko E (2008) Database resources of the National Center for Biotechnology Information. *Nucleic Acids Research* 36, D13-21.

Whitfield ML, George LK, Grant GD & Perou CM (2006) Common markers of proliferation. *Nature Reviews Cancer* 6, 99-106.

Wilting SM, Snijders PJ, Meijer GA, Ylstra B, van den Ijssel PR, Snijders AM, Albertson DG, Coffa J, Schouten JP, van de Wiel MA, Meijer CJ & Steenbergen RD (2006) Increased gene copy numbers at chromosome 20q are frequent in both squamous cell carcinomas and adenocarcinomas of the cervix. *The Journal of pathology* 209, 220-230.

Wong YF, Cheung TH, Tsao GS, Lo KW, Yim SF, Wang VW, Heung MM, Chan SC, Chan LK, Ho TW, Wong KW, Li C, Guo Y, Chung TK & Smith DI (2006) Genome-wide gene expression profiling of cervical cancer in Hong Kong women by oligonucleotide microarray. *International journal of cancer* 118, 2461-2469.

Wong YF, Selvanayagam ZE, Wei N, Porter J, Vittal R, Hu R, Lin Y, Liao J, Shih JW, Cheung TH, Lo KW, Yim SF, Yip SK, Ngong DT, Siu N, Chan LK, Chan CS, Kong T, Kutlina E, McKinnon RD, Denhardt DT, Chin KV & Chung TK (2003) Expression genomics of cervical cancer: molecular classification and prediction of radiotherapy response by DNA microarray. *Clinical cancer research* 9, 5486-5492.

Woodman CBJ, Collins SI & Young LS (2007) The natural history of cervical HPV infection: unresolved issues. *Nature Reviews Cancer* 7, 11-22.

Woodworth CD, Michael E, Marker D, Allen S, Smith L & Nees M (2005) Inhibition of the epidermal growth factor receptor increases expression of genes that stimulate inflammation, apoptosis, and cell attachment. *Molecular cancer therapeutics* 4, 650-658.

Yamashita T, Honda M & Kaneko S (2008) Application of Serial Analysis of Gene Expression in cancer research. *Current pharmaceutical biotechnology* 9, 375-382.

Yen CC, Chen YJ, Pan CC, Lu KH, Chen PC, Hsia JY, Chen JT, Wu YC, Hsu WH, Wang LS, Huang MH, Huang BS, Hu CP, Chen PM & Lin CH (2005) Copy number changes of target genes in chromosome 3q25.3-qter of esophageal squamous cell carcinoma: TP63 is amplified in early carcinogenesis but down-regulated as disease progressed. *World journal of gastroenterology : WJG* 11, 1267-1272.

Yim EK & Park JS (2006) Role of proteomics in translational research in cervical cancer. *Expert review of proteomics* 3, 21-36.

Yuan J, Yan R, Kramer A, Eckerdt F, Roller M, Kaufmann M & Strebhardt K (2004) Cyclin B1 depletion inhibits proliferation and induces apoptosis in human tumor cells. *Oncogene* 23, 5843-5852.

Zimmermann CR, Orr WC, Leclerc RF, Barnard EC & Timberlake WE (1980) Molecular cloning and selection of genes regulated in Aspergillus development. *Cell* 21, 709-715.

zur Hausen H (2002) Papillomaviruses and cancer: from basic studies to clinical application. *Nature Reviews Cancer* 2, 342-350.

zur Hausen H (2009) The search for infectious causes of human cancers: Where and why (Nobel lecutre). *Angewandte Chemie International Edition* 48, 5798-5808.

12

Evaluation of p53, p16^{INK4a} and E-Cadherin Status as Biomarkers for Cervical Cancer Diagnosis

M. El Mzibri[1,*], M. Attaleb[1], R. Ameziane El Hassani[1], M. Khyatti[2], L. Benbacer[1], M. M. Ennaji[3] and M. Amrani[4]

[1]*Unité de Biologie et Recherche Médicale, Centre National de l'Energie, des Sciences et Techniques Nucléaires (CNESTEN), Rabat*

[2]*Laboratoire d'Onco-Virologie, Institut Pasteur du Maroc, Casablanca*

[3]*Laboratoire Virologie Hygiène and Microbiologie, Faculté des Sciences et Techniques Mohammédia*

[4]*Service d'Anatomie Pathologique, Institut National d'Oncologie, Rabat*

Morocco

1. Introduction

Worldwide, carcinoma of the uterine cervix is one of the most common malignancies among women. Incidence rates of this disease vary from about 5 cases per 100 000 women per year in many industrialized countries to more than 50 per 100 000 in some developing nations. Approximately 80% of all cases occur in less-developed countries, because prevention programs are either non-existent or poorly conducted (WHO, 2009). Furthermore, in the less developed areas of the world, cervical cancer begins to strike significantly among women as young as 25-30 years of age, clearly identifying this disease as the cancer priority in women.

Clinical epidemiology have clearly identified that the association between infection with high-risk types of human papillomavirus (HPV) and high-grade cervical cancer precursors as well as cervical cancer is very strong (Wright Jr., 2006). However, even high-risk HPV infection are widespread in the world, the majority of HPV-associated lesions such as cervical intraepithelial neoplasia (CIN) will remain stable or spontaneously regress over time (zur Hausen, 2000; Ferenczy, 2001; Holowaty, 1999; Syrjanen, 1996), suggesting that other genetic and epigenetic events are likely to be involved in cervical carcinogenesis. Indeed, genomic alterations leading to tumor suppressor gene inactivation and/or oncogene activation are the critical pathways in the development and progression of cervical cancer as well as the other types of cancer. In this field, p53, p16 and E-cadherin are important proteins that play critical role in the development and the progression of cervical cancer.

* Corresponding Author

2. Human papillomavirus and cervical cancer

Association between HPV and cervical lesions and cancer has started in 1970s' years after the hypothesis that cervical cancer may arise from infections with the virus found in condylomata acuminata (zur Hausen, 1975; 1976). Then epidemiological and clinical studies have clearly demonstrated that HPV are the major etiologic agents of neoplasia of the cutaneous and mucosal epithelia; HPV positivity in cervical cancer is estimated to be between 90% and 95% (zur Hausen, 1991; Munoz, 2003). Currently, there is compelling evidence to indicate that the development of human cervical cancer without involvement of the specific HPV is exceptional.

Up to now, more than 200 HPV genotypes were recensed, but the interest is focused only on 30 types that are closely associated to cervical lesions. Among them, 15 HPV types have been classified as high risk types (16, 18, 31, 33, 35, 39, 45, 51, 52, 56, 58, 59, 68, 73, and 82); three have been classified as probable high risk types (26, 53, and 66); and 12 have been classified as low risk types (6, 11, 40, 42, 43, 44, 54, 61, 70, 72, 81, and CP6108) (Munoz, 2003). Among the high risk HPV genotypes, HPV-16 is the most common in squamous cell carcinoma of the cervix (50–60%), followed by HPV-18, which is present in about 11–15% of cervical cancer cases (Munoz, 2003, Saranath, 2002).

HPV genomes code for at least six different early and two late proteins. The structure of the genome and the characteristic properties of individual viral proteins have been well reviewed (zur Hausen, 2000; Stanley, 2010; Moody & Laimins, 2010). High-risk HPVs code for at least three proteins with growthstimulating and transforming properties (E5, E6, and E7).

In the pathogenesis of cervical carcinoma we can identify three major factors. Two of them are related to the HPV presence, the effects of viral E6 and E7 proteins, and the consequences of HPV DNA integration in the cellular genome. The third factor is the accumulation of cellular genetic damage, not related to HPV, needed for tumour development (Lazo, 1999).

Viral DNA integrated into host genome is found in all cases of cervical carcinoma (Bosch, 1995), their metastasis and derivative cell lines (Cullen, 1991).

HPV DNA integration into host chromatin is usually a necessary event in the pathogenesis of HPV-related cervical cancer. It is one of the key stages in malignant progression and is therefore a potential biomarker that precedes invasive disease.

Many studies have demonstrated that the integrated HPV DNA is linearized between the E1 and L1 genes. Upon viral integration, variable parts of the HPV genome are disrupted; fragments containing E2 and E4 ORFs are missing whereas the entire E1, E6 and E7 ORFs are integrated and retained (Raybould, 2011).

HPV viral integration is made in such way that the viral regulatory region and the E6 and E7 genes are expressed from viral promoters, but with a different regulation, in which cellular factors might play an important role (Lazo, 1999; Raybould, 2011). In the normal HPV life-cycle expression of E5, E6 and E7 is tightly regulated within cells that are destined to be lost from surface epithelial layers, such that they do not pose a carcinogenic threat (Raybould, 2011)

E5 expression enhances oncogenic potential (Stoppler, 1996; Maufort, 2010) but the exact function of E5 remains poorly understood. E6 and E7 expression is essential for maintenance of the transformed state and malignant progression (Bosch, 1990; von Knebel Doeberitz, 1988).

The implication of E6 and E7 proteins in cervical cancer progression is mainly due through their interactions with hTERT, p53 and Retinoblastoma protein (pRB). hTERT is a catalytic subunit of Telomerase that acts to synthesise telomere ends of linear chromosomes during DNA replication. p53 is a transcription factor that regulates cell cycle arrest, apoptosis, senescence, DNA repair and cell metabolism; p53 activity is inhibited by ubiquitin ligase which also ubiquitinates p53 to initiate p53 degradation (Figure 1). In addition to inducing the rapid degradation of p53, E6 also binds to and degrades FADD, preventing the transmission of apoptotic signals via the Fas pathway (Filippova, 2004).

pRB is a tumour suppressor protein and interacts with transcription factor E2F to repress the transcription of genes required for the S phase of the cell cycle (Figure 1). E7 can also bind to other connected proteins such as p107 and p130 (Raybould, 2011).

Currently vaccination based strategy is an alternative method showed to be amore effective and practical approach than the implementation of regular and periodic cytological screening. Today it is very well established that intervention with vaccines permits already the statement that essential precursor lesions of this cancer are efficiently prevented (Zur Hausen, 2009).

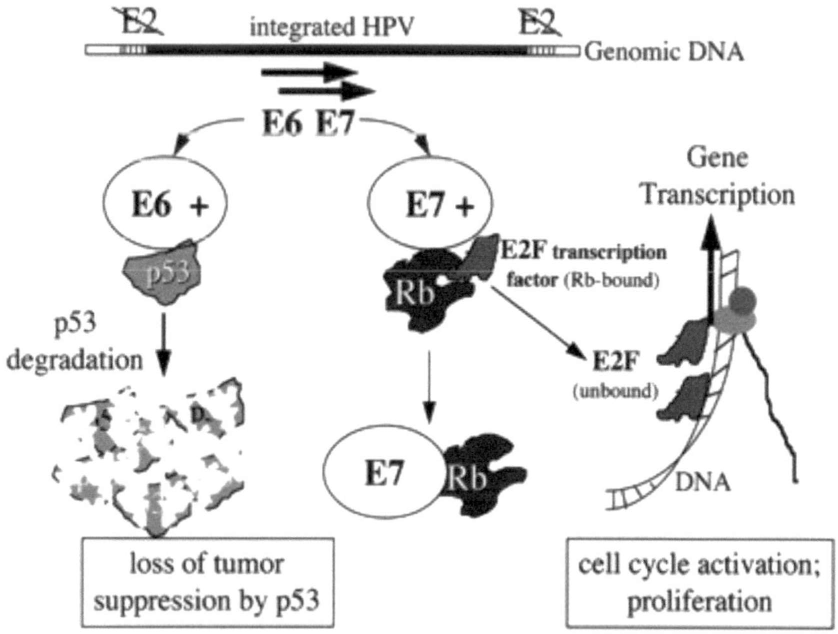

Fig. 1. Schematic representation of E6 and E7 activities in cervical cells

3. p53 expression and polymorphism in cervical cancer

The human tumour suppressor gene p53 plays a key role in the cell's response to genotoxic stress and loss of this 'guardian of the genome' is an important step in carcinogenesis. The highly significant tumour suppressor gene, p53, is implicated in a wide range of human cancers, and is a multifunctional protein that plays critical roles in cellular responses to DNA damage, cellular senescence and apoptosis to maintain genomic stability of a cell (Kashima, 2007). p53 encodes a transcription factor at the centre of a network that maintains cellular integrity by the inhibition of cell growth and stimulation of apoptosis in response to cellular stresses such as DNA damage (Scheffner, 1990).

Because mutation of the p53 gene is a relatively rare event in cervical cancer, p53 activity is mainly inhibited by the viral oncoprotein E6. It's clearly identified that abrogation of p53 function by the E6 protein of HPV is thought to be one of the major events in cervical carcinogenesis (Soussi, 2001). The viral E6 protein interacts with protein p53 and inhibits its activity, followed by proteolytic degradation through the ubiquitin pathway (Scheffner, 1990; Werness, 1990).

As shown if Figure 2, expression of p53 on cervical cancer biopsies showed that the p53 immunoreactivity is detected especially in nuclei. The expression is greater in the peripheral cells of tumours.

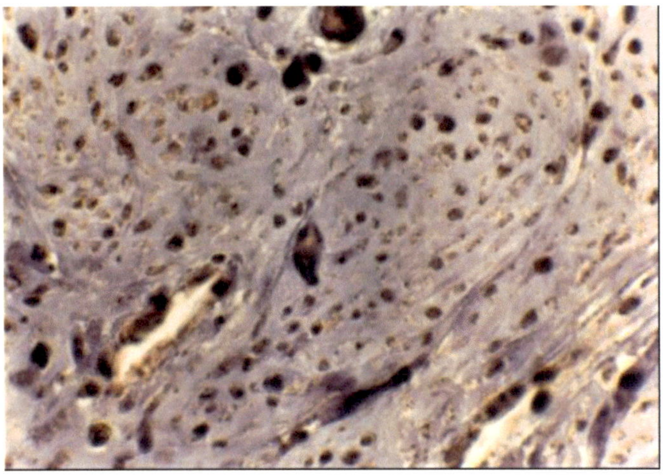

Fig. 2. Representative p53 immunohistochemical staining in epidermoid carcinoma

Different studies showed that p53 expression did not correlate with tumour recurrence demonstrating that immunohistochemistry for p53 protein appears to provide no prognostic information for all patients with cervical cancer (Abd El All, 1999; Vasilescu, 2009; Abrahao, 2011). However, it still remains a prognostic factor for the aggressive behavior of the tumour, when it exceeds more than 30% positivity in tumour cells nuclei (Vasilescu, 2009). Many studies, using different p53 monoclonal antibodies, have reported the lack of any association between p53 IHC expression and staging (Abd El All, 1999). Indeed, in HPV positive cervical carcinoma, the wild type p53 complex with E6 of HPV 16 or 18, is degraded and cannot be detected by IHC. In other cancers, Overexpression of p53 in tissues has generally been assumed to reflect accumulation of p53 mutations.

Several polymorphisms have been identified within the p53 gene, both in non-coding and coding regions and may represent an important contribution to cancer susceptibility and tumour behaviour (Costa, 2008). The common polymorphism is known at codon 72, with two alleles encoding either arginine (p53 Arg) or proline (p53 Pro) (Matlashewski, 1987). The genotype of p53 gene at codon 72 is detected by PCR with allele specific primers "ASP" that especially detects either the p53Pro or p53Arg allele. DNA is amplified in separate reactions with p53 Pro and p53 Arg primers. Example of resulting amplifications is reported in Figure 3.

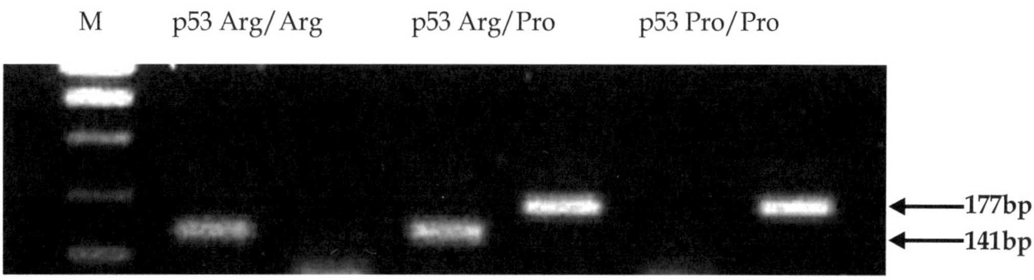

Fig. 3. Analysis of p53 codon 72 polymorphism by PCR using allele specific primers
Arg allele specific primers: 141 bp and Pro allele specific primers: 177 bp. M: 100 bp ladder.

The Pro/Pro, Pro/Arg, and Arg/Arg frequencies have been reported in human cancers including lung, colorectal, breast, stomach, bladder, head and neck and oral, for their association with predisposition and subsequent increased susceptibility to the cancer. These studies have shown that the presence of Arg/Arg genotype has been associated with increased susceptibility to cervical cancer and Pro/Pro genotype is more frequent in lung cancers (Storey, 1998; Hamel, 2000; Tandle, 2001).

This polymorphism occurs in the proline-rich domain of the p53 protein, which is necessary for the protein to fully induce apoptosis (Zhu, 2007). The functional difference between the 2 alleles of this polymorphism is that the Arg/Arg genotype induces apoptosis with faster kinetics and suppresses transformation more efficiently than the Pro/Pro genotype (Kuroda, 2007). In cervical cancer, different studies have investigated the effect of the codon 72 polymorphism of p53 on the susceptibility to E6-mediated degradation. They reported that individuals homozygous for p53 Arg are more susceptible to HPV-associated carcinogenesis of the cervix than heterozygotes (Storey, 1998). However the relationship between the p53 polymorphism and susceptibility of HPV infection as well as cervical cancer development is still unclear.

Storey *et al.* (1998) showed that the codon 72 arginine variant of *p53* encodes a protein that is more sensitive to HPV16 and HPV18 degradation than the proline variant. The biological and biochemical differences between the two p53 genotypes at codon 72 were demonstrated by a study showing that the arginine form of the protein was much more susceptible to HPV E6 mediated degradation than the proline form (Mitra, 2005; Oliveira, 2008). Moreover, Thomas *et al.* (1999), presented evidence that, *in vitro*, the p53 arginine variant induces apoptosis with faster kinetics and suppresses transformation more efficiently than the p53 proline variant. These observations may have implications for the development of cancer in subjects harbouring p53 modified sequences and for the responsiveness of tumours to therapy.

The case-control study conducted in 113 cancerous lesions and 100 healthy women from Morocco highlighted the absence of any association between p53 polymorphism at codon 72 and cervical cancer development (Meftah El Khair, 2009). However reported data on the prevalence of p53 polymorphism in cervical cancer patients are controversial and the ethnic group characteristics seem to be an important reason for discrepancies in the frequency of this polymorphism (Brenna, 2004; Wang, 1999; Wu, 2004; Pegoraro, 2002; Klug, 2001; Szarka, 2000; Agorastos, 2000; Hildesheim, 1998; Bhattacharya, 2002). Moreover, other potential confounding factors should be also considered including the sample size, the source of DNA and the detection techniques used. Another important reason for these discrepant results could be misclassification of the p53 polymorphism, due to inter-laboratory variations in protocols, affecting the ability to detect p53 polymorphisms (Brenna, 2004; Govan, 2007; Sousa, 2007).

4. Epigenetic alteration and cervical cancer

Cancer is a multi-factor process. Molecular analysis of tumours reveals genetic and epigenetic abnormalities. Genetic mutations, which alter DNA sequence, lead to constitute activation of some oncogenes (as RAS and RAF genes) and inhibition of some tumour suppressors (as p53 gene). Epigenetic mutations (epimutations) lead often to gene silencing without altering the DNA sequence. Alteration in expression of key genes through aberrant epigenetic regulation can lead to initiation, promotion and maintenance of carcinogenesis, and is even implicated in the generation of drug resistance. The significance of epigenetic alterations is used as predictive biomarkers and as new targets of anticancer therapy.

Genetic information may not be the only relevant source of information in order to understand the molecular basis of disease. Epigenetic information may hold the key to a better understanding of various pathological conditions (Chahwan, 2011).

Epigenetic mechanisms are essential for normal development and maintenance of tissue-specific gene expression patterns in mammals. These include embryonic development, transcription, chromatin structure, X-chromosome inactivation, genomic imprinting, and chromosome stability (Watanabe, 2010). Epigenetic dysregulation, which may be passed from one generation to the next, are believed to be implicated in the promotion of tumorigenesis in cancers through the downregulation of tumour repressor genes (Hidemi, 2011). Epigenetic aberrations, often observed in tumours, include changes in DNA methylation and histone modifications that influence the chromatin states and impact gene expression patterns. Methylation of cytosine bases in DNA is the main epigenetic event and is involved in most cellular physiopathological processes (Watanabe, 2010).

The CpG islands, where Cytosine and Guanine are connected by a phosphodiester bond, are shorts stretches of DNA in which the frequency of the CG sequence is higher than other regions. CpG islands are mostly located in the upstream promoter and exon 1 region of over half of human genes (Lo, 2008). In mammals, the methylation process is achieved by the DNA methyltransferase (DNMT), that catalyses the transfer of the methyl group from S-adenosyl L-methionine (SAM) to the cytosine in 5'-CG-3' sequence.

In cancer, abnormal hypermethylation of gene promoter CpG islands induces transcriptional silencing of tumour suppressor genes (Lo, 2008) and is by far the best-categorised epigenetic change.

Inactivation of tumour suppressor genes by promoter hypermethylation has been recognized to be at least as common as gene disruption by mutation in tumorigenesis (Jones, 2002).

Multiple genes are hypermethylated in primary carcinomas as well as in carcinoma cell line and the methylation profile has strong associations with genetic and clinicopathological features (Lind, 2004).

HPV regulates the methylation status of genes involved in the cell cycle regulation, apoptosis, DNA repair, cell adhesion and migration, development and differentiation, cellular signalling and metabolism (Anita Szalmás, 2009).

The HPV oncoprotein E7 control cellular proliferation pathways through epigenetic mechanisms. Recently, it has been shown that E7 bind directly to the DNMT1 and activate its DNA methyltransferase activity. This direct association may lead to aberrant methylation of the genome followed by cellular transformation as a result of tumour suppressor gene silencing (Burgers, 2007). E7 can induce viral replication also through epigenetic changes. E7 inhibits HDAC (histone deacetylase) binding to the E2F promoter resulting in activation of expression and facilitates HPV replication (Longworth, 2005).

HPV can epigenetically regulate cell cycle via down regulation of p16INK4A, an inhibitor of cyclin dependent phosphorylation and inactivation of Rb (retinoblastoma) tumour suppressor protein. The occurrence of p16INK4A promoter hypermethylation is very low in low grade of cervical cancer and it increases moderately with the severity of the carcinogenetic stages (Wong, 1999; Gustafson, 2004).

Cyclin A1 (CCNA1) is involved in cell cycle regulation and in repair of DNA doublestrand breaks. Kitkumthorn *et al.* (2006) have evaluated the epigenetic status of cyclin A1 in HPV-associated cervical cancer. The authors demonstrated that cyclin A1 methylation is common in cervical cancer and is specific to the invasive phenotype indicating that hypermethylation of promoter of cyclin A1 is a potential tumour marker for early diagnosis of invasive cervical cancer (Kitkumthorn, 2006)

E-cadherin is a transmembrane glycoprotein that mediates interactions between adjacent epithelial cells. Hypermethylation of CpG islands in E-cadherin promoter regions is associated with suppressed transcriptional activity and it is particularly found in various in invasive cervical cancers (Kang S 2006).

5. Study of gene promoter methylation

For gene-specific methylation analysis, a large number of techniques have been developed. Most early studies used methylation sensitive restriction enzymes to digest DNA followed by Southern detection or PCR amplification. Recently, bisulfite reaction based methods have become very popular. In these techniques, analysis of DNA methylation is based on bisulfite treatment of genomic DNA, which converts cytosine to uracil, but methylated cytosines remain unaltered in this process. Several techniques have been applied to analyse bisulfite-modified DNA, with variation in sensitivity, amount of DNA needed. However, PCR based techniques are the fast, simple and reliable methods to assess the methylation status of DNA. After PCR amplification, uracil will be converted to thymidine, which will be determined by direct PCR sequencing (bisulfite sequencing) or methylation specific PCR

(MSP-PCR) (Figure 4). In bisulfite sequencing, primers are designed not to contain any CpGs to avoid discrimination against methylated or unmethylated DNA. In MSP-PCR, two pairs of primers are designed, one of which is specific for methylated DNA (M) and the other for unmethylated DNA (U).

After pyrosequencing or MSP-PCR, amplified fragments are usually cloned to determine the degree of methylation (Herman, 1996).

Additionally, in order to identify unknown methylation hot-spots or methylated CpG islands in the genome, several of genome-wide screen methods have been invented such as Restriction Landmark Genomic Scanning for Methylation (RLGS-M), and CpG island microarray.

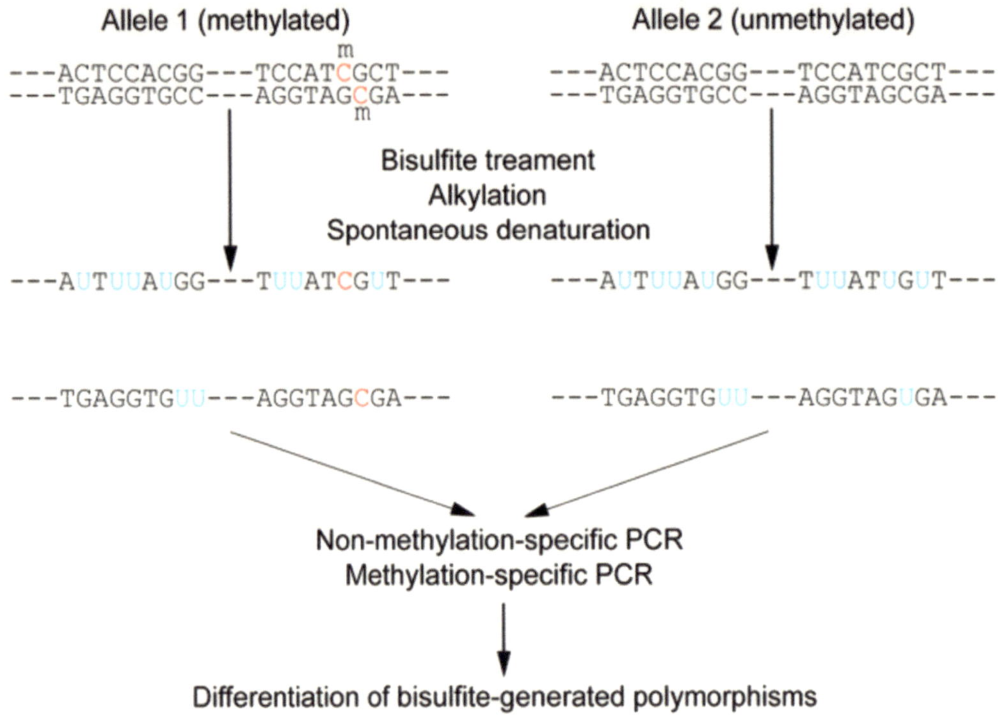

Fig. 4. Schematic representation of bisulfite based modifications

6. p16^{INK4a} expression in cervical cancer

The cellular tumour suppressor protein p16 has a central function in the regulation of cell cycle activation. The p16^{INK4a}, the product of *CDKN2A* gene is a negative regulatory protein that regulates the progression of eukaryotic cells through the G1 phase of the cell cycle (Serrano, 1997). p16^{INK4a} is a component of p16^{INK4a}-Cdk4-6/CyclinD-pRb signalling pathway and is perturbed in many cancers. In these tumours, the functions of p16^{INK4a} may be lost due to mutations or suppression of its transcription by promoter methylation (Gonzalgo, 1998). In high risk-HPV positive cervical cancer, the oncogene E7 disrupts pRb/E2F interaction, releases active E2F and induces the pRb degradation (Liuet, 2006). The existence of the regulatory feedback in the pRb/p16 pathway leads to an overexpression of p16^{INK4a} in cervical tumours (Ivanova, 2007). Klaes *el al.* (2001) have shown that overexpression of p16^{INK4a} is a specific marker for dysplastic and neoplastic epithelial cells in the cervix. They have clearly demonstrated that use of p16^{INK4a} immunostaining allows precise identification of cervical lesions and significantly reduce false-negative and -positive interpretation in cervical cancer screening. For theses reasons, p16^{INK4a} expression is usually used in cervical neoplasia diagnosis (Klaes, 2001).

Many studies have analyzed the presence of p16^{INK4a} in cervical neoplasia and have found a relationship between p16^{INK4a} expression and cervical neoplasia; raising hope that p16^{INK4a} could represent a specific and sensitive marker for cervical neoplasia (Klaes, 2001; Milde-Langosch, 2001; Riethdorf, 2004). A representative p16^{INK4a} immunohistochemical staining in epidermoid carcinoma is given in Figure 5. It is generally believed that p16^{INK4a} functions as Cdk-inhibitor in the nucleus. Klaes *et al.* have showed that 58 of 60 invasive cervical carcinomas expressed p16^{INK4a} both in nuclei and cytoplasm (Klaes, 2001). Theses findings were corroborated with published data from Moroccan cases. Indeed, p16^{INK4a} staining by IHC in 53 cervical cancer biopsies from Morocco showed that 92.4% had high level of p16^{INK4a} expression with a predominance of both nuclear and cytoplasmic staining (El Hamdani, 2010).

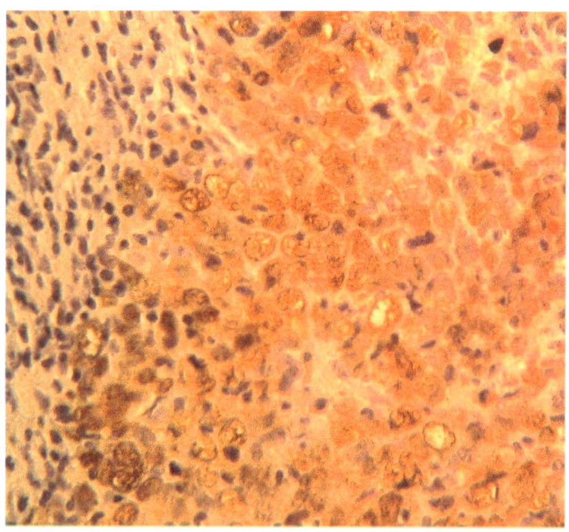

(Intense Nuclear staining of p16^{INK4a})

Fig. 5. Representative p16 immunohistochemical staining in epidermoid carcinoma sample

On the other hand, Ivanova *et al.* (2007) have clearly demonstrated that in normal cells p16^{INK4a} localizes mainly in nuclei, the loss of p16^{INK4a} nuclear staining in favour of cytoplasmic staining have been observed earlier in different tumours including cervical carcinomas and cervical cancer cell lines.

Loss of p16^{INK4a} protein expression, leading to overcome cell cycle arrest at senescence and immortalization, could be studied by evaluating the methylation status of its promoter (Ivanova, 2007).

Indeed, hypermethylation of the promoter region of a tumour suppressor gene has been increasingly recognized as an alternative mechanism for inactivation of function of a tumour suppressor gene. In this topic, hypermethylation of the *p16* gene has been suggested to be a shared epigenetic alteration in multiple human cancers, including cervical cancer (Esteller, 2001).

An example of MSP analysis of the promoter regions of p16INK4a after bisulfite treatment is given if Figure 6. Using MSP and/or bisulfite sequencing, hypermethylation of p16^{INK4a} gene was observed in 19 to 61% of invasive cervical carcinoma (Ivanova, 2007, Nehls, 2008; Attaleb, 2009). However, hypermthylation of p16^{INK4a} promoter region is absent in DNA specimens from normal cervical swabs as well as cervical cell lines such as SiHa, HeLa, C33A and Caski (Attaleb, 2009).

Moreover, the increased risk for disease progression was independent from clinical and pathological factors, suggesting that p16^{INK4a} gene promoter methylation is an early event in cervical cancer development.

Moreover, in HPV induced cervical cancer, the cell cycle activation is not mediated by Cdks but by E7-related Rb disruption. The p16 inactivation would not confer any further growth promoting effect, because in this cancer the HR-HPV oncogene E7 induces a permanent release of E2F from its binding to pRb, leading to continuous cell cycle activation (Nehls, 2008).

Thus, hypermethylation of p16^{INK4a} promoter gene may be a result of genetic and epigenetic events produced during the carcinogenesis steps of cervical cancer development, and when occurs, it did not affect the regulation of p16^{INK4a} expression. Moreover, the high p16^{INK4a} immunoreactivity with partial promoter hypermethylation needs to be further investigated.

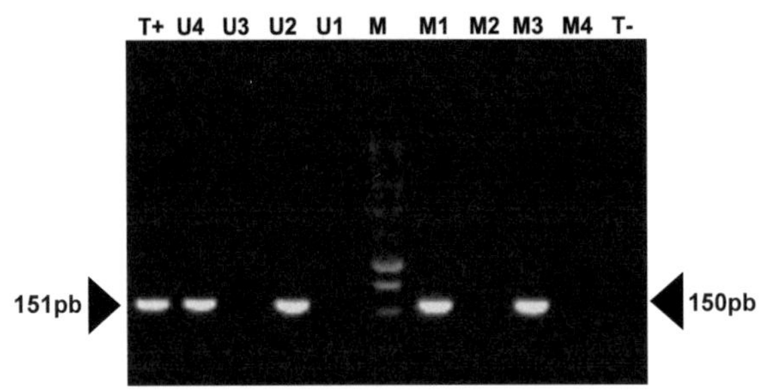

Fig. 6. MSP analysis of the promoter regions of p16^{INK4a}
The presence of a visible PCR product in lane U indicates the presence of unmethylated genes; the presence of a PCR product in lane M indicates the presence of methylated genes. Normal lymphocytes DNA (T) was used as a negative control for methylation. Cases 1 and 3 were methylated at p16^{INK4a}. M: 100 bp ladder.

7. Expression of E-cadherin in cervical cancer

Cadherins are a family of cell–cell adhesion molecules which can modulate epithelial phenotype and morphogenesis in a variety of tissues. E-cadherin is the major cadherin expressed on the surface of normal epithelial cells and plays a pivotal role in maintenance of normal adhesion in epithelial cells but has also been shown to suppress tumour invasion and participate in cell signalling (Chen, 2003; Virmani, 2001; Ziober, 2001). Cell adhesion is mediated through Ca^{2+}-dependent homotypic binding. This transmembrane glycoprotein is encoded by *CDH1* gene.

Based on its biological functions, E-cadherin is regarded as an invasion and metastasis suppressor. Loss of E-cadherin expression or function correlates with increased invasiveness and metastasis in carcinomas of several anatomical sites (Chen, 2003; Virmani, 2001). E-cadherin-mediated cell adhesion system is inactivated by multiple mechanisms. It may be inactivated as a result of genetic alteration, reduced gene expression, changes of other cadherin–catenin complexes or posttranslational modification of the protein leading to cytoplasmic delocalization (Widschwendter, 2004; Oki, 2007).

The expression of E-cadherin is impaired as squamous intraepithelial lesions progress to squamous cervical carcinoma (Laird, 2003). In cervical cancer, the presence and localisation of cytoplasmic E-cadherin were significantly correlated with CIN grade. In invasive types, the expression of E-cadherin was significantly reduced (Hirohashi, 1998) and this is mainly due to gene silencing by methylation processes (Nehls, 2008).

E-cadherin expression, as well as p16INK4a expression, is usually used in cervical neoplasia diagnosis. In squamous cervical epithelium, E-cadherin is predominantly found at the cell-to-cell borders in the basal and parabasal cell layers (Laird, 2003). However, E-cadherin expression is reduced during tumour progression and metastasis, and associated with poor prognosis in a variety of cancers (Karayiannakis, 1998; Sulzer, 1998; Zheng, 1999). A representative E-cadherin immunohistochemical staining in epidermoid carcinoma is given in Figure 7.

Reported data showed that E-cadherin is moderately expressed in about 85% of informative cases with a main localisation at the cell membrane and cytoplasm (El Hamdani, 2010). Decrease or loss of E-cadherin expression is a common feature of many human epithelial cancers, including cervical cancer, although a decreased expression of this molecule has been described in metastasis, but not primary tumours (Carico, 2001).

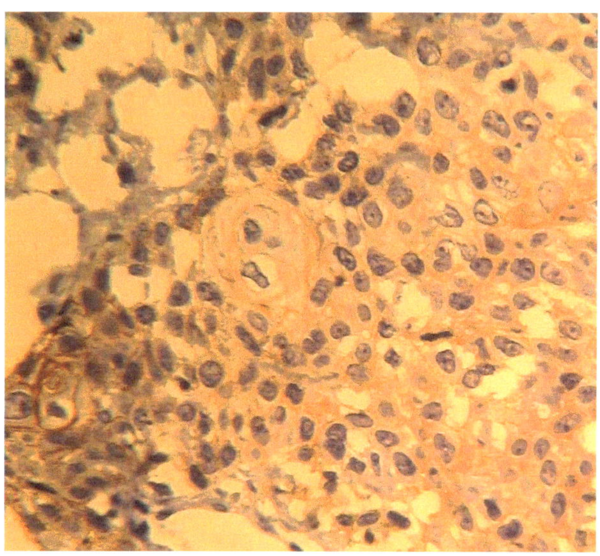

Moderate membranous staining of E-cadherin

Fig. 7. Representative E-cadherin immunohistochemical staining in epidermoid carcinoma sample

It's widely accepted that hypermethylation plays a critical role in gene silencing. Promoter hypermethylation has been proposed as an explanation for the decrease of *E-cadherin* expression (Chen, 2003, Graff, 2000) and was even suggested as a potential marker for identifying cervical cancer patients at high risk for relapse (Widschwendter, 2004).

Thus, methylation status of E-cadherin promoter has been studied to understand the implication of this gene silencing in cervical cancer development. Methylatio status was mainly studied using MSP analysis, as shown in Figure 8. Reported data showed that less than 50% of cervical cancer cases exhibited E-cadherin promoter hypermethylation at their CpG islands (Chen, 2003, Dong, 2001; Narayan, 2003; Attaleb, 2009). Moreover, E-cadherin promoter was also hypermethylated in 3 cervical cell lines (HeLa, SiHa and C33A) (Attaleb, 2009). Thus, partial methylation of the E-cadherin gene promoter leads to down-regulate the gene expression.

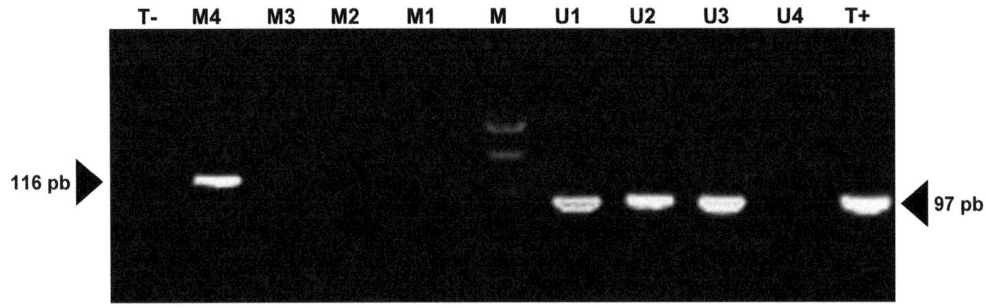

Fig. 8. MSP analysis of the promoter regions of p16^{INK4a}
The presence of a visible PCR product in lane U indicates the presence of unmethylated genes; the presence of a PCR product in lane M indicates the presence of methylated genes. Normal lymphocytes DNA (T) was used as a negative control for methylation. Case 4 was unmethylated at E-cadherin. M: 100 bp ladder.

8. Epigenetic based therapy

In tumours, epigenetic silencing of genes involved in DNA damage response pathways, such as cell cycle control, apoptosis signalling and DNA repair, has the potential to influence drug resistance and clinical outcome following therapy (Teodoridis, 2004).

Promoter hypermethylation and histone hypoacetylation contribute to this transcriptional inactivation. It is possible to reverse silencing using small molecule inhibitors. Such compounds, that can reverse this epigenetic inactivation, show anti tumour activity and can increase the sensitivity of drug resistant preclinical tumour models (Teodoridis, 2004). Hypomethylating and hyperacetylating drugs, HDAC (histone deacetylase) and DNMT inhibitors, can reverse epigenetic silencing and improve the cancer therapy (Hidemi, 2011).

The targeting of epigenetic pathways is an attractive therapeutic strategy and current clinical trials aim to improve efficacy of DNA hypomethylating drugs for e.g. by combination with standard chemotherapy. Key components in the regulation of DNA methylation are DNA methyltransferases (DNMT1, 2, 3A and 3B) and methyl CpG-binding proteins, which recognize methyl cytosine residues and recruit transcriptional repressor complexes, including histone deacetylases (HDAC). Because of the interdependence of epigenetic processes, combinations of these approaches may have maximum clinical efficacy (Ferguson, 2011).

Epigenetic therapy leads to gene reactivation in primary tumours of cervical cancer patients. A number of these reactivated genes have a definitive role as tumour suppressors (De la Cruz-Hernández, 2011).

Hydralazine, a demethylating agent, was administrated in different doses to cohorts of previously untreated patients with histological diagnosis of cervical cancer in a phase I study. Hydralazine at doses between 50 and 150 mg/day is well tolerated and effective to demethylate and reactivate the expression of tumour suppressor genes without affecting global DNA methylation (Zambrano, 2005).

Valproic acid, an HDAC inhibitor, exerted a growth inhibitory effect on cervical cancer cell line: HeLa, SiHa and CaSki (De la Cruz-Hernandez, 2007; Chen, 2006). These drugs led to an increase of p53 transcription, and increase its stabilisation due to acetylation at lysines 273 and 282, protecting it from degradation by E6 (CruzHernandez, 2007). Valproic acid impede Akt1 and Akt2 expression, which leads to Akt deactivation and apoptotic cell death mediated through the caspase dependent pathway (Chen, 2006).

The combined antineoplastic effect of the DNA methylation inhibitor hydralazine and the histone deacetylase inhibitor valproic acid leads to increase in the cytotoxicity of cisplatin, adriamycin or gemcitabine in human cervical cancer cell lines (ChavezBlanco, 2006).

Also, epigenetic profiling using DNA methylation and histone analysis, can provide useful information for translational purposes, with a special emphasis on the potential use of DNA methylation marks for early disease detection and prognosis (Park, 2011) and for effective treatment strategies (Watanabe, 2010).

9. Conclusion

Identification of relevant biomarkers for early and specific diagnosis as well as the identification of promising therapeutic targets for molecular targeted therapy is a key role to improve cancer management worldwide.

In cervical cancer, even the importance of combined cytology and HPV testing, the use of epigenetic alterations as biomarkers will be of a great interest to enhance cervical diagnosis. Since alterations of the cellular epigenome usually precede morphologic changes and genetic alterations, identification of related aberrant DNA methylation profiles according to specific anatomopathologic status may serve as a reasonable early diagnostic marker for cervical cancer diagnosis.

Moreover, the crucial role of epigenetic alterations at an early stage in the carcinogenesis may be promising targets for the prevention or treatment of cancer. Thus, understanding the epigenetic derepression of oncogenes, or cancer-promoting genes, would be important for the development of epigenetic-based therapies used in combination with other therapies for cervical cancer treatment.

10. References

Abd El All, H., Rye, A., Duvillard P. 1999. p53 Immunohistochemical Expression of Egyptian Cervical Carcinoma. Pathology Oncology Research. 5 : 280 - 284.

Abrahao AC, Bonelli BV, Nunes FD, Dias EP, Cabral MG. 2011. Immunohistochemical expression of p53, p16 and hTERT in oral squamous cell carcinoma and potentially malignant disorders. Braz Oral Res. 25 : 34-41.

Agorastos T, Lambropoulos AF, Constantinidis TC, et al. p53 codon 72 polymorphism and risk of intra-epithelial and invasive cervical neoplasia in Greek women. Eur J Cancer Prev. 2000; 9:113–18.

Anita Szalmás, József Kónya. Seminars in Cancer Biology 19 (2009) 144–152

Attaleb, M., W. El hamadani, M. Khyatti, L. Benbacer, N. Benchekroun, A. Benider, M. Amrani and M. El Mzibri. 2009. Status of $p16^{INK4a}$ and E-Cadherin genes promoter methylation in Moroccan patients with cervical carcinoma. Oncol. Res. 18: 185-192.

Bhattacharya P, Duttagupta C, Sengupta S. Proline homozygosity in codon 72 of p53: a risk genotype for human papillomavirus related cervical cancer in Indian women. Cancer Lett. 2002;188(1-2):207-11.

Bosch FX, Manos MM, Munoz N, Sherman M, Jansen AM, Peto J, Schiffman MH, et al. Prevalence of human papillomavirus in cervical cancer: a worldwide perspective. International biological study on cervical cancer (IBSCC) study group, J. Natl. Cancer. Inst. 1995; 87: 796–802.

Bosch FX, Schwarz E, Boukamp P, Fusenig NE, Bartsch D, zur Hausen H. Suppression *in vivo* of human papillomavirus type 18 E6-E7 gene expression in nontumorigenic HeLa X fibroblast hybrid cells. J Virol. 1990. 64: 4743-54.

Brenna SM, Silva ID, Zeferino LC, Pereira JS, Martinez EZ, Syrjänen KJ. Prevalence of codon 72 P53 polymorphism in Brazilian women with cervix cancer. Genet Mol Biol. 2004; 27(4): 496-499.

Burgers WA, Blanchon L, Pradhan S, de Launoit Y, Kouzarides T, Fuks F. Oncogene. 2007 Mar 8;26(11):1650-5.

Carico, E.; Atlante, M.; Bucci, B.; Nofroni, I.; Vecchione, A. E-cadherin and a-catenin expression during tumor progression of cervical carcinoma. Gynecol. Oncol. 80:156-161; 2001.

Chahwan R, Wontakal SN, Roa S. Discov Med. 2011 Mar;11(58):233-43.

Chavez-Blanco A, PerezPlasencia C, PerezCardenas E, CarrascoLegleu C, RangelLopez E, SeguraPacheco B, et al. Antineoplastic effects of the DNA methylation inhibitor hydralazine and the histone deacetylase inhibitor valproic acid in cancer cell lines. Cancer Cell Int 2006;6:2.

Chen J, Ghazawi FM, BakkarW, Li Q. Valproic acid and butyrate induce apoptosis in human cancer cells through inhibition of gene expression of Akt/protein kinase B. Mol Cancer 2006;5:71.

Chen, C.L.; Liu, S.S.; Ipb, S.M.; Wongb, L.C.; Ng, T.Y.; Nganb, H.Y.S. E-cadherin expression is silenced by DNA methylation in cervical cancer cell lines and tumours. Eur. J. Cancer. 39:517-523; 2003.

Costa S, Pinto D, Pereira D, Rodrigues H, Cameselle-Teijeiro J, Medeiros R, Schmitt F. 2008. Importance of TP53 codon 72 and intron 3 duplication 16bp polymorphisms in prediction of susceptibility on breast cancer. BMC Cancer. 29 : 32 - 38

Cullen AP, Reid R, Campion M and AT, Lr. Analysis of the physical state of different human papillomavirus DNAs in intraepithelial and invasive cervical neoplasia. *J Virol* 1991. 65: 606–612

De la Cruz-Hernandez E, Perez-Cardenas E, Contreras-Paredes A, Cantu D, Mohar A, Lizano M, et al. The effects of DNA methylation and histone deacetylase inhibitors on human papillomavirus early gene expression in cervical cancer, an in vitro and clinical study. Virol J 2007;4:18.

De la Cruz-Hernández E, Perez-Plasencia C, Pérez-Cardenas E, Gonzalez-Fierro A, Trejo-Becerril C, Chávez-Blanco A, Taja-Chayeb L, Vidal S, Gutiérrez O, Dominguez GI, Trujillo JE, Duenas-González A. Oncol Rep. 2011 25: 399-407.

Dong, S.M.; Kim, H.S.; Rha, S.H.; Sidransky, D. Promoter hypermethylation of multiple genes in carcinoma of the uterine cervix. Clin. Cancer Res. 7:1982-1986; 2001.

El Hamdani W., M. Amrani, M. Attaleb, N. Laantri, M.M. Ennaji, M. Khyatti and M. El Mzibri. 2010. EGFR, p16INK4a and E-Cadherin immuno-histochemistry and EGFR point mutations analyses in invasive cervical cancer specimens from Moroccan women. Cellular and Molecular Biology (Noisy-le-grand). 56 : 1373-1384.

Esteller, M.; Corn, P.G.; Baylin, S.B.; Herman, J.G: A gene hypermethylation profile of human cancer. Cancer Res. 61:3225-3229; 2001

Ferguson LR, Tatham AL, Lin Z, Denny WA. Curr Cancer Drug Targets. 2011 Feb;11(2):199-212.

Filippova M, Parkhurst L, Duerksen-Hughes PJ. The human papillomavirus 16 E6 protein binds to Fas-associated death domain and protects cells from Fastriggered apoptosis. J Biol Chem. 2004. 279: 25729–44.

Gonzalgo, M.L., Hayashida, T., Bender, C.M., Pao, M.M., Tsai, Y.C., Gonzales, F.A., Nguyen, H.D., Nguyen, T.T. and Jones, P.A. The role of DNA methylation in expression of the p19/p16 locus in human bladder cancer cell lines. *Cancer Res.* 1998, 58: 1245 1252.

Govan VA, Loubser S, Saleh D, Hoffman M, Williamson AL. No relationship observed between human p53 codon-72 genotype and HPV-associated cervical cancer in a population group with a low arginine-72 allele frequency. Int J Immunogenet. 2007; 34:213–217.

Graff, J.R.; Gabrielson, E.; Fujii, H. Methylation patterns of the Ecadherin 5′CpG island are unstable and reflect the dynamic, heterogeneous loss of E-cadherin expression during metastatic progression. J. Biol. Chem. 275:2727–2732; 2000.

Gustafson KS, Furth EE, Heitjan DF, Fansler ZB, Clark DP. DNA methylation profiling of cervical squamous intraepithelial lesions using liquidbased cytology specimens: an approach that utilizes receiveroperating characteristic analysis. Cancer 2004;102:259–68.

Hamel N, Black MJ, Ghadirian P, Foulkes WD. No association between p53 codon 72 polymorphism and risk of squamous cell carcinoma of the head and neck. Br J Cancer. 2000; 82:757–9.

Herman JG, Graff JR, Myöhänen S, Nelkin BD, Baylin SB: Methylation-specific PCR: a novel PCR assay for methylation status of CpG islands. Proc Natl Acad Sci U S A 1996, 93:9821-9826.

Hidemi Rikiishi 2011 Journal of Biomedicine and Biotechnology Volume 2011, 830 : 260-268.

Hildesheim A, Schiffman M, Brinton LA, Fraumeni JF Jr, Herrero R, Bratti MC, Schwartz P, Mortel R, Barnes W, Greenberg M, McGowan L, Scott DR, Martin M, Herrera JE, Carrington M. p53 polymorphism and risk of cervical cancer. Nature. 1998; 396(6711):531-2.

Hirohashi, S. Inactivation of the E-cadherin-mediated cell adhesion system in human cancers. Am. J. Pathol. 153: 333–339; 1998.

Ivanova, T.A., Golovina, D.A., Zavalishina, L.E., Volgareva, G.M., Katargin, A. N., Andreeva, Y.Y., Frank, G.A., Kisseljov, F.L. and Kisseljova, N.P. Up-regulation of expression and lack of 5' CpG island hypermethylation of p16 INK4a in HPV-positive cervical carcinomas. *BMC Cancer*. 2007, 7: 47-56.

Jones PA, Baylin SB: The fundamental role of epigenetic events in cancer. Nat Rev Genet 2002, 3:415-428.

Kang S, Kim JW, Kang GH, Lee S, Park NH, Song YS, et al. Comparison of DNA hypermethylation patterns in different types of uterine cancer: cervical squamous cell carcinoma, cervical adenocarcinoma and endometrial adenocarcinoma. Int J Cancer 2006;118:2168–71.

Karayiannakis, A.J.; Syrigos, K.N.; Chatzigianni, E.; Papanikolaou, S.; Alexiou, D.; Kalahanis, N.; Rosenberg, T.; Bastounis, E. Aberrant E-cadherin expression associated with loss of differentiation and advanced stage in human pancreatic cancer. Anticancer Res. 18:4177-4180; 1998.

Kashima T, Makino K, Soemantri A, Ishida T. 2007. TP53 codon 72 polymorphism in 12 populations of insular Southeast Asia and Oceania. J Hum Genet. 2007; 52(8): 694-697.

Kitkumthorn N, Yanatatsanajit P, Kiatpongsan S, Phokaew C, Triratanachat S, Trivijitsilp P, Termrungruanglert W, Tresukosol D, Niruthisard S, Mutirangura A. BMC Cancer. 2006 Mar 8;6:55.

Klaes, R., Friedrich, T., Spitkovsky, D., Ridder, R., Rudy, W., Petry, U., Dallenbach-Hellweg, G., Schmidt, D. and von Knebel Doeberitz, M. Overexpression of p16(INK4A) as a specific marker for dysplastic and neoplastic epithelial cells of the cervix uteri. *Int J Cancer*. 2001, 92: 276–284.

Klug SJ, Wilmotte R, Santos C, et al. TP53 polymorphism, HPV infection, and risk of cervical cancer. Cancer Epidemiol Biomarkers Prev. 2001; 10: 1009–12.

Kuroda Y, Nakao H, Ikemura K, Katoh T. 2007. Association between the TP53 codon72 polymorphism and oral cancer risk and prognosis. Oral Oncol. 43: 1043- 1048.

Laird, P.W. The power and the promise of DNA methylation markers. Nat. Rev. Cancer. 3:253-266; 2003.

Lazo PA. The molecular genetics of cervical carcinoma. Br J Cancer 1999; 80: 2008-2018

Lind GE, Thorstensen L, Løvig T, Meling GI, Hamelin R, Rognum TO, Esteller M, Lothe RA.Mol Cancer. 2004 Oct 11;3:28.

Liu, X., Clements, A. and Zhao, K. Structure of the human papillomavirus E7 oncoprotein and its mechanism for inactivation of retinoblastoma tumor suppressor. J. B. C. 2006, 281: 578-586.

Lo PK, Sukumar S. Pharmacogenomics. 2008 Dec;9(12):1879-902.

Longworth MS, Wilson R, Laimins LA. EMBO J. 2005 May 18;24(10):1821-30.

Matlashewski GJ, Tuck S, Pim D, Lamb P, Schneider J, Crawford LV. Primary structure polymorphism at amino acid residue 72 of human p53. Mol Cell Biol. 1987; 7(2):961-3

Maufort JP, Shai A, Pitot HC, Lambert PF. A role for HPV16 E5 in cervical carcinogenesis. Cancer Res. 2010. 70: 2924-31.

Meftah El khair, M., MM. Ennaji, R. El kebbaj, R. Ait Mhand, M. Attaleb and M. El Mzibri. 2009. p53 codon 72 polymorphism and risk of cervical carcinoma in Moroccan Women. Medical oncology. Septembre 23.

Milde-Langosch, K., Riethdorf, S., Kraus-Poppinghaus, A., Riethdorf, L. and Loning, T. Expression of cyclin-dependent kinase inhibitors p16MTS1, p21WAF1, and p27KIP1 in HPV-positive and HPV-negative cervical adenocarcinomas. *Virchows Arch.* 2001, 439: 55–61.

Mitra S, Misra C, Singh R K, Panda C K, Roychoudhury S. Association of specific genotype and haplotype of p53 gene with cervical cancer in India. J Clin Pathol. 2005; 58:26-31.

Moody CA, Laimins LA. Human papillomavirus oncoproteins: pathways to transformation. Nat Rev Cancer. 2010. 10 : 550-60.

Muñoz N, Bosch FX, de Sanjosé S, Herrero R, Castellsagué X, Shah KV, Snijders PJ and CJ. Meijer. Epidemiologic classification of human papillomavirus types associated with cervical cancer. Engl J Med. 2003. 348: 518-27.

Narayan, G.; Arias-Pulido, H.; Koul, S.; Vargas, H.; Zhang, F.F.; Villella, J.; Schneider, A.; Terry, M.B.; Mansukhani, M.; Murty, V.V. Frequent promoter methylation of CDH1, DAPK, RARB, and HIC1 genes in carcinoma of cervix uteri: its relationship to clinical outcome. Molecular Cancer. 2: 24-35; 2003.

Nehls, K.; Vinokurova, S.; Schmidt, D.; Kommoss, F.; Reuschenbach, M.; Kisseljov, F.; Einenkel, J.; von Knebel Doeberitz, M.; Wentzensen, N. p16 methylation does not affect protein expression in cervical carcinogenesis. Eur. J. Cancer. 44:2496-2505; 2008.

Oki, Y.; Aoki, E.; Issa, J.P: Decitabine – bedside to bench. Crit. Rev. Oncol. Hematol. 67:140-152, 2007.

Oliveira S, Sousa H, Santos AM, Pinto D, Pinto-Correia AL, Fontoura. The p53 R72P polymorphism does not influence cervical cancer development in a Portuguese population: a study in exfoliated cervical cells. J Med Virol. 2008; 80(3):424-9.

Park YJ, Claus R, Weichenhan D, Plass C.Prog Drug Res. 2011;67:25-49.Genome-wide epigenetic modifications in cancer.

Pegoraro RJ, Rom L, Lanning PA, et al. p53 codon 72 polymorphism and human papillomavirus type in relation to cervical cancer in South African women. Int J Gynecol Cancer. 2002; 12:383–8.

Raybould R., A. Fiander and S. Hibbitts. Human Papillomavirus Integration and its Role in Cervical Malignant Progression. The Open Clinical Cancer Journal. 2011. 5 : 1-71.

Riethdorf, S., Neffen, E.F., Cviko, A., Loning, T., Crum, C.P. and Riethdorf, L. P16INK4A expression as biomarker for HPV 16-related vulvar neoplasias. *Hum Pathol.* 2004, 35: 1477 - 1483

Saranath D, Khan Z, Tandle AT, Dedhia P, Sharma B, Contractor R, Shrivastava S, Dinshaw K. HPV16/18 prevalence in cervical lesions/cancers and p53 genotypes in cervical cancer patients from India. Gynecol Oncol. 2002. 86: 157-62.

Scheffner M, Werness BA, Huibregtse JM, et al. The E6 oncoprotein encoded by human papillomavirus types 16 and 18 promotes the degradation of p53. Cell. 1990; 63:1129-36.

Serrano, M.; Lin, A.W.; McCurrach, M.E.; Beach, D.; Lowe, S.W. Oncogenic ras provokes premature cell senescence associated with accumulation of p53 and p16INK4a. Cell. 88:593-602; 1997.

Sousa H, Santos AM, Pinto D, Medeiros R. Is the p53 codon 72 polymorphism a key biomarker for cervical cancer development? A meta-analysis review within European populations. Int J MolMed. 2007; 20:731-741.

Soussi T, Béroud C. Assessing TP53 status in human tumours to evaluate clinical outcome. Nat Rev Cancer. 2001; 1 (3):233-40.

Stanley M. Pathology and epidemiology of HPV infection in females. Gynecol Oncol. 2010. 117 : S5-10.

Stoppler MC, Straight SW, Tsao G, Schlegel R, McCance DJ. The E5 gene of HPV-16 enhances keratinocyte immortalization by fulllength DNA. Virology. 1996. 223: 251-4.

Storey A, Thomas M, Kalita A, Harwood C, Gardiol D, Mantovani F et al. Role of a p53 polymorphism in the development of human papillomavirus-associated cancer. Nature.1998; 393(6682):229-34.

Sulzer, M.A.; Leers, M.P.; van Noord, J.A.; Bollen, E.C.; Theunissen, P.H. Reduced E-cadherin expression is associated with increased lymph node metastasis and unfavorable prognosis in non-small cell lung cancer. Am. J. Resp. Crit. Care Med. 157:1319-1323; 1998.

Szarka K, Veress G, Juhasz A, et al. Integration status of virus DNA and p53 codon 72 polymorphism in human papillomavirus type 16 positive cervical cancers. Anticancer Res. 2000; 20:2161–7.

Tandle AT, Sanghvi V, Saranath D. Determination of p53 genotypes in oral cancer patients from India. Br J Cancer. 2001; 84:739–42.

Teodoridis JM, Strathdee G, Brown R.Drug Resist Updat. 2004 Aug-Oct;7(4-5):267-78.

Thomas M, Kalita A, Labrecque S, Pim D, Banks L, Matlashewski G. Two polymorphic variants of wild-type p53 differ biochemically and biologically. Mol Cell Biol. 1999; 19: 1092–1100.

Vasilescu F, Ceauşu M, Tănase C, Stănculescu R, Vlădescu T, Ceauşu Z. 2009. P53, p63 and Ki-67 assessment in HPV-induced cervical neoplasia. Rom J Morphol Embryol. 50(3): 357-361.

Virmani, A.; Muller, C.; Rayhi, A.; Zoechbauer-Mueller, S.; Mathis, M.; Gazdar, A. Aberrant methylation during cervical carcinogenesis. Clin. Cancer Res. 7:584-589; 2001.

von Knebel Doeberitz M, Oltersdorf T, Schwarz E, Gissmann L. Correlation of modified human papilloma virus early gene expression with altered growth properties in C4-1 cervical carcinoma cells. Cancer Res. 1988. 48: 3780-6.

Wang NM, Tsai CH, Yeh KT, et al. p53 codon 72Arg polymorphism is not a risk factor for carcinogenesis in the Chinese. Int J Mol Med. 1999; 4:249–52.

Watanabe Y, Maekawa M.. Methylation of DNA in cancer. Adv Clin Chem. 2010;52:145-67.

Werness BA, Levine AJ, Howley PM. Association of human papillomavirus types 16 and 18 E6 proteins with p53. Science. 1990; 248:76–9.

Widschwendter, A.; Gattringer, C.; Ivarsson, L.; Fiegl, H.; Schneitter, A.; Ramoni, A.; Müller-Holzner, M.; Wiedemair, A.; Jerabek, S.; Müller-Holzner, E.; Goebel, G.; Marth, C.; Widschwendter, M. Analysis of aberrant DNA methylation and human papillomavirus DNA in cervicovaginal specimens to detect invasive cervical cancer and its precursors. Clin. Cancer Res. 10:3396-400; 2004.

Widschwendter, A.; Muller-Holzner, M.; Fiegl, H.; Ivarsson, L.; Wiedemair, A.; Muller-Holzner, E.; Goebel, G.; Marth, C.; Widschwendter, M.. DNA methylation in serum and tumors of cervical cancer patients. Clin. Cancer Res. 10:565-571; 2004.

Wong YF, Chung TK, Cheung TH, Nobori T, Yu AL, Yu J, et al. Methylation of p16INK4A in primary gynecologic malignancy. Cancer Lett 1999;136:231–5.

World Health Organisation (WHO). Strengthening cervical cancer prevention and control. Report of the GAVI-UNFPA-WHO meeting /RHR/10.13.

Wu MT, Liu CL, Ho CK, et al. Genetic polymorphism of p53 and XRCC1 in cervical intraepithelial neoplasm in Taiwanese women. J Formos Med Assoc. 2004; 103:337–43.

Zambrano P, Segura-Pacheco B, Perez-Cardenas E, Cetina L, Revilla-Vazquez A, Taja-Chayeb L, Chavez-Blanco A, Angeles E, Cabrera G, Sandoval K, Trejo-Becerril C, Chanona-Vilchis J, Duenas-González A.BMC Cancer. 2005 Apr 29;5:44.

Zheng, Z.; Pan, J.; Chu, B.; Wong, Y.C.; Cheung, A.L.; Tsao, S.W. Downregulation and abnormal expression of E-cadherin and b-catenin in nasopharyngeal carcinoma: close association with advanced disease stage and lymph node metastasis. Hum. Pathol. 30:458–466; 1999.

Zhu ZZ, Wang AZ, Jia HR, Jin XX, He XL, Hou LF, Zhu G. 2007. Association of the TP53 codon 72 polymorphism with colorectal cancer in a Chinese population. Jpn J Clin Oncol.; 37: 385-90.

Ziober, B.L.; Silverman, S.S.; Kramer, R.H. Adhesive mechanisms regulating invasion and metastasis in oral cancer, Crit. Rev. Oral. Biol. Med. 12:499-510; 2001.

zur Hausen H, Gissmann L, Steiner W, Dippold W, Dreger I. Human papilloma viruses and cancer. Bibl Haematol. 1975. 43: 569-71.

zur Hausen H. Condylomata acuminata and human genital cancer. Cancer Res. 1976. 36: 794.

zur Hausen H. Human papillomaviruses in the pathogenesis of anogenital cancer. Virology. 1991. 184: 9-13.

zur Hausen H. Papillomaviruses causing cancer: evasion from host-cell control in early events in carcinogenesis. J Natl Cancer Inst. 2000. 92: 690-8.
zur Hausen H. Papillomaviruses in the causation of human cancers - a brief historical account. Virology. 2009. 384: 260-5.

13

New Biomarkers for Cervical Cancer – Perspectives from the IGF System

Martha-Lucía Serrano, Adriana Umaña-Pérez,
Diana J. Garay-Baquero and Myriam Sánchez-Gómez*
Hormone Laboratory, Department of Chemistry,
Faculty of Science, Universidad Nacional de Colombia, Bogotá
Colombia

1. Introduction

The insulin-like growth factor (IGF) family is organized in a complex regulatory network at the cellular and sub-cellular levels. In the human the IGF system has a key physiological role in the development of the organism and maintenance of normal cellular function during foetal and postnatal life. The IGF system consists of three ligands, IGF-I, IGF-II and Insulin; three cell membrane receptors, IGF-I receptor (IGF-IR), insulin receptor (IR), and IGF-II receptor (IGF-IIR); six high-affinity IGF binding proteins, IGFBP-1 through -6, their specific proteases (IGFBP proteases) and membrane receptors (IGFBP-R) (Fig. 1).

IGF-I and IGF-II share a 62% homology in amino acid sequence and there is a 40% homology between the IGFs and proinsulin (Furstenberger & Senn, 2002). IGF-IR is a member of the family of the tyrosine kinase growth factor receptors and is highly homologous at the amino acid sequence level to the IR. The mature membrane receptor is a tetramer made of two α-chains and two β-chains, with several disulfide bridges (LeRoith et al., 1995). The extracellular α-subunits form the ligand binding domain and several lines of evidence suggest that the binding sites for IGF-I and IGF-II may be distinct (Samani et al., 2007). IGF-I and IGF-II bind to IGF-IR with high affinity, however, ligand affinities may vary with cell type and experimental conditions. IGF-II can also bind to the insulin receptor isoform A (IR-A) with an affinity similar to that of insulin. IR-A is expressed in certain tumours and has a more mitogenic effect than the IR-B isoform, the latter having a more metabolic function (Pandini et al., 2002). In cells expressing both IR and IGF-IR, IR hemireceptors may heterodimerize with IGF-IR hemireceptors, leading to the formation of hybrid receptors (IR/IGF-IR). The proportion of hybrid receptors is a function of the mole fractions of each receptor. Early studies carried out with purified hybrid receptors indicate that these receptors mostly bind IGF-I and that they bind insulin with a much lower affinity (Belfiore et al., 2009).

IGF-II can also bind to a second receptor, IGF-IIR, which is a multifunctional single transmembrane glycoprotein, identical to the cation-independent mannose 6-phosphate receptor. It is composed of a large extracytoplasmic domain and a short cytoplasmic tail that lacks intrinsic cytoplasmic activity (El-Shewy & Luttrell, 2009). IGF-IIR perform diverse

* Corresponding Author

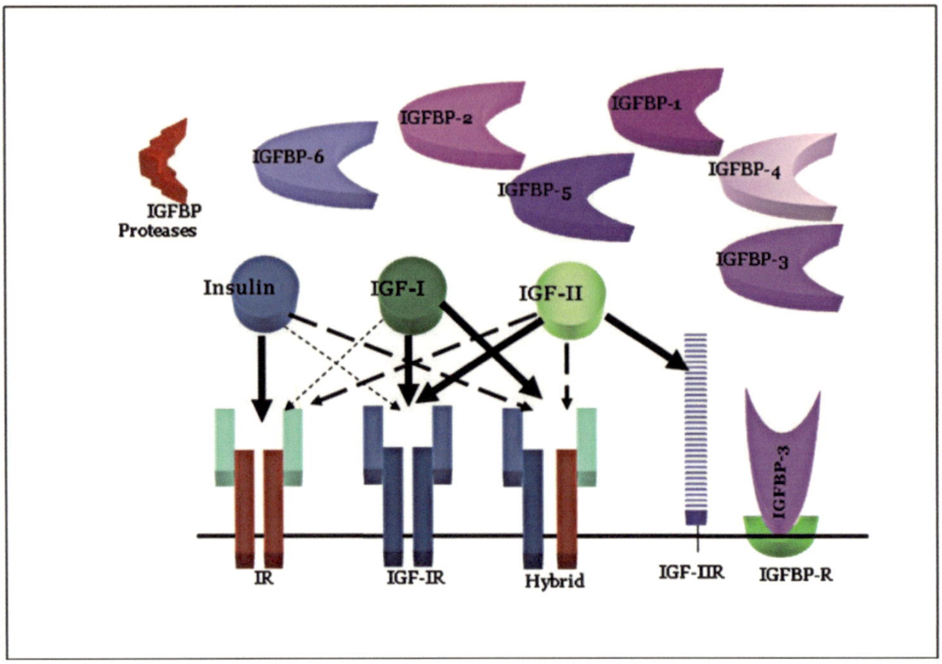

Fig. 1. The IGF system. The IGF system consists of the receptors (IR, IGF-IR, IGF-IR/IR hybrids and IGF-IIR), the peptides (IGF-I, IGF-II and insulin), six high affinity IGFBPs (-1 to -6), IGFBP proteases and IGFBP receptors (IGFBP-R).

cellular functions related to lysosome biogenesis and the regulation of growth and development. The IGF-IIR receptors recycle continuosly between two cellular pools and at steady state most of the receptor localize in endosomes and the remainder (approx. 10%) on the plasma membrane. Traditionally, the IGF-IIR was considered a scavenger receptor, regulating the extracellular IGF-II concentrations, but recent studies suggest that the IGF-IIR also functions in signal transduction and may play an important role in tumour progression (El-Shewy et al., 2006,).

To add more complexity to the system, the IGFs in circulation and in the tissues, are associated with a family of six high affinity IGF-binding proteins (IGFBPs) that regulate the bioavailability of the IGFs (Baxter, 2000). The IGFBPs regulate the interaction of IGFs with the receptors. In human about 80% of circulating IGF-I is carried by IGFBP-3/acid label subunit complex (Lewitt et., 1994). All IGFBPs inhibit IGF action by sequestering IGFs and some IGFBPs (IGFBP-1, -3, -5) can also potentiate IGF action. The resulting change in the ratio of IGF to IGFBP modulates IGF/IGFBP/IGF receptor interactions and may play a role in normal and abnormal tissue proliferation (Mohan & Baylink, 2002).

Overexpression of growth factors and/or their receptors is a common event in malignancy and provides the underlying mechanism for uncontrolled proliferation, one of the hallmarks of cancer (Hanahan & Weinberg, 2000). The IGF signalling system network is tightly controlled under normal physiological conditions and alterations that disrupt the delicate balance of the system can trigger a number of molecular events that can lead to malignancy. Many studies have involved the IGF system in carcinogenesis and tumour progression of different cell types (LeRoith & Roberts, 2003). Many cancers have been shown to overexpress the IGF-I receptor and/or the ligands (IGF-I and IGF-II) and some combinations of the six IGF binding proteins (IGFBPs) (Samani et al., 2007). It appears that abnormal IGF-IR activation can result in oncogene activation leading to increased cellular proliferation and malignancy. Although the IGFs are not in themselves tumorigenic factors, it has been shown that overexpression of IGF-II, as in the case of loss of imprinting (LOI) (Pavelic et al, 2002), can contribute to gynaecological malignancies like ovarian cancer (Murphy et al., 2006) and choriocarcinoma (Diaz et al., 2007).

Compared to other types of cancer, like breast, colon, prostate, and lung, little research has been done on the relationship between the IGF family and cervical neoplasias, and by now, much remains to be learned. In this review, we will discuss some of the studies focused on the role of the components of the IGF system in the progression of cervical cancer and its potential utility as a diagnostic biomarker.

2. The IGF system and cervical cancer

Cervical cancer is the third most commonly diagnosed cancer and the fourth leading cause of cancer death in females worldwide, accounting for 9% (529,800) of the total new cancer cases and 8% (275,100) of the total cancer deaths among females in 2008. More than 85% of these cases and deaths occur in developing countries. Worldwide, the highest incidence rates are in Eastern, Western and Southern Africa, as well as South-Central Asia and South America (Jemal et al., 2011). In Colombia, cervical cancer is one of the most common causes of cancer mortality among women (Ferlay, 2010).

Persistent infection with high-risk types of HPV (HR HPV) has been identified as the main risk factor for the development of cervical cancer and its precursor lesions, squamous intraepithelial lesions (SIL) (Walboomers et al., 1999; Muñoz et al., 2003). SILs precede the development of cervical cancer and are classified in two groups: low-grade SIL (LSIL), and high-grade SIL (HSIL) (Solomon et al., 2002) (Fig. 2). Although HPV infections are among the most frequent sexually transmitted diseases, infections are usually self-limited and revert spontaneously, with only a small group of women developing cervical cancer (Woodman et al., 2001). The evolution of infection to LSIL, HSIL and cancer is dependent on several factors, many of which remain to be identified. Despite intensive investigation, the tumor biology of this disease is still largely unknown. Although prognostic factors such as pelvic lymph node metastasis affects the outcome of cervical cancer, the variability in progression-free and overall survival (OS) among patients with similar clinical and pathological characteristics, makes it difficult to predict the outcome reliably (Huang et al., 2008). Current research strives to determine why certain HPV-positive women develop cervical cancer while others do not (Schaffer et al., 2007).

2.1 Serum levels of IGFs as cervical cancer biomarkers

IGF-I is a potent mitogenic growth factor that plays a critical role during embryogenesis and development in human and animal species. Together with Growth Hormone (GH) constitute an axis that regulate postnatal growth and development in an endocrine, paracrine and autocrine mode of action. IGF-I is produced by numerous adult organs, with major contribution of liver to overall circulating IGF-I levels. After puberty, circulating IGF-I

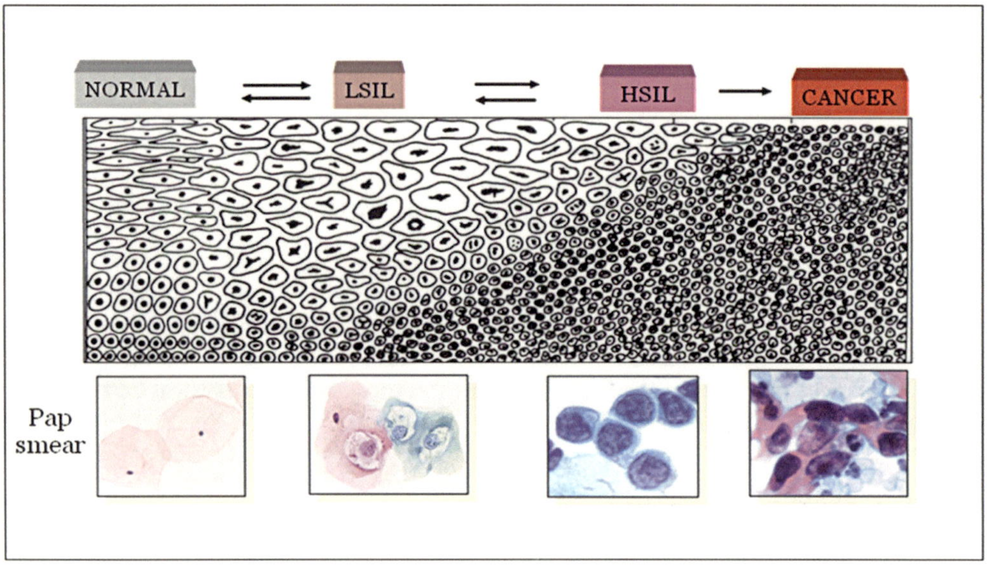

Fig. 2. Schematic representation of cervical cancer and its precursor lesions. Low-grade squamous intraepithelial lesions (LSIL), High-grade squamous intraepithelial lesions (HSIL).

levels decline, in contrast to IGF-II levels that remain elevated throughout adult life (Bang & Hall, 1992).

The proliferative and anti-apoptotic effects of IGF-I observed in animal and cell cultures, made it an obvious risk factor candidate in cancer development. In attempt to find a reliable serum biomarker to predict occurrence, progression or prognosis of human cancer, scientists have investigated the correlation of serum IGF-I or IGFBP-3, the most abundant IGFBP in circulation, to the prevalence of a variety of cancers. Prospective and retrospective studies have demonstrated an association between high concentrations of serum IGF-I and increased risk for prostate and premenopausal breast cancer (Renehan et al., 2004), whereas an inverse association has been reported for certain types of cancer, including gastric (Lee et al., 1997), endometrial (Lacey et al., 2004), liver (Stuver et al., 2000), and contradictory results for lung cancer (Yu et al, 1999; Mazzoccoli et al., 1999; Renehan, 2004).

With respect to cervical cancer, results have not shown consistency. Mathur et al. found that serum IGF-II levels were elevated, whereas IGFBP-3 levels were decreased, across the cervical lesion spectrum, and proposed that this could be used as an aid for early diagnosis and predicting prognosis of cervical cancer (Mathur et al., 2000, 2003, 2005). Two other epidemiological studies (Lee et al., 2010; Wu et al., 2003) did not find an association between IGFBP-3 levels and risk of squamous intraepithelial lesions, but on the other hand, a strong significant increase in the risk of low-grade or high-grade squamous intraepithelial lesions was observed for women with IGF-I serum levels in the highest versus the lowest quartiles.

We conducted a case-control study on Colombian women with SIL and cervical cancer, and our findings illustrated an inverse association between cervical cancer risk and IGF-I circulating levels. In accordance to this result, IGF-I/IGFBP-3 molar ratio was also inversely associated with cervical carcinoma (Serrano et al., 2006). Similar results were obtained in a study conducted in patients with diagnosed pre-cancer lesions where levels of IGF-I were inversely associated with risk of high-grade cervical intraepithelial neoplasia (Schaffer et al, 2007).

A recent prospective study reported a possible influence of the IGF axis on the natural history of oncogenic HPV and the development of cervical neoplasia (Harris et al., 2008). A high IGF-I/IGFBP-3 ratio was associated with increased persistence of oncogenic HPV infection [adjusted hazard ratio (AHR), 0.14; 95% confidence interval (95% CI), 0.04-0.57], whereas IGFBP-3 was inversely associated with both the incident detection of oncogenic HPV (AHR, 0.35; 95%CI, 0.13-0.93) and the incidence of oncogenic HPV positive cervical neoplasia (that is, squamous intraepithelial lesions at risk of progression; AHR, 0.07; 95% CI, 0.01-0.66). We conducted a case-control study with in a prospective populational-based cohort of 2200 women, followed-up during 10 years. Results adjusted by age, menarche, smoking, parity and hormonal contraceptives, showed that high IGF-I serum levels were associated with persistence (lower vs. higher quartile: RR 2.60 95% CI 0.61–10.94) and prevalent (lower vs. higher quartile: RR 2.67, 95% CI 0.37–19.09) HPV infection, however, no significance was achieved, and no association can be demonstrated (Serrano et al., 2010b).

A recent nested case-control study (151 cervical cancer cases, 443 controls), found an inverse correlation between IGFBP-3 serum levels in pregnant women and risk of cervical cancer [OR 0.43 (95% CI 0.21-0.86)], suggesting that IGFBP-3 measured in pregnancy may be a marker of lower risk of cervical cancer (Jeffreys et al., 2011). In early-stage cervical cancer patients, lower IGF-I levels seemed to be associated with worse overall survival rate, but was not of an independent value, and there was no relationship between IGFBP-3 levels and survival (Huang et al., 2008).

It is unclear why increased serum IGF-I levels may have a protective effect on development of cervical cancer, whereas in breast and prostate cancer it has the opposite effect. One of the theories is that the natural history to cervical cancer, where infection with HPV plays a crucial role, differs from sex hormone-related cancers (Schaffer et al., 2007). Larger prospective investigations are indicated to better clarify these associations, including any potential HPV type-specific differences in the effects of IGFs.

2.2 Aberrant expression of IGFs in cancer

Several lines of evidence support an important role for the IGF system in tumor tissue. IGF-IR activation is involved in several processes associated to oncogenic transformation, such as proliferation, migration and invasion (Coppola et al, 1994; Pavelic et al., 2002; Samani et al., 2007; Sell et al., 1994). IGF-I expression rarely occurs in tumoral cells, but can be produced by stromal cells surrounding the tumor. IGF-II, IGF-IR and certain IGFBPs are overexpressed in many primary tumors and cancer cell lines (Cullen et al., 1990; Hellawell et al., 2002; Werner & LeRoith, 1996). IGFBP-3 generally has, with some exceptions, a rather inhibiting effect on IGF action in tumor tissues (LeRoith & Roberts, 2003).

Increased expression of IGF-I, IGF-II, IGF-IR, or combinations thereof have been documented in various malignancies including glioblastomas, neuroblastomas, meningiomas, medulloblastomas, carcinomas of the breast, malignancies of the gastrointestinal tract, such as colorectal and pancreatic carcinomas, and ovarian cancer (Samani et al., 2007). These data show that whereas a correlation between IGF-I/ IGF-II expression levels and tumor progression could be consistently documented in some malignancies (*e.g.*, colorectal, hepatocellular, and pancreatic carcinomas), no consistent correlation was seen in others (*e.g.*, breast cancer). Moreover, in some cases, conflicting results were obtained in different studies that analyzed the same types of cancers (*e.g.*, gliomas) (Samani et al., 2007). Overexpression of IGF-II has been reported in several malignancies. A study identified the loss of imprinting (LOI) of the gene, frequently observed in the colonic mucosa of colorectal carcinoma patients, as a risk factor for developing colorectal carcinoma (Cui et al., 2003). Overexpression of IGF-II and IGF-IR, was observed in gestational trophoblastic neoplasias, including hydatidiform moles and choriocarcinoma, correlating with the elevated IGF-II levels in the circulation (Díaz et al., 2007), Taken as a whole, these studies suggest that the IGFs can play a paracrine and/or autocrine role in promoting tumor growth.

IGF-IR may also form hybrid receptors with one α- and β- subunit from the IR. There are two IR isoforms formed by alternative splicing of exon 11, IR-A which lacks exon 11 and IR-B which contains exon 11. IGF-I and IGF-II, bind to hybrid receptors IGF-IR/IR-A leading to mitogenic signaling. IGF-II and insulin bind to IR-A leading also to mitogenic signaling, whereas, activation of IR-B by insulin, or the hybrid IGF-IR/IR-B by IGF-I, results mostly in metabolic signaling. After *in vitro* and *in vivo* studies demonstrating that insulin may also play a significant and independent role in tumorigenesis, insulin is now receiving more attention in this regard (Gallagher & LeRoith, 2011).

In the past few decades, accumulating evidence has established that insulin receptors (IRs) are usually abnormally expressed in cancer cells, where they mediate both the metabolic and nonmetabolic effects of insulin. Most recently, it was observed that splicing of the IR gene is altered in cancer cells, thus increasing IR-A/IR-B ratio, which affects the cell response to circulating IGFs and insulin (Belfiore et al., 2009). As it was mentioned earlier, many tumors overexpress IGF-II, which also signals through the IR-A isoform. An important role of the IGF-II/IR-A loop has been observed in gestational trophoblastic diseases. Both IGF-I and IGF-II stimulated JEG-3 choriocarcinoma cell invasion, although they signal through different receptors: IGF-I through IGF-IR, and IGF-II through IR-A. In JEG-3 cells, which predominantly express IR-A, IGF-II stimulated cell invasion more potently than insulin (Diaz et al., 2007). The effects of IGF-II may also be mediated by the IGF-IIR, as reported in trophoblast cells (MacKinnon et al., 2001), giving more relevance to the role of this receptor in signaling and tumorigenesis.

2.2.1 Tissue expression of IGFs as risk or prognosis biomarkers in cervical cancer

In a recent study the expression levels and activated status of IGF-IR were measured by immunohistochemistry in formalin-fixed and paraffin-embedded specimens. IGF-IR levels and phosphorylation status were significantly high in cervical intraepithelial neoplasia (CIN III) and invasive cancer specimens (Kuramoto et al., 2008). An interesting retrospective analysis of patients with early-stage cervical cancer evaluated IGF-IR expression levels by immunoflorescent stain. Authors found that high-grade expression of IGF-IR, is an independent predictor of cervical cancer death and recurrence, and when combined with elevated squamous cervical cancer antigen (SCC Ag) serum level, could further help identify the subgroup of patients at higher death risk. Colocalisation of IGF-I and IGF-IR in the cancerous tissues, and the lack of correlation between circulating IGF-I or IGFBP-3, and

IGF-IR overexpression in cervical cancer tissue, give support to a paracrine or autocrine function of the IGF system in early-stage cervical cancer, with the corresponding adverse IGF-I stimulation of IGF-IR signaling (Huang et al., 2008).

Only few studies have addressed the analysis of gene expression on exfoliated cells. The remaining cellular material after preparation of routine Pap smear can be used for the search of new biomarkers at both the mRNA and protein levels. The use of cervical scrapes instead of biopsies for biomarker studies has several advantages, since this is a noninvasive procedure, the material obtained is not affected by stroma or other contaminants, as is the case in the analysis of tissue homogenates and can be the base for molecular epidemiology studies.

In a study on cervical scrapes from SIL and cancer patients, we found no difference in IGF-II mRNA levels between cancer and normal cells, whereas at the protein level, IGF-II expression was reduced in cancer cervical scrapes (Serrano et al., 2007, 2010a). There is ample evidence that the levels of IGF-II mRNA differ from the protein. While IGF-II transcripts were higher than in normal tissue in prostate cancer (Tennant et al., 1996), Wilms tumors (Haselbacher et al., 1987), and glioblastomas and astrocytomas (Hultberg et al., 1993), it was not the case for the protein. High levels of IGF-II protein, but not mRNA were found in pheocromocytomas (Haselbacher et al., 1987). These evidences indicate that regulation of IGF-II expression involves transcriptional mechanisms, as genomic imprinting, but also post-transcriptional regulation, that can occur through malignant progression. A member of the IGF-II mRNA binding protein family (IMP), IMP-3, has been reported to be an activator of IGF-II mRNA translation and therefore may play a critical role in IGF-II-dependent cellular proliferation (Liao et al., 2005). IMPs were detected in various cancers; increased levels were found in ovarian cancer and correlated with prognosis. There are no studies about IMP in cervical cancer.

Few studies have examined the expression of hybrid receptors in cervical cancer cells. In a recent study, we found that IR-A, IR-B and hybrid receptors coexist with IGF-IR in human papillomavirus-positive cervical cancer cells. Tyrosine phosphorylation of the receptors and activation of the MAPK and PI3-K pathways were observed upon ligand binding, which may explain the anti-apoptotic effect mediated by IGF-I in these cells (Serrano et al., 2008). Further studies are required to fully understand the significance of the hybrid receptors, especially IGF-IR/HR-A in cervical carcinogenesis and for the design of therapies to target their effects.

2.2.2 The role of IGF in radioresistance in cervical cancer

The crucial role of IGF-IR in promoting resistance to cancer treatments, such as radiation and chemotherapy, is well documented for several cancer types (Samani, et al., 2007). IGF-IR down-regulation by antisense nucleotides or its inhibition by tyrosine kinase inhibitors increases cancer cell sensitivity to both radiation and chemotherapy in a variety of malignancies. Some studies indicate an important role of IGF-IR in several pathways involved in the induction of radioresistance (Belfiore et al., 2009).

The identification of the mechanisms underlying the effects of IGF-II/IGF-IR signaling in the induction of resistance to oxidative stress in cancer cells may provide useful information for the selection of the appropriate treatment strategy. In a study with advanced cervical cancer patients (CIN I-III), we found that tumor tissues co-expressing IGF-IR and IGF-II, showed an increase (4.6-fold) in the risk of developing resistance to radiotherapy. The increased expression of the glycolitic enzyme glyceraldehyde 3-phosphate dehydrogenase (GAPDH) in these cancer tissues, demonstrated the metabolic shift to glycolisis under hypoxic conditions (Moreno-Acosta et al., 2010). Therefore, targeting IGF-II/IGF-IR signaling may be a desirable option in the treatment of tumors overexpressing the IGF-IR.

3. Biomarkers for cervical cancer

Biomarkers used for screening in cancer, usually consist of biomolecules that are released from tumors or precancerous lesions into the bloodstream, urine, or other means, they should have the property to survive the metabolic degradation to be measurable (Ahlquist, 2010). Molecular changes that occur in the development of tumors may take several years; some biomarkers can be used to detect early stage disease. However, biomarkers are usually found at relatively low level compared to other biomolecules; research and validation as possible diagnostic tests depend critically on the ability to achieve measurements with high precision and sensitivity.

Several biologic markers or indexes have been studied as potential tools to determine the prognosis and biological behaviour of various types of gynaecological neoplasias. From years the search of cervical cancer biomarkers has been fed through different techniques, such as immunohistochemistry (IHC), probably the most affordable and simple technology to detect many such biomarkers (McCluggage, 2002; Munoz et al., 2003). This fact prompted investigators to develop and test antibodies in a widespread range of neoplasic lesions. In this approach, some researchers found a two component system, denominated MaTu, consisting of an exogenous transmissible MX agent (coding for p58X protein) and an endogenous MN (coding for MN-protein) in HeLa cells (Závada et al., 1993). The association between MN protein (MN-p) expression and oncogenesis was suggested by its presence in neoplasms, and not in benign tissue (Brewer et al., 1996; Liao et al., 1994). Because HeLa is a cultured human uterine cervix carcinoma cell line, these authors concluded that MN-p had great use as a tumour marker in the evaluation of cervical carcinoma and could predict progression in precursor cervical intraepithelial neoplasic (CIN) lesions. Nonetheless, its utility was questioned as MN-p inmunostaining was not limited to neoplastic tissue, but found in adjacent basal cell hyperplasia, metaplasias and benign glandular epithelium (Liao et al., 1994; Resnick et al., 1996).

Ki67, a nuclear proliferation associated antigen is expressed in the growth and synthesis phases of the cell cycle (G1, S, G2, and mitosis) but not in the resting phase, G0. The proportion of cells which express Ki67 (Ki67 index) is an excellent measure of neoplasm proliferation. Production of specific antibodies against recombinant DNA Ki67 antigen (MIB-1) confirmed the definite use of MIB-I immunoreactivity, exhibiting close correlation with CIN grade and providing additional risk prediction beyond HPV type (Resnick et al., 1996). In low-grade CIN, anti-MIB-1 staining is not detected in superficial levels of epithelium, whereas in high-grade CIN full thickness staining is present. The authors´ hypothesis was that viral gene expression undergoes programmed cessation in superficial layers of low-grade CIN; therefore viral E6/E7 protein is no longer present to inhibit p53 and the cells stop cycling (so Ki67 detection through anti-MIB-1 disappears). In high-grade CIN, viral expression of E6/E7 proceeds unabated often in absence of vegetative viral functions leading to inhibition of p53 and uninhibited cell cycling (so Ki67 detection through anti-MIB-1 continues). In contrast with MN-p expression, anti-MIB-1 shows consistent results by most investigators and exhibits definitive, important associations with clinical outcome and basic carcinogenesis hypotheses in the uterine cervix (Costa, 1996).

For several years, it has been known that high vascularity is characteristic of grade 3 CIN and invasive lesions, and angiogenesis has been associated as indicator of prognosis. The onset of angiogenesis in human cervical cancer occurring during the premalignant dysplastic stage is unique. An association between lymphatic high microvessel density with vascular invasion and a lower global survival rate has been described. There is a study demonstrating that microvessel density in carcinomas of the uterine cervix is a factor associated with poor prognosis (Tjalma et al., 1999). The authors showed that during the progression from noninvasive to microinvasive cervical carcinoma, the microvessel density increases significantly. However, the vessel density does not predict recurrence of noninvasive lesions. Once the tumour cells have passed the basal membrane, the tumour apparently switches to an angiogenic phenotype. Angiogenesis becomes a tumour initiator with prognostic potential (Tjalma et al., 1999). Measures of factor VIII, CD31, and vimentin, showed no association between microvessel count and lymph node invasion, depth of invasion, and histological differentiation. Nevertheless, these studies found an association between lymphatic vessel invasion and a larger number of newly formed vessels (Di Leo et al., 1998).

Other studies have proposed anti-CD34 as a marker for evaluating angiogenesis in cervical cancer (Vieira et al., 2004, 2005). Anti-CD34 antibody is a highly sensitive marker for endothelial cell differentiation and has also been studied as a marker for vascular tumours (Stross et al., 1989; Traweek et al., 1991). Vieira et al. (Vieira et al., 2005) showed that this antibody was able to detect a number of microvessels on neoplasm of the uterine cervix better than anti-factor VIII. They suggested that anti-CD34 antibody reactivity in cervical carcinoma is associated with pathoanatomical features, as microvessel density or invasion, indicative of poorer prognosis and greater risk of recurrence (Vieira et al., 2005). Briefly, they showed lymphatic invasion in 40% of the cases, while vascular and perineural invasion was observed in 24% and 19% of the cases, in a population of 62 patients diagnosed with invasive cervical carcinoma, stages Ib and IIa. They also observed that 55% of women whose carcinoma presented high microvessel density had an undifferentiated type of cancer, suggesting that the presence of lymphatic invasion may associate with higher microvessel density. In general, different markers for angiogenesis may or may not present a statistically significant association with different pathoanatomic features of cervical cancer. These possible markers should be tested prospectively as a prognostic and predictive factor of the response to different therapies used in cervical carcinoma.

On the other hand, a recent study explored the power of serum markers such as squamous cell carcinoma antigen (SCC), CYFRA 21-1, CA 125, immunosuppressive acidic protein (IAP) and vascular endothelial growth factor (VEGF) in patients with cervical cancer (Gadducci et al., 2008). Squamous cell carcinoma antigen comprises two similar proteins, SCC-1 and SCC-2, that posses protease inhibitory property: SCC-1 inhibits chymotrypsin and cathepsin L, while SCC-2 inhibits cathepsin G and mast cell chymase. Both proteins exert anti-apoptotic effects. The mechanism of protection of tumour cells from apoptosis involves the inhibition of caspase-3 activity and/or upstream proteases. SCC-1 and SCC-2 reside in the citosol of squamous cells, and their presence in the sera of patients with advanced squamous cell carcinomas is mainly due to a passive release rather than an active secretory process into the circulation. Increased SCC levels have been observed in 28-88% of patients with squamous cell cervical cancer. Pre-treatment SCC levels reflect tumour stage and size, cervical stoma invasion, lymph-vascular space status, parametrial involvement and lymph node status; however, its clinical relevance is still debated.

CA 125, an antigenic determinant of a high molecular weight glycoprotein, is recognized by a monoclonal antibody developed against a human ovarian cancer cell line. Elevated CA 125 levels are detectable in 20-75% of patients with cervical adenocarcinoma and have been associated with advanced tumour stage, large tumour size, high histological grade, lymph node involvement and status. CA 125 is detected in normal adult fallopian tube, endometrium, endocervix and peritoneum, and *in vitro* studies showed that CA 125 secretion by human mesothelial cell monolayers may be enhanced by the inflammatory cytokines interleukin-1 and tumour necrosis factor. However, the specificity of the antigen is not yet optimal, since elevated serum CA 125 can be found in benign gynaecological conditions, such as endometriosis and pelvic inflammatory disease, benign non-gynaecological conditions, such as hepatitis, pancreatitis, renal failure and pleural effusion and non-gynaecological malignancies, including lung cancer, pancreatic cancer and non-Hodgkin's lymphoma.

Serum levels of vascular endothelial factor (VEGF) are often elevated in patients with cervical cancer, and decrease significantly after successful treatment. However, the clinical relevance of serum VEGF is still investigational (Gadducci et al., 2008).

New predictive biomarkers for cervical cancer are still necessary to improve the accuracy of screening and thereby reduce overtreatment and possibly improve cost-effectiveness of the treatment. Advances in molecular biology and high throughput technologies have heralded a new era in identification of biomarkers and molecular targets related to carcinogenesis to improve our understanding of the disease and will facilitate screening, early detection, management, and individualized targeted therapy.

3.1 Proteomic studies

Proteomics has emerged as a promising tool for unravelling protein signatures that are associated with a particular malignancy that can be useful biomarkers of the disease. High-throughput technologies like surface-enhanced laser desorption and ionization-time of flight mass spectrometry (SELDI-TOF MS), nanoHPLC-MS/MS or the combination of one- or two-dimensional gel electrophoresis (1-DE, 2-DE) methods with multidimensional chromatographic separation and MS provide a snapshot of the proteome. Validated protein biomarkers could be useful in early detection of disease, monitoring disease progression or monitoring response to treatment.

3.1.1 Proteomic studies on body fluids

After exploring markers in tissue, several studies have focused on biomarker discovery in body fluids which would be advantageous for eventual clinical implementation. Cervical mucous or cervical vaginal fluid (CVF) is potentially an ideal sample to screen for biomarkers for early detection of cervical cancer. As cervical mucous is produced in the microenvironment where cervical neoplasia arises, it is likely to include proteins produced by the lesion as well as by the host in response to the lesion. Several studies have analyzed peptides and proteins present in human cervical mucous (Dasari et al., 2007; Pereira et al., 2007; Tang et al., 2007). A recent study identified 151 new proteins that included proteins present in the lower female genital tract, such as HBD-2 and cathelicidin, two proteins that play an important role in the innate immunity of the cervicovagina (Zegels et al., 2009). Another recent study on cervical mucous proteome indicated that plasma proteins were abundant in cervical mucous (Panicker et al., 2010). The majority of proteins identified were categorized under metabolism and immune-response functional groups.

In contrast to plasma samples, some authors discuss the advantages of cervical mucous as a potential source of concentrated biomarkers due to lesser dilution of the sample in CVF-vaginal washings (volume ±50 mL) in comparison to plasma volume (±3 L) (Good et al., 2007). In addition, altered biomarker expression patterns in plasma are often not very specific, as they may be associated with different pathologies, because plasma comes in contact with all organs of the body. In contrast, when using CVF samples, it is expected that expression patterns will directly correlate with gynaecological pathologies (Zegels et al., 2009). However, it should be taken into account that CVF is a body fluid that can be highly influenced by many biological factors including menstruation, age, infection, sexual intercourse, usage of contraceptives, pregnancy, etc. Moreover, conditions of CVF collection and the experimental proteomic strategy could affect the proteome results. Although there are promising results, studies in biomarkers in body fluids have not reached consensus on peptides or proteins that have this feature.

3.1.2 Membrane proteomic studies

The main potential of proteomics in cancer research is not only derived from individual experiments, but from comparative studies between different types and states of cancer. There is a need to integrate proteomics, genomics and metabolomics with the aim of achieving a functional and comprehensive interpretation of clinical and pathological data. Comparative proteomic studies have provided tools for establishing some molecular mechanisms of cancer progression, either from normal to neoplasic cells, or from cancer models with different malignant phenotypes. Information obtained through proteomic analysis allows building extensive and comprehensive databases leading to discovery of tumor biomarkers.

Metastasis represents the main cause of death in cancer patients; this multi-step process involves the acquisition of migrating and invasive phenotypes, where the plasma membrane displays a fundamental role. Membrane proteomic studies constitute an analytical challenge due to its heterogeneous composition, dynamic physicochemical characteristics and hydrophobicity; however, 60% of therapeutic targets are directed against membrane proteins. The study of well established cancer cell lines with different phenotypes allows the correlation between the IGF axis expression/activation with membrane protein expression measurements. In particular, cellular motility depends on the adaptive response to environment that extensively relies on key molecular elements of the plasma membrane and cytoskeleton, and therefore usually considered as tumour targets.

Here we present novel results of studies on membrane proteomes of cervical cancer cell lines, differing in viral status and invasive phenotypes: HeLa, an invasive HPV positive cell line, and C33-A, a non-invasive HPV negative cell line (Garay et al., 2010). C33-A cells express almost exclusively IR-A while HeLa express IGF-IR, IR-A and IR-B. Functional assays showed that IGF-I and IGF-II stimulate migration and invasion in HeLa but not in C33-A cervical cancer cells. In order to make comparisons between proteomic maps, we obtained proteomic maps of the two cell lines by two–dimensional electrophoresis (2-DE), and used the PDQuest (Bio-Rad®) and Progenesis SameSpot (Nonlinear Dynamics Ltd) softwares, to perform between-gel spot comparisons (Fig. 3 A,B). A total of 641 spots in C33-A and 493 spots in HeLa proteomes were identified, with 399 spots matching between the two cell lines. This means that the whole proteomic profiles of cervical adenocarcinoma and cervical carcinoma cells share 80% of similarity, suggesting that the differences in occurrence, prognosis, dissemination and recurrence after treatment, may be related to a limited number of proteins and their relative distribution and expression.

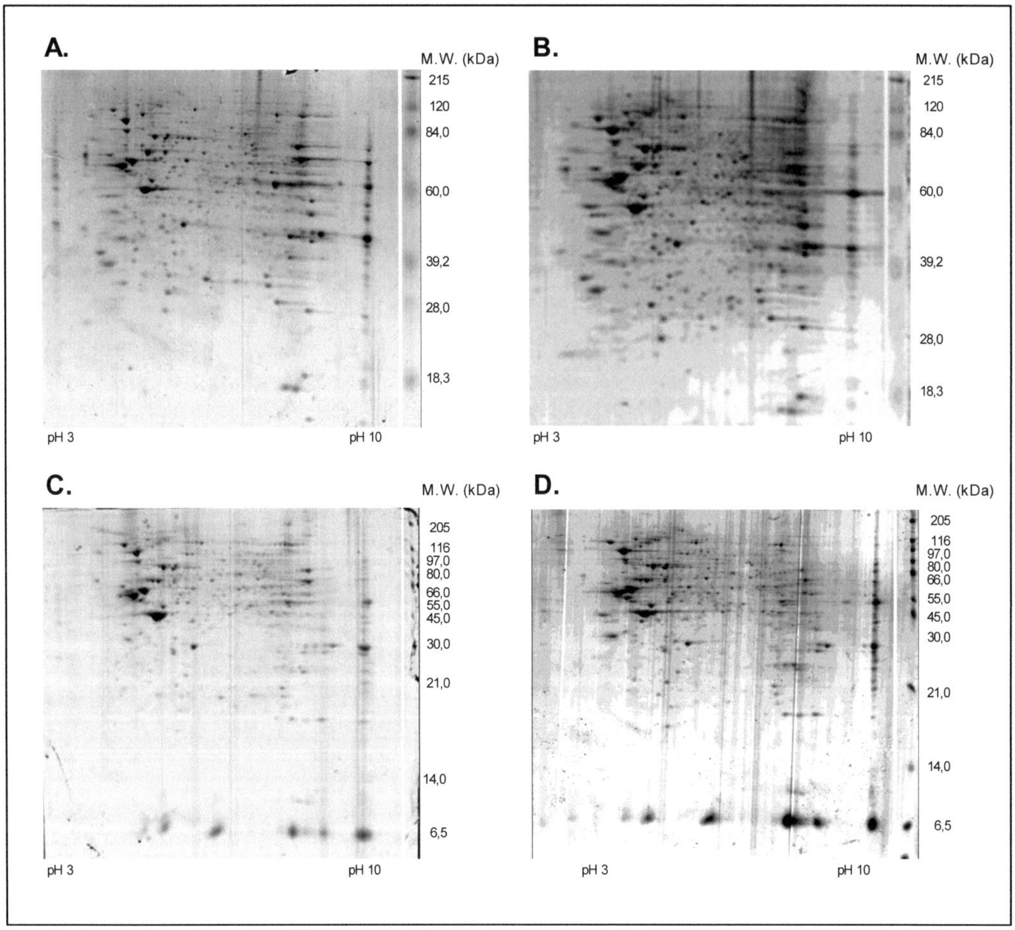

Fig. 3. Proteomes and sub-proteomes of cervical cancer cells. Whole protein extracts from HeLa (A) and C33-A (B) and enriched membrane extracts from HeLa (C) and C33-A (D) were separated by two-dimensional electrophoresis (2-DE) on IPG NL strips pH 3-10 followed by SDS-PAGE and stained with colloidal Coomassie Blue.

Frequently, whole proteomic profiles do not represent the complete map of the expressed proteins in a cell at a given moment; the concentration of some proteins can mask others less abundant but with pivotal biological roles. Study of sub-cellular compartments could improve the identification of a higher number of proteins and consequently a more efficient detection of therapeutic targets. We obtained enriched protein membrane extracts from HeLa and C33-A cells by cell surface biotin labelling followed by avidin purification and separation by 2-DE to obtain the corresponding membrane proteomes (Fig. 3 C, D).

We detected 351 spots in HeLa sub-proteome, out of which 207 spots (41%) were present in the whole proteome and 144 spots corresponded to new proteins not visualized in the total proteome. With respect to C33-A, 395 spots were found in the membrane proteome where 170 spots (43%) matched with the total proteome; additionally 255 new spots were detected. Furthermore, comparison of membrane-enriched proteomes, showed a 58% match between the two cell lines with 272 common proteins, out of which, 86 proteins were found to be differentially expressed (>3-fold). The invasive abilities of HeLa in opposition to C33-A cells, may be related to the observed differences in the membrane protein profile.

In order to identify a higher number of proteins and overcome the limitations associated with the separation of membrane proteins by bi-dimensional electrophoresis, we conducted a multidimensional analysis of enriched membrane fractions. Proteins were separated by SDS-PAGE, each lane in the gel was cut and divided in equal fragments and digested with trypsin. The peptides were separated by reversed-phase liquid chromatography (LC) and analyzed in a hybrid quadrupole mass spectrometer–time of flight (Q-TOF) instrument. Bioinformatics analysis was performed using Mascot Distiler® and Proteome Software Scaffold, which allowed the identification of 44 and 56 proteins in HeLa and C33-A fractions, respectively.

Results showed a differential or exclusive protein expression profile that correlated with cell phenotype. We identified 33 proteins exclusively expressed in C33-A cells that corresponded to cell cycle regulation, metabolism, stress response and immune system evasion, more related to a proliferative non-invasive phenotype. Meanwhile, 22 proteins exclusively expressed in HeLa cells, where mainly involved in cytoskeleton remodelling and associated with cell motility, according to the invasive phenotype. Among the new identified proteins, the more relevant in the regulation of metastatic properties, include: Filamin A and B, Myoferlin and the CD44 - Moesin complex, which have been previously associated with cell adhesion and tumour progression (Feng & Walsh, 2004; Ravid et al., 2008; Bernatchez et al., 2007).

To explore the relationships between the identified proteins and the IGF system, we used the STRING 8.3 database to examine the known or predicted protein-protein interactions among them. The interaction network was built including all the previously identified proteins in the membrane proteome and the members of the IGF system. The interaction network obtained for HeLa cells is visualized in Fig. 4. This analysis confirmed the interaction of some components of the membrane with members of the IGF family, and suggests a potential role in the promotion of the invasive phenotype display by these cells. In particular, this analysis confirmed a direct interaction between IGFBP-3 and the CD44 - Moesin complex, associated with cell adhesion and tumor progression, meaning a promising target for cervical cancer invasion and metastasis control. In conclusion, our

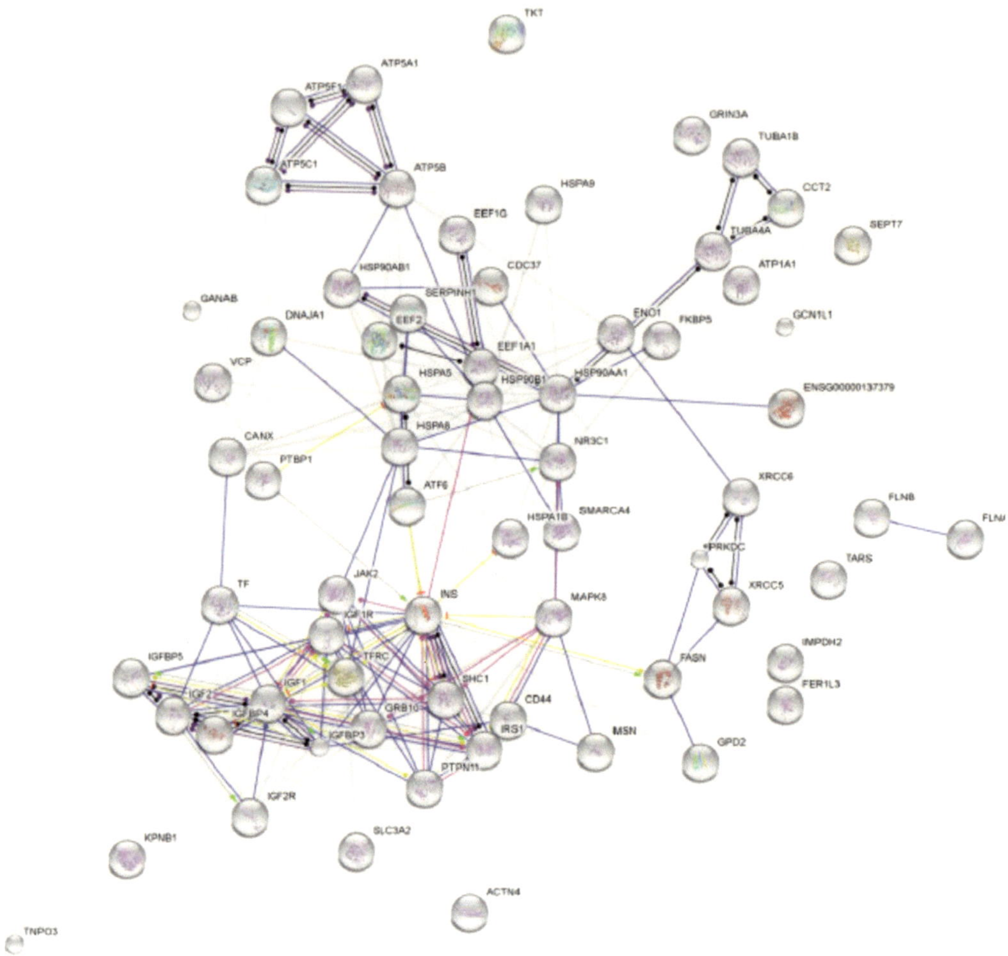

Fig. 4. Protein-protein interaction network representing the associations between the IGF system and identified membrane proteins expressed by the cervical cancer HeLa cell line. The network is visualized by STRING 8.3 database. Each circle represents an individual protein with the recognized abbreviated name. Connecting lines represent association.

approach is unique as it considers the IGF receptors in a wider context within a protein network, and shows that the membrane is a rich reservoir for potential targets for cancer.

4. Conclusion

The evidence reviewed above shows that the IGF system plays a central role in many aspects of the development and progression of cervical cancer. The effects of components of the IGF axis in cervical carcinogenesis share some similarities with those observed in other types of cancer, however, clear differences exist that reflect specificities, possibly due to associations with oncogenic and nononcogenic HPV. The available data support dysregulation of the IGF system expression and signaling, that could promote the progression to a malignant phenotype. It is plausible to consider these molecules as promising targets for cervical cancer invasion and metastasis control and source of valuable biomarkers of the disease, as deduced from the proteomic approach of membrane targets. Advances in molecular biology and high throughput technologies will improve our understanding of the disease and the search for reliable biomarkers that will facilitate screening, early detection, management, and individualized targeted therapy.

5. Acknowledgment

This work was supported by the Research Council of the Universidad Nacional de Colombia (Grants No. 9173 and 9478) and Colciencias, Colombia (Grant 110145221052). We thank Dr. Patricia Cuervo, Instituto Oswaldo Cruz, Fiocruz, Rio de Janeiro, Brazil and Dr. Gilberto B. Domont, Universidade Federal de Rio de Janeiro, Brazil, for the helpful support with the proteomic studies.

6. References

Ahlquist, D.A. (2010). Molecular detection of colorectal neoplasia. *Gastroenterology*, Vol.138, No.6, (June 2010), pp.2127-2139, ISSN 0016-5085

Bang, P. & Hall, K. (1992). Insulin-like growth factors as endocrine and paracrine hormones. In: *The Insulin-like Growth Factors. Structure and Biological Functions*. Ed. P.N. Schofield, pp.151-177, Oxford University Press, ISBN 0-19-854270-4, Oxford, UK

Baxter, R.C. (2000). Insulin Like growth factor (IGF)-binding proteins: interactions with IGFs and intrinsic bioactivities. *American Journal of Physiology-Endocrinology and Metabolism*, Vol.278, No. 6 41-6, pp.E967-E976, ISSN 0193-1849

Belfiore, A., Frasca, F., Pandini, G., Sciacca, L. & Vigneri, R. (2009). Insulin receptor isoforms and insulin receptor/insulin-like growth factor receptor hybrids in physiology and disease. *Endocrine Reviews*, Vol.30, No.6, (September 2009),pp.586-623, ISSN 002-972X

Bernatchez, P.N., Acevedo, L., Fernandez-Hernando, C., Murata, T., CHalouni, C., Kim, J., Erdjument-Bromage, H., Shah, V., Gratton, J.P., McNally, E.M., Tempst, P. & Sessa, W.C. (2007). Myoferlin regulates vascular endothelial growth factor receptor-2 stability and function. *Journal of Biological Chemistry*, Vol. 282, No.42, (October 2007), pp.30745-30753, ISSN 0021-9258

Brewer, C.A., Lia, S.Y., Wilczynski, S.P., Pastorekova, S., Pastorek, J., Zavada, J., Kurosaki, T., Manetta, A., Berman, M.L., DiSaia, P.J. & Stanbridge, P.J. (1996). A study of biomarkers in cervical carcinoma and clinical correlation of the novel biomarker MN. *Gynecological Oncology*, Vol.63, No.3, (December 1993), pp.337-344, ISSN 0090-8258

Coppola, D., Ferber, A., Miura, M., Sell, C., D´Ambrosio, C., Rubin, R. & Baserga, R. (1994). A functional insulina-like growth factor receptor I is required for the mitogenic and transforming activities of the epidermal growth factor receptor. *Molecular and Cellular Biology*, Vol.14, No.7, (July 1994), pp.4588-4595, ISSN 0270-7306

Costa, M.J. (1996). MN and Ki67 (MIB-1) in uterine cervix carcinoma: novel biomarkers with divergent utility. *Human Pathology*, Vol.27, No.3, (March 1996), pp.217-219, ISSN 0046-8177

Cui, H, Cruz-Correa, M., Giardiello, F.M., Hutcheon, D.F., Kafonek, D.R., Brandenburg, S., Wu,Y., He,X., Powe, N.R. & Feinberg, A. P. (2003). Loss of IGF2 imprinting: a potential marker of colorectal cancer risk. *Science*, Vol.299, No.5613, (March 2003), pp.1753–1755, ISSN 0036-8075

Cullen, K..J., Yee, D., Sly, W.S., Perdue, J., Hampton, B., Lippman, M.E. & Rosen, N. (1990). Insulin-like growth factor receptor expression and function in human breast cancer. *Cancer Research*, Vol. 50, No.1, (January 1990), pp.48-53, ISSN 0008-5472

Dasari, S., Pereira, L. Reddy, A.P., Michaels, J.E., Lu, X., Jacob, T., Thomas, A., Rodland, M., Roberts, C.T.Jr, Gravett, M.G. & Nagalla, S.R. (2007). Comprehensive proteomic analysis of human cervical-vaginal fluid. *Journal of Proteome Research*, Vol.6, No.4, (April 2007), pp.1258-1268, ISSN 1535-3893

Di Leo, S., Caschetto, S., Garozzo, G., Nuciforo, G., Cassaro, N., Meli, M.T., DiMaur, R. & Caragliano, L. (1998). Angiogenesis as a prognostic factor in cervical carcinoma. *European Journal of Gynecological Oncology*, Vol.19, No.2, pp.158-162, ISSN 0392-2936

Díaz, L.E., Chuan, Y.C., Lewitt, M., Fernández-Pérez, L., Carrasco-Rodríguez, S., Sánchez-Gómez, M. & Flores-Morales. A. (2007). IGF-II regulates metastatic properties of choriocarcinoma cells through the activation of the insulin receptor. *Molecular Human Reproduction*, Vol 13, No.8, (June 2007), pp.567-576, ISSN 1360-9947

El-Shewy, H.M., Johnson, K.R., Lee, M.-H., Jaffa, A.A., Obeid, L.M. & Luttrell, L.M. (2006). Insulin-like growth factors mediate heterotrimeric G Protein-dependent ERK1/2 activation by transactivating sphingosine 1-Phosphate receptors. *Journal of Biological Chemistry*, Vol.281, No.42, (October 2006),pp.31399-31407, ISSN 31399-31407

El-Shewy, H.M. & Luttrell, L.M. (2009). Insulin-like growth factor-2/Mannose-6 phosphate receptors. In: *Vitamins and Hormones*, Vol. 80. T.P. Begley, A.R. Means, B.W. O´Malley, L. Riddiford & A.H. Tashjian, Jr. Editors, pp.667-697, Elsevier Academic Press, ISBN 978-0-12-374408-1, Oxford, UK

Feng, Y. & Walsh, C.A. (2004). The many faces of filamin: a versatile molecular scaffold for cell motility and signalling. *Nature Cell Biology*, Vol.6, No.11, (November 2004), pp. 1034-1038, ISSN 1465-7392

Ferlay, J., Shin, H.R., Bray, F., Forman, D., Mathers, C. & Parkin DM. (2010). Estimates of worldwide burden in cancer in 2008: GLOBOCAN 2008. *International Journal of Cancer.* Vol. 127, No. 12, (June 2010), pp.2893-2917, Online ISSN 1097-0215

Furstenberger, G. & Senn, H.J. (2002). Insulin-like growth factors and cancer. *Lancet Oncology*, Vol.3, No.5, (May 2002), pp.298-302, ISSN 1470-2045

Gadducci, A., Tana, R., Cosio, S. & Genazzani, A. R. (2008). The serum assay of tumour markers in the prognostic evaluation, treatment monitoring and follow-up of patients with cervical cancer: a review of the literature. *Critical Reviews in Oncology Hematology*, Vol. 66, No. 1, (Apr 2008), pp. 10-20, ISSN 1040-8428

Gallagher, E. J. & LeRoith, D. (2011). Minireview: IGF, Insulin and Cancer, *Endocrinology*, Vol. 152, No.7, (July 2011), pp.2546-2551, ISSN 0013-7227

Garay-Baquero, D.J., Vallejo, A.F., Umaña-Pérez, A., García, C., Nogueira, F.S.C., Domont, G.B., Cuervo, P. & Sánchez-Gómez, M. (2010). A comparative proteomic study of cervical cancer invasion. In: *Human Proteome Organization Annual World Congress 2010*, Sydney, Australia, October 2010. Available from: http://posters.f1000.com/P566

Good, D.M., Thongboonkerd, V., Novak, J., Bascands, J.L., Schanstra, J.P., Coon, J.J., Dominiczak, A. & Mischak, H. (2007). Body fluid proteomics for biomarker discovery: lessons from the past hold the key to success in the future. *Journal of Proteome Research*, Vol.6, No.12, (December 2007), pp.4549-4555, ISSN 1535-3893

Hanahan, D. & Weinberg, R.A. (2000). The hallmarks of cancer. *Cell*, Vol.100, No.1, (January 2000), pp.57-70, ISSN 0092-8674

Harris, T.G., Burk, R.D., Yu, H., Minkoff, H., Massad, L.S., Watts, D.H., Zhong, Y., Gange, S., Kaplan, R.C., Anastos, K., Levine, A.M., Moxley, M., Xue, X., Fazzari, M., Palefsky, J.M. & Strikler, D. (2008). Insulin-like growth factor axis and oncogenic human papillomavirus history. *Cancer Epidemiology, Biomarkers & Prevention*, Vol.17, No.1, (January 2008), pp.245-248, ISSN 1055-9965

Haselbacher, G. K., Irminger, J.C., Zapf, J., Ziegler, W.H. & Humber, R.E. (1987). Insulin-like growth factor II in human adrenal pheochromocytomas and Wilms tumors: expression at the mRNA and protein level. *Proceedings of the National Academy of Sciences of the United States of America*, Vol.84, No.4, (February 1987), pp.1104-1106, ISSN 0027-8424

Hellawell, G. O., Turner, G.D., Davies, D.R., Poulsom, R., Brewster, S.F. & Macaulay, V.M. (2002). Expression of the type 1 insulin-like growth factor receptor is up-regulated in primary prostate cancer and commonly persists in metastatic disease. *Cancer Research*, Vol. 62, No.10, (May 2002), pp.2942-2950, ISSN 0008-5472

Huang, Y-F., Shen, M-R., Hsu, K-F, Cheng, Y-M. & Chou, C-Y. (2008). Clinical implications of insulin-like growth factor I system in early stage cervical cancer. *British Journal of Cancer*, Vol.99, No.7, (September 2008), pp.1096-1102, ISSN 0007-0920

Hultberg, B.M., Haselbacher, G., Nielsen, F.C., Wulff, B.S. & Gammeltoft, S. (1993). Gene expression of insulin-like growth factor II in human intracraneal meningiona. *Cancer*, Vol.72, No.11, (December 1993), 3282-3286, Online ISSN 1097-0142

Jemal, A., Bray, F., Center, M.M., Ferlay, J., Ward, E. & Forman, D. (2011). Global cancer statistics. *CA: A Cancer Journal for Clinicians*, Vol. 61, No.2, (February 2011), pp.69-90, Online ISSN 1542-4863

Jeffreys, M., Northstone, K., Holly, J., Emmett, P. & Gunnell, D. (2011). Levels of insulin-like growth factor during pregnancy and maternal cancer risk: a nested case-control study. *Cancer Causes And Control*, Vol.22, No.7, (July 2011), pp.945-953, ISSN 0957-5243

Kuramoto, H., Hong, A., Liu, Y.X., Ojima, Y., Nakamura, K., Seki, N., Kodama, J. & Hiramatsu, Y. (2008). Immunohistochemical evaluation of insulin-like growth factor I receptor status in cervical cancer specimens. *Acta Medica Okayama*, Vol.62, No.4, (August 2008), pp.251-259, ISSN 0386-300X

Lacey, J.V. Jr., Potischman, N., Madigan, M.P., Berman, M.L., Mortel, R., Twiggs, L.B., Barrett, L.J., Wilbanks, G.D., Lurain, J.R., Fillmore, C.M., Sherman, M.E. & Brinton, L.A. (2004). Insulin-like growth factors, insulin-like growth factor-binding proteins, and endometrial cancer in postmenopausal women: results from a U.S. case-control study. *Cancer Epidemiology, Biomarkers & Prevention*, Vol.13, No.4, (April 2004), pp.607-612, ISSN 1055-9965

Lee, D.Y., Yang, D.H., Kang, C.W., Kim, S.J., Joo, C.U., Cho, S.C. & Kim, J.S. (1997). Serum insulin-like growth factors (IGFs) and IGF binding protein (IGFBP)-3 in patients with gastric cancer: IGFBP-3 protease activity induced by surgery. *Journal of Korean Medical Science*, Vol. 12, No.1, (February 1997), pp.32-39, ISSN 1011-8934

Lee, S.W., Lee, S.Y., Lee, S.R., Wu, W. & Kim, S.C. (2010). Plasma levels of insulin-like growth factor-1 and insulin-like growth factor binding protein-3 in women with cervical neoplasia. *Journal of Gynecologic Oncology*, Vol.21, No.3, (September 2010), pp.174-180, ISSN 2005-0380

LeRoith, D., Werner, H., Neuenschwander, S., Kalebic, T. & Helman, L.J. (1995). The role of the insulin-like growth factor-I receptor in cancer. *Annals of the New York Academy of Sciences*, Vol.766, (September 1995), pp.402-406, Online ISSN 1749-6632

LeRoith, D. & Roberts Jr, C.T. (2003). The insulin-like growth factor system and cancer. *Cancer Letters*, Vol.195, No.2, (May 2003),pp.127-137, ISSN 0304-3835

Lewitt, M. S., Saunders, H., Phuval, J.L. & Baxter, R.C. (1994). Complex formation by Insulin-like growth factor binding protein-3 and human acid-labile subunit in growth hormone-deficient rats. *Endocrinology*, Vol.134, No.6, (June 1994), pp.2404-2409, ISSN 0013-7227

Liao, B., Hu, H., Herrick, D.J. & Brewer, G. (2005). The RNA-binding protein IMP-3 is a translational activator of insulin-like growth factor II leader-3 mRNA during proliferation of human K562 leukemia cells. *Journal of Biological Chemistry*, Vol.280, No.18, (March 2005), pp.18517-18524, ISSN 0021-9258

Liao, S.Y., Brewer, C., Závada, J., Pastorek, J., Pastorekova, S., Manetta, A, Berman, M.L., DiSaia, P.J., Stanbridge, E.J. (1994). Identification of the MN antigen as a diagnostic biomarker of cervical intraepithelial squamous and glandular neoplasia and cervical carcinomas. *American Journal of Pathology*, Vol.145, No.3, (September 1994), pp.598-609, ISSN 0002-9440

MacKinnon, T., Chakraborty, C., Gleeson, L.M., Chidiac, P. & Lala, P.K. (2001). Stimulation of human extravillous trophoblast migration by IGF-II is mediated by IGF type 2 receptor involving inhibitory G protein(s) and phosphorylation of MAPK. *Journal of Clinical Endocrinology and Metabolism*, Vol.86, No.8, (August 2001), pp. 3665-3674, ISSN 0021-972X

McCluggage, W.G. (2002). Recent advances in immunohistochemistry in gynaecological pathology. *Histopathology*, Vol.40, No.4, (April 2002), pp.309-326, ISSN 0309-0167

Mathur, S.P., Mathur, R.S. & Young, R.C. (2000). Cervical epidermal growth factor-receptor (EGF-R) and serum insulin-like growth factor-II (IGF-II) levels are potential markers for cervical cancer. *American Journal of Reproductive Immunolgy*, Vol.44, No.4, (October 2000), pp.222-230, ISSN 1046-7408

Mathur, S.P., Mathur, R.S., Underwood, P.B., Kohler, M.F., Creasman, W.T. (2003), Circulating levels of insulin-like growth factor-II and IGF-binding protein 3 in cervical cancer. *Gynecologic Oncology*, Vol.91, No.3, (December 2003), pp.486–493, ISSN 0090-8258

Mathur, S.P., Mathur, R.S., Gray, E.A., Lane, D., Underwood, P.B., Kohler, M.F., Creasman, W.T. (2005). Serum vascular endothelial growth factor C (VEGF-C) as a specific biomarker for advanced cervical cancer: Relationship to insulin-like growth factor II (IGF-II), IGF binding protein 3 (IGF-BP3) and VEGF-A. *Gynecologic Oncology*, Vol.98, No.3, (September 2005), pp.467–83, ISSN 0090-8258

Mazzoccoli, G., Giuliani, A., Bianco, G., De Cata, A., Balzanelli, M., Carella, A.M., La Viola, M. & Tarquini, R. (1999). Decreased serum levels of insulina-like growth factor (IGF)-I in patients with lung cancer: temporal relationship with growth hormone

(GH) levels. *Anticancer Research*, Vol.19, No.2B, (March-April 1999), pp.1397-1399, ISSN 0250-7005

Mohan, S & Baylink, D.J. (2002). IGF binding proteins are multifunctional and act via IGF-dependent and independent mechanisms. *Journal of Endocrinology*, Vol.175, No.1 (October 2002), pp. 19-31, ISSN 0022-0795

Moreno-Acosta, P., Cendales, R., Sánchez de Gómez, M., García-Carrancá, A., Gamboa, O., Conrado, Z. & Magne, N. (2010). IGF-IR gene expression as a predictive marker of ionizing radiation response for patients with locally advanced cervical cancer. *International Conference on Frontiers in Cancer Prevention Research*, Houston, USA, December 2009, *Cancer Prevention Research*, Vol.3, No.1, Suppl 1, (January 2010), B85, ISSN 1940-6207

Muñoz, N., Bosch, F.X., De Sanjosé, S., Herrero, R., Castellsagué, X, Shah, K.V., Snijders, P.J., Meijer, C.J., International Agency for Research on Cancer Multicenter Cervical Cancer Study Group. (2003). Epidemiologic classification of human papillomavirus types associated with cervical cancer. *New England Journal of Medicine*, Vol.348, No. 6, (February 2003), pp. 518–527, ISSN 0028-4793

Murphy, S.K., Huang, Z., Wen, Y., Spillman, M.A., Whitaker, R.S., Simel, L.R., Nichols, T.D., Marks, J.R. & Berchuck, A. (2006). Frequent IGF2/H19 domain epigenetic alterations and elevated IGF2 expression in epithelial ovarian cancer. *Molecular Cancer Research*, Vol.4, No.4, (April 2006), pp.283-292, ISSN: 1541-7786

Pandini, G., Frasca, F., Mineo, R., Sciacca, L., Vigneri, R. & Belfiore, A. (2002). Insulin/insulin-like growth factor I hybrid receptors have different biological characteristics depending on the insulin receptor isoform involved. *Journal of Biological Chemistry*, Vol.277, No.42, (October 2002), pp.39684-39695, ISSN 31399-31407

Panicker, G., Ye, Y., Wang, D. & Unger, E.R. (2010). Characterization of the human cervical mucous proteome. *Clinical Proteomics*, Vol. 6, No.1-2, (June 2010), pp.18-28, ISSN 1542-6416

Pavelic, K., Bukovic, D. & Pavelic J. (2002). The role of Insulin-like growth factor 2 and its receptors in human tumors. *Molecular Medicine*, Vol. 8, No. 12, (December 2002), pp. 771-780, ISSN 1076-1551

Pereira, L., Reddy, A.P., Jacob, T., Thomas, A., Schneider, K.A., Dasari, S., Lapidus, J.A., Lu, X., Rodland, M., Roberts, C.T.Jr, Gravett, M.G. & Nagalla, S.R. (2007). Identification of novel protein biomarkers of preterm birth in human cervical-vaginal fluid. *Journal of Proteome Research*, Vol.6, No.4, (April 2007), pp.1269-1276, ISSN 1535-3893

Ravid, D., Chuderland, D., Landsman, L., Lavie, Y., Reich, R. & Liscovitch, M. (2008). Filamin A is a novel caveolin-1-dependent target in IGF-I-stimulated cancer cell migration. *Experimental Cell Research*, Vol. 314, No.15, (June 2008).pp. 2762-2773, ISSN 0014-4827

Renehan, A.G., Zwahlen, M., Minder, C., O'Dwyer S.T., Shalet, S.M. & Egger, M. (2004). Insulin-like growth factor (IGF)-I, IGF binding protein-3, and cancer risk: systematic review and meta-regression analysis. *Lancet*, Vol.363, No.9418, (April 2004), pp.1346-1353, ISSN 0140-6736

Resnick, M., Lester, S., Tate, J.E., Sheets, E.E., Sparks, C. & Crump, C.P. (1996). Viral and histopathologic correlates of MN and MIB-1 expression in cervical epithelial neoplasia. *Human Pathology*, Vol.27, No.3, (March 1996), pp.234-239, ISSN 0046-8177

Samani, A.A., Yakar, S., LeRoith, D. & Brodt, P. (2007). The role of the IGF system in cancer growth and metastasis: Overview and recent insights. *Endocrine Reviews*, Vol.28, No. 1, (February 2007),pp.20-47, ISSN 0163-769X

Schaffer, A., Koushik, A., Trotier, H., Duarte-Franco, E., Mansour, N., Arseneau, J., Provencher, D., Gilbert, L., Gotlieb, W., Ferenczy, A., Coutleé, F., Pollak, M.N., Franco, E.L. & The Biomarkers of Cervical Cancer Risk Study Team. (2007). Insulin-like growth factor-I and risk of high-grade cervical intraepithelial neoplasia. *Cancer Epidemiology, Biomarkers & Prevention*, Vol.16, No.4, (April 2007), pp.716-722, ISSN 1055-9965

Sell, C., Dumenil, G., Deveaud, C., Miura, M., Coppola, D., DeAngekis, T., Rubin, R., Efstratiadis, A. & Baserga, R. (1994). Effect of a null mutation of the insulin-like growth factor I receptor gene on growth and transformation of mouse embryo fibroblast. *Molecular and Cellular Biology*, Vol.14, No.6, (June 1994), pp.3604-3612, ISSN 0270-7306

Serrano, M.L., Romero, A., Cendales, R., Sánchez-Gómez, M. & Bravo, M.M. (2006). Serum levels of insulin-like growth factor-I and –II and insulin-like growth factor binding protein 3 in women with squamous intraepithelial lesions and cervical cancer. *Biomédica*, Vol.26, No. 2, (July 2006), pp.258-268, ISSN 0120-4157

Serrano, M-L., Sánchez-Gómez, M. & Bravo, M-M. (2007). Insulin-like growth factor gene expression in cervical scrapes from women with squamous intraepithelial lesions and cervical cancer. *Growth Hormone & IGF Research*, Vol. 17, No. 4, (August 2007), pp.492-499, ISSN 1096-6374

Serrano, M-L., Sánchez-Gómez, M., Bravo, M-M., Yakar, S. & LeRoith, D. (2008). Differential expression of IGF-I and insulin receptor isoforms in HPV positive and negative human cervical cancer cell lines. *Hormone and Metabolic Research*, Vol.40, No.10, (August 2008), pp.661-667, ISSN 0018-5043

Serrano, M-L., Sánchez-Gómez, M. & Bravo, M-M. (2010a). Cervical scrapes levels of insulin-like growth factor –II and insulin-like growth factor binding protein 3 in women with squamous intraepithelial lesions and cervical cancer. *Hormone and Metabolic Research*, Vol.42, No.13, (October 2010), pp.977-981, ISSN 0018-5043

Serrano, M.L., Hernández, G. & Sánchez-Gómez, M. (2010b). Serum levels of insulin-like growth factor-I and oncogenic human papillomavirus natural history. *The Fifth International Congress of the GRS and IGF Society*, New York, USA, October 2010, *Growth Hormone & IGF Research*, Vol.20, (October 2010), pp.S54, ISSN 1096-6374

Solomon, D., Davey, D., Kurman, R., Moriarty, A., O´Connor, D., Prey, M., Raab, S., Sherman, M., Wilbur, D., Wright, T.Jr., Young, N. & Forum Group Members Bethesda 2001 Workshop. (2002). The 2001 Bethesda System: terminology for reporting results of cervical cytology. *Journal of the American Medical Association*, Vol.287, No.16, (April 2002), pp.2114-2119, ISSN 0098-7484

Stross, W.P., Warnke, R.A., Flavell, D.J., Flavell, S.U., Simmons, D., Gatter, K.C. & Mason, D.J. (1989). Molecule detected in formalin fixed tissue by antibodies MT-1, DF-T1, and L60(Leu-22) corresponds to CD43 antigen. *Journal of Clinical Pathology*, Vol.42, No.9, (September 1989), pp.953-961, ISSN 0021-9746

Stuver, S.O., Kuper, H., Tzonou, A., Lagiou, P., Spanos, E., Hsieh, C.C., Mantzoros, C. & Trichopoulos D. (2000). Insulin-like growth factor 1 in hepatocellular carcinoma and metastatic liver cancer in men. *International Journal of Cancer,* Vol.87, No.1, (July 2000), pp.118-121, Online ISSN 1097-0215

Tang, J.L., De Seta, F., Odreman, F., Venge, P., Piva, C., Guaschino, S. & Gracia, R.C. (2007). Proteomic análisis of human cervical-vaginal fluids. *Journal of Proteome Research,* Vol.6, No.7, (July 2007), pp.2874-2883, ISSN 1535-3893

Tennant, M-K., Thrasher, J.B., Towmey, P.A., Drivdahl, R.H., Birnbaum, R.S. & Plymate, S.R. (1996). Protein and messenger ribonucleic acid (mRNA) for the type 1 insulin-like growth factor (IGF) receptor is decreased and IGF-II mRNA is increased in human prostate carcinoma compared to benign prostate epithelium. *Journal of Clinical Endocrinology and Metabolism,* Vol.81, No.10, (October 1996), pp. 3774-3782, ISSN 0021-972X

Tjalma, W. Sonnemans, H., Weyler, J., Van Mark, E., Van Daele, A. & van Dam, P. (1999). Angiogenesis in cervical epithelial neoplasia and the risk of recurrence. *American Journal of Obstetrics & Gynecology,* Vol.181, No.3, (September 1999), pp.554-559, ISSN 0002-9378

Traweek, S.T. Kandalaft, P.L., Mehta, P. & Battifora, H. (1991). The human hematopoietic progenitor cell antigen (CD34) in vascular neoplasia. *American Journal of Clinical Pathology,* Vol.96, No.1, (July 1991), pp.25-31, ISSN 0002-9173

Vieira, S.C., Seferino, L.C., Da Silva, B.B., Aparecida Pinto, G., Vasallo, J., Carvasan, G.A. & De Moraes N.G. (2004). Quantification of angiogenesis in cervical câncer: a comparison among three endothelial cell markers. *Gynecological Oncology,* Vol.93, No.1, (April 2004), pp.121-124, ISSN 0090-8258

Vieira, S.C. , Silva, B.B., Pinto, G.A., Vasallo, J., Moraes N.G., Santana, J.O., Santos, L.G., Carvasan, G.A. & Seferino, L.C. (2005). CD34 as a marker for evaluating angiogenesis in cervical cancer. *Pathology, Research & Practice,* Vol.201, No.4, pp.313-318, ISSN 0344-0338

Walboomers, J.M., Jacobs, M.V., Manos, M.M., Bosch, F.X., Kummer, J.A., Shah, K.V., Snijders, P.J., Peto, J., Meijer, C.J. & Muñoz, N. (1999). Human papilloma virus is a necessary cause of invasive cervical cancer worldwide. *The Journal of Pathology,* Vol.189, No.1, (September 1999), pp.12-19, Online ISSN 1096-9896

Werner, H. & LeRoith, D. (1996). The role of the insulin-like growth factor system in human cancer. In: *Advances in Cancer Research,* Vol.68, G.F. Vande Woude & G. Klein, Eds. Academic Press, pp.183-223, ISBN 978-0-12-0066681

Woodman, C.B., Collins, S., Winter, H., Bailey, A., Ellis, J., Prior, P., Yates, M., Rollason, T.P. & Young, L.S. (2001). Natural history of cervical human papillomavirus infection in young women: a longitudinal cohort study. *Lancet,* Vol.357, No.9271, (June 2001), pp.1831-1836, ISSN 0140-6736

Wu, X., Tortolero-Luna, G., Zhao, H., Phatak, D., Spitz, M.R. & Follen, M. (2003).Serum levels of insulin-like growth factor I and risk of squamous intraepithelial lesions of the cervix. *Clinical Cancer Research,* Vol.9, No.9, (August 2003), pp.3356-3361, ISSN 1078-0432

Yu, H., Spitz, M.R., Mistry, J., Gu, J. Hong, W.K. & Wu, X. (1999). Plasma levels of insulin-like growth factor-I and lung cancer risk: a case-control analysis. *Journal of the National Cancer Institute,* Vol.91, No.2, (January 1999), pp.151-156, ISSN 1460-2105

Závada, J., Závadová, Z., Pasterokevá, S., Ciampor, F., Pastorek, J. & Zelnik, V. (1993). Expression of MaTu-MN protein in human tumor cultures and in clinical specimens. *International Journal of Cancer*, Vol.54, No.2, (May 1993), pp.268-274, Online ISSN 1097-0215

Zegels, G., Van Raemdonk, G.A., Coen, E.P., Tjalma, W.A., Van Ostade, X.W. (2009). Comprehensive proteomic analysis of human cervical-vaginal fluid using colposcopy samples. Proteome Science, Vol.7, (April 2009), pp.17, ISSN 1477-5956

14

HPV Bioinformatics: In Silico Detection, Drug Design and Prevention Agent evelopment

Usman Sumo Friend Tambunan and Arli Aditya Parikesit
Department of Chemistry, Faculty of Mathematics and Science,
University of Indonesia
Indonesia

1. Introduction

Viral infection is a very serious threat to humanity. It causes malicious diseases, such as HIV/AIDS, dengue, and Avian Influenza, therefore, novel method in virology to combat the viral infection is necessary. Bioinformatics provides outstanding tools for developing vaccines, PCR primers, mutation detection and drugs based design on genetic engineering principles. Those tools are mostly freeware. Algorithm from the computer science has made major contribution to them. Bioinformatics experiment greatly reduces the cost and time in wet laboratory experiment. Our lab has successfully designed PCR primers, vaccine, and mutations prediction. The vaccine design is elaborated for Dengue and HPV. The design has BLAST homology of more than 90%, and RSMD value of 0.1. Those data shown, that the design have identical structure with the native viral protein.

However, their efficacy should be verified in the wet laboratory experiment. The future of medicine will greatly be shaped by advancement in bioinformatics (Tambunan et al, 2010). Moreover, we need to emphasize the needs to understand more about HPV genome and its protein expression.

The human papillomavirus (HPV) is a family of sexually transmitted, double-stranded DNA viruses with over 100 different genotypes identified till date. It is associated with many different types of cancers including cervical, vaginal, head and neck, penile and anal cancer. With approximately 450,000 newly diagnosed cases each year and a 50% mortality rate, cervical cancer is the second most common cause of cancer-related death in women worldwide and it is almost always associated with HPV. Cervical cancer is the most common cancer of women in most developing countries, where it may account for as many as one fourth of female cancers.

HPV genotypes are divided into the low risk and high risk categories based on the spectrum of lesions they induce. The low-risk types induce only benign genital warts and include HPV 6 and 11. The high-risk group containing HPV 16, 18, 31, 33, 45 and 56 is associated with the development of anogenital cancers and can be detected in 99% of cervical cancers , with HPV16 found in 50% of cases.

A consistently effective and safe treatment for HPV infections is currently not yet available. Present therapeutic options are more directed at surgical eradication and/or by destroying malignant lesions via physical or chemotherapeutical intervention. A majority of these treatments have been developed empirically, few have been thoroughly tested, but none of them are completely satisfactory. In attemps to find additional drugs in the treatment of cervical cancer, inhibitors of the histone deacetylases have received much attention due to their low cytotoxic profiles (Tambunan et al, 2010).

Elaborating a methodological comparison between our computational approaches with the other bioinformatics labs. We will not compare our method directly with wet labs, because our method is developed to supplement it. Our objective is to find the optimal in silico HPV therapeutic design, and implement it in the wet laboratory.

2. In silico HPV related research

2.1 Detection of HPV genome

This section will elaborate more on HPV Genome Annotation. The conserved region of HPV Genome needs to be annotated, in order to design a useful detection tools. Conventional method of detecting cervical cancer is done by carrying out cytological examination, which is more widely known as Pap smear. Due to rapid advancement of molecular biology, molecular based diagnostic and early detection methods on cervical cancer has been highly developed to replace conventional method of detection. Examples include polymerases chain reaction (PCR) and hybrid capture 1, 2 and 3. Hybrid capture 1 is liquid hybridization assaying method designed to detect 14 types of HPV, 9 of which are high risk (type 16, 18,31, 33, 35, 45, 51, 52, 56), while the other 5 are low risk (type 6, 11, 42, 43, and 44). Hybrid capture 2 is a development of hybrid capture 1 which uses microtitre plates instead of tubes and is capable of detecting four additional types of viral oncogenic (type 39, 58, 59, and 68) (Clavel *et al*, 1998). Hybrid capture 3, similar to previous hybrid capture tests, relies on the formation of target HPV DNA-RNA probe heteroduplexes during the hybridization step in specimens containing sufficient HPV DNA. The chemiluminescent detection of these hybrids is by adding an alkaline phosphatase-conjugated monoclonal antibody, specific to the DNA-RNA complexes with dioxetane substrate in a 96-well enzyme-linked immunosorbent assay format (Lorinze and Anthony, 2001). Most of the above mentioned methods are spesific, sensitive, reliable, and easy to perform. Moreover, its routine application has been very much improved by the use of non-radioactive enzyme immunoassay detection procedure (Clavel *et al*, 1998). Modification of the Hybrid Capture method is expected to be achieved through the use of a customized oligonucleotide probe able to detect multiple high-risk HPV infection.

There are 10 genes encoded in HPV genome. These gene may be classified into two groups, namely Gene E (early) which encodes regulatory proteins and Gene L (late) which encodes structural proteins. The region of L1 and L2 of Gene L is responsible for encoding capsid protein to be used as DNA envelope in HPV. The capsid protein will serves as protection system to HPV genetic materials. It is generally assumed that there are many nucleotides sequence in the region of L1 and L2 that is conserved throughout the evolution process of HPV (Dahlgren, 2005).

2.1.1 Other labs approach

Mendez-Tenorio and his group were using DNA fingerprinting. Identification of microorganisms by whole genome DNA fingerprinting was tested "in silico". 94 HPV genome sequences were submitted to virtual hybridization analysis on a DNA chip with 342 probes. This Universal Fingerprinting Chip (UFC) constitutes a representative set of probes of all the possible 8-mer sequences having at least two internal and non-contiguous sequence differences between all them. A virtual hybridization analysis was performed in order to find the fingerprinting pattern that represents the signals produced for the hybridization of the probes allowing at most a single mismatch. All the fingerprints for each virus were compared against each other in order to obtain all the pairwise distances measures. A match-extension strategy was applied to identify only the shared signals corresponding to the hybridization of the probes with homologous sequences between two HPV genomes. A phylogenetic tree was constructed from the fingerprint distances using the Neighbor-Joining algorithm implemented in the program Phylip 3.61. This tree was compared with that produced from the alignment of whole genome HPV sequences calculated with the program Clustal_X 1.83. The similarities between both trees are suggesting that the UFC-8 is able to discriminate accurately between viral genomes. A fingerprint comparative analysis suggests that the UFC-8 can differentiate between HPV types and subtypes (Méndez-Tenorio *et al,* 2006)

Kaladhar and his group are working on annotation HPV-92 genome. Most of the biologists focus to explore innovations of their research in faster rate using developments in Information technology. The gene identification, characterization and modeling of the proteins in HPV 92 is done using bioinformatics tools. A complete genome of HPV-92 with NCBI's accession number NC_004500 was submitted to FGENES V0, a viral gene prediction server, predicts six genes. These six genes are characterized as E6 oncoprotein, E7 oncoprotein, E1 Replication protein, E2 Regulatory protein, L1 major capsid protein and L2 minor capsid protein. Isoelectric points and Molecular weights of all the six proteins vary largely and the modeled structures are shown. The research can provide characterization and modeling of genome which can further implemented in drug designing methods using bioinformatics tools (Kaladhar et al, 2010).

Eom and his group has interesting approach towards mapping HPV genome. They are using genetic mining algorithm. Classifying the type of HPV is very important to the treat of cervical cancer. The machine learning approach to mine the structure of HPV DNA sequence for effective classification of the HPV risk types has been introduced. The most informative subsequence segment sets and its weights with genetic algorithm to classify the risk types of each HPV has been determined and learnt. To resolve the problem of computational complexity of genetic algorithm, distributed intelligent data engineering platform based on active grid concept called IDEA@Home was used. The proposed genetic mining method, with the described platform, shows about 85.6% classification accuracy with relatively fast mining speed (Eom et al, 2004).

Lee and his groups are using in silico DNA microarry for detecting HPV genome. DNA microarrays are widely used techniques in molecular biology and DNA computing area. It consists of the DNA sequences called probes, which are DNA complementaries to the genes of interest, on solid surfaces. And its reliability seriously depends on the quality of the probe sequences. Therefore, one must carefully choose the probe sets in target sequences. The probe design for DNA microarrays was formulated as the multi-objective optimization problem. Multi-objective evolutionary approach was proposed, which is known to be suitable for this kind of optimization problem. Since a multi-objective evolutionary algorithm can find multiple solutions at a time, thermodynamic criteria was used to choose the most suitable one. For the experiments, the probe set generated by the proposed method is compared to the sequences used in commercial microarrays, which detects a set of Human Papillomavirus (HPV). The comparison result supports that the approach can be useful to optimize probe sequences (Lee et al, 2004).

2.1.2 Our approach

The aim of our study was to determine the conserved regions of late genes L1 and L2 from 74 sequenced and published HPV genome (Icenogle, 1995). The result was used to predict candidate template for oligonucleotide probes that are specific on types of HPV, which cause cervical cancer. Nevertheless, the spesific purpose of this study is to design primer that is able to detach on the open reading frame region and also to develop a new assay for the detection of high risk HPV DNA.

This study was carried out to determine the conserved regions of late genes from sequenced HPV types. HPV genome sequences were collected from the Los Alamos National Laboratory *papillomavirus* database. There are 74 types of HPV in the database, which have completely documented genome sequences as well as their translation product. Specific types of HPV, which may cause cervical cancer, are grouped into high risk or low risk, according to their risk potential. This classification may differ from one research methodology to another. In order to access a representative classification, three sets of classification were studied for this research. HPV type 16 and 18 are consistently grouped as high risk, while other types of HPV varied randomly. Sequence alignment was taken and the result shows 62 conserved regions as a primer template for L1 and L2 genes. These conserved regions were then subjected to BLASTn operation in order to search the conserved region with least similarity to low risk HPV and human genome.

Finally, 7 selected conserved regions were examined for secondary structures using NetPrimer program. From this operation, only region 52 (5′-ACAGGCTATGGTGCTATGGA-3′) met the criteria to be used as an oligonucleotide primer (Tambunan et al, 2007).

Oligonucleotide primers are considered based upon certain properties, namely: they must not have potential secondary structures such as hairpins or dimmers have a GC content of 45-60%; have a Tm between 52-58%; their 5' ends stability has to be greater than the stability of their 3' ends; be 17-25 nucleotides in length. From NetPrimer analysis results of seven regions, only region 52 meet with the above mentioned criteria. with a NetPrimer rating of 100 (maxium) (Tambunan et al, 2007). The result is shown in table 1. Based on sequence similarity, 62 conserved regions were found. Out of the 62, 7 regions were then used as templates for primers used in detection of high and low risk HPV. From the 7 template candidates, only one met the criteria to be used as an oligonucleotide primer, namely region 52. From the study, region 52 is predicted to be selective to be used in the detection of oncogenic Human *papillomavirus.*

2.2 HPV vaccine design and its post translation studies

A new paradigm of vaccine design is now emerging, following essential discoveries in immunology and the development of bioinformatics tools for T-cell epitope prediction from

Nucleotide sequence	Alignment	Region	BLASTn result and Position on Genome according to HPV type
	Type	1	Type 16 (5734-5751)
TATCATGCA	16;18;31;45		Type 31 (5647-5660)
			Type 33 (1920- 1929)
			Type 35 (5703-5719)
			Type 45 (5703-5726)
			Type 51 (5616-5639)
			Type 52 (5742-5761)
			Type 53 (7424-7434)
			Type 56 (5693-5715)
			Type 59 (5714-5724)
			Type 66 (5743-5759)
	Type	21	Type 11 (6350-6372)
ATATGGTTG	11;16;18;3T		Type 16 (6227-6246)
	35;68		Type 31 (6143-6165)
			Type 68 (2205-2229)
	Type	31	Type 16 (4907-5003)
	11;16;18;31;		Type 33 (4960-4976)
	35;68		Type 35 (4950-4974)
			Type 50 (4994-5004)
			Type 59 (6143-6165)
	Type	43	Type 16 (5933-5945)
GTTTGGGCCT	11;16;18;		Type 31(5046-5061)
	31;35;68		Type 35 (5009-5906)
			Type 39 (7001-7014)
			Type 45 (2951-2961)
			Type 52 (7096-7003)
			Type 68 (4997-4907)
	Type	45	Type 06 (6063-6001)
	11;16;18		Type 18 (5096-5915)
	35;68		Type 31 (5040-5057)
			Type 39 (5926-5944)
			Type 45 (2951-2961)
			Type 52 (7069-7004)
	Type	46	Type 16 (5979-5909)
TAGTGGCCAT-3	11;16;18		Type 31 (2303-2393)
	31; 35;68		Type 42 (6176-6193)
	Type	52	Type 16 (6240-6264)
	16;18;52		Type 61 (6373-6303)
			Type 68 (2223-2242)
			Type 70 (6190-6209)

Table 1. Conserved regions selected as templates

primary protein sequences. One rationale for this new paradigm is that following exposure to a pathogen, epitope-specific memory T-cell clones are established. These clones respond rapidly and efficiently upon any subsequent infection, elaborating cytokines, killing infected host cells, and marshalling humoral and cellular defences against the pathogen. The most efficient immune response to some pathogens is derived from a number of different T cells that respond to an ensemble of pathogen-derived short peptides called epitopes. Whether an immune response is directed against a single immunodominant epitope or against many epitopes, the generation of a protective immune response does not require the development of T-cell memory to every possible peptide in the entire pathogen. T-cell response to the ensemble of epitopes, not the whole pathogen, is the source from which a protective immune response is derived. Similarly, if an individual is previously exposed to a language, upon hearing just a few words of that language he/she will usually recognize, for example, that French or English is being spoken. Complete mastery of the language is not required for this recognition. Using this analogy to describe epitopes, one could say that they are pathogen-specific 'words' that alert the immune system to the presence of a pathogen. It is now possible to envisage the design of vaccines based on an ensemble of epitopes (a string of words, a few sentences, a paragraph, or a chapter) derived from the genome of a pathogen, using tools that have been developed in the field of immuno-informatics (De Groot et al, 2002). Knowledge about immunology is crucial in designing vaccine. Immunoinformatics, which is a branch of Bioinformatics, is a flourishing field.

The significant breakthrough in HPV vaccine research was accomplished, when capsid protein L1 and L2 was found to be able to assemble themselves to be Virus Like Particles (VLP) during cell expression. VLP is very similar to the native HPV particle, and it includes the conformation epitope that induce the viral neutralization antibody. This is very crucial for the immune system, in order to detect VLP as viral infection, and giving the proper response. Because VLP is coreless and didn't contain the viral DNA, then it is expected that it won't create infection. The produced VLPs are type 6,11, 16, 18, 31, 33, 35, 39, 45,and 58). One VLP Chimeric (cVLP) model has sucessfully induced Mice Cytotoxic T Cell, by joining E6 and E7 capsid protein in the VLP. Some scientist believes, that cVLP has huge potentials to be utilized as infection prevention (Kolls et al, 2000).

Protein must be folded like its native conformation, in order to be activated as mature protein. The protein modification into its native conformation is called as post-translation modification. The polypeptide chain, which consisted of more than 200 residues, is usually folded into two or more globular domain. Most of the domain has 100 until 200 amino acid residues, and having diameter of ~25 Å (Voet *et al*, 1995).

DNA vaccine is designed using choice of a suitable expression vector, ensuring optimal expression by codon optimization, engineering CpG motifs for enhancing immune responses and providing additional sequence signals for efficient translation. DNA vaccines have been one of the latest developments in vaccine technology. DNA vaccines are essentially plasmids capable of expressing an antigenicpeptide in the host. These expressed proteins are recognized as foreign in the cells of the body. They are processed by the host cells and displayed on their surface to alert the immune system and trigger body's immune responses. DNA vaccines have become anattractive alternative to conventional methods due to the fact that it can elicit sustained cell-mediated as well as humoral immun responses, which is very much important in combating pathogenic organisms, especially intracellular pathogens. Vaccine efficacy can be assessed by correlating the vaccine's immunogenicity such as its ability to induce CD8+ or CD4+ T cells to the HPV oncoproteins with its ability to protect vaccinated animals against formation of tumors or to cause clearance of already established tumors. Recently several techniques like optimizing codons, CpG optimization and promoter and resistance gene insertion have been tried to enhance the immunogenicity of DNA vaccines (Gupta et al, 2009).

2.2.1 Other labs approach

Gupta and his group are working with DNA vaccine. There is a need to develop a new prophylactic DNA vaccine, which can work against different strains of HPVs and may lead to protection of cervical cancer against new pandemicviruses. Potential prophylactic DNA vaccine has been designed by using all the consensus epitopic sequences of HPVs L2 capsid protein and performed in silico cloning of multiepitopic antigenic DNA sequence in pVAX-1 vector. Immunogenicity of vaccine has been enhanced by techniques like codon optimization, engineering CpG motifs, introducing promoters and co-injection with plasmids expressing immune-stimulatory molecules (Gupta et al, 2009).

2.2.2 Our approach

Unlike others, our laboratory is using chimeric protein for designing the vaccine. The cVLP HPV-16 ANN1, ANN2, HMM1, and HMM2 in silico vaccine design were discovered. The BLAST test towards them was generating 96% identity with native L1 HPV-16 protein. Therefore, it is expected that the vaccines could cause same level of immunogenicity with the native protein. The Ramacandran Plot of them showed that the disallowed region plot of non-glycine residue was less than 15%. Henceforth, the quality of the vaccine could be structuraly good. The VAST test toward them showed the RMSD of 0,1 Å, which shows that they have a high structural similarity.

Based upon in silico predition, it was found that post-translational modification could occur at cVLP. During the formation of cVLP, the possible occurred post-translational modification is N-Glicocylation. It is because this modification has N-Xaa-S/T motif which found at our in silico detection method. Although it is expected to happen, it is predicted that this modification wouldn't affect the tability of the cVLP, because its epitope did not affected.

Chimeric virus like particles (cVLP) has been developed as vaccine candidate for preventing cervical cancer. cVLPs are improvement of Virus Like Particles (VLP) by substituting the epitope of L1 HPV -18 and -52 protein to L1 HPV -16 protein. They are ANN1, ANN2, HMM1, and HMM2. The impact of post translation modification will be determined. Based on In Silico study, the dominant post translation modification is glycosylation (Tambunan et al 2007).

However, the next step is to develop in silico plasmid vector for expressing cVLP at the euchariotic host cell. The necessary step is to conduct in vitro experimentation to construct the cVLP HPV L1 at the proper host cell. After the cVLP has sucessfully produced, we could conduct in vivo research to determine the immunogenicity of cVLP at the animal testing, for example at rabbits or mice. Figure 1 shows the amino acid sequence of our vaccine design, while figure 2 shows its 3D visualization.

>SequenceANN1:

KVVSTDEYVARTNIYYHAGTSRLLAVGHPYFPIKKPNNNKILVPKVSGLQYRVFRIHLPDP
NKFGFPDTSFYNPDTQRLVWACVGVEVGRGQPLGVGISGHPLLNKLDDTENASAYAAN
AGVDNRECISMDYKQTQLCLIGCKPPIGEHWGKGSPCTQVAVQPGDCPPLELINTVIQDG
DMVDTGFGAMDFTTLQANKLFLRNVNVFSICKYPDYIKMVSEPYGDSLFFYLRREQMFVR
HLFNRAGTVGENVPDDLYIKGSGSTANLASSNYFPTPSGSMVTSDAQIFNKPYWLQRAQ
GHNNGICWGNQLFVTVVDTTRSTNMSLCAAISTSETTYKNTNFKEYLRFYILVIFYYIFQLC
KITLTADVMTYIHSMNSTILEDWNFGLQPPPGGTLDTYRFVTSQAIACQKHTPPAPKEDPL
KKYTFWEVNLKEKFSADLDQFPLGRKFLLQLGL

Fig. 1. The sequence of Our ANN1 cVLP L1 HPV Vaccine design.

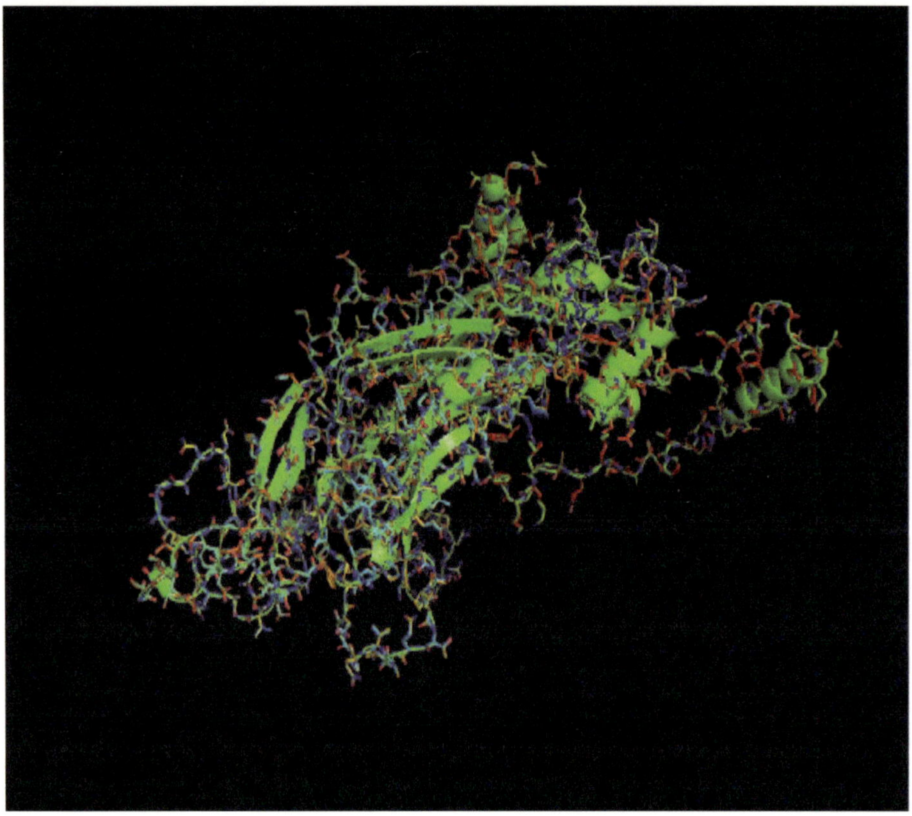

Fig. 2. Our ANN1 cVLP L1 HPV Vaccine Design. The vaccine was visualized by using MacPymol application. The ribbons inside the chains are the vaccine backbone (Tambunan et al, 2010).

2.3 HPV drugs design

This section will elaborate more on Drugs design. Knowledge about protein receptor-inhibitor interaction is very important for designing drugs. Computational Chemistry is the major supporting science in it. The structural modification of histones is playing important roles in the knowledge of HPV drug design.

However, we are going to explain more about drug design biochemistry background. The structural modification of histones is regulated mainly by acetylation/deacetylation of the N-terminal tail and is crucial in modulating gene expression, because it affects the interaction of DNA with transcription-regulatory non-nucleosomal protein complexes. The balance between the acetylated/deacetylated states of histones is mediated by two different sets of enzymes: histone acetyltransferases (HATs) and histone deacetylases (HDACs). HATs prefentially acetylate specific lysine substrates among other non-histones protein sub- strates and transcription factors, affecting DNA-binding properties and, in turn, altering gene transcription. HDACs restore the positive charge on lysine residues by removing acetyl groups and thus are involved primarily in the repression of gene transcription by compacting chromatin structure. Therefore, open lysine residues attach firmly to the phosphate backbone of the DNA, preventing transcription. In this tight conformation, transcription factors, regulatory complexes, and RNA polymerases cannot bind to DNA Acetylation relaxes the DNA conformation, making it accessible to transcription machinery. High levels of acetylation of core histones are seen in chromatin-containing genes, which are highly transcribed genes; genes that are silent are associated with low levels of acetylation. Inappropriate silencing of critical genes can result in one or both hits of tumor suppressor gene inactivation in cancer. Members of the classical HDAC family fall into two different phylogenetic classes, namely class I and class II. The class I HDACs (HDAC1, HDAC2, HDAC3, and HDAC8) are most closely related to the yeast (*Saccharomyces cerevisiae*). Class II HDACs (HDAC4, HDAC5, HDAC6, HDAC7, HDAC9, and HDAC10) share domains with similarity to HDA1, another deacetylase found in yeast (de Ruitter et al, 2003).

The inhibition of HDAC activity by a specific inhibitor induces growth arrest, differentiation, and apoptosis of transformed cells as well as several cancer cells (Subha et al, 2008). Recent studies were directed to investigate the molecular effects of HDAC inhibition on cervical carcinoma cells as well as on primary human foreskin keratinocytes, separately immortalized with amphotropic retroviruses that carry the open reading frames of HPV 16 E6, E7 or E6/E7. In these experiments one could show that E6/E7 oncogene function of human papillomavirus can be completely bypassed by HDAC inhibition. Both malignant and immortalized HPV 16/18-positive cells became blocked in G1/S transition despite ongoing viral gene expression. G1 arrest was accompanied by a down-regulation of cyclin D and cyclin A and a concomitant up regulation of the cyclin kinase inhibitors (CKI) p21 and p27. Binding of both CKIs led to a complete block of the cyclin-dependent kinase (cdk2) activity and in turn prevented binding of E7. This was intriguing with respect to the reversibility of HPV transformation process, since it is thought that the abrogation of the growth inhibitory function of p21 and p27 through E7 represents a key event in HPV-induced carcinogenesis. HDAC inhibitors also trigger pRb degradation, while E2F expression remained unaffected. pRb degradation is an E7-specific phenomenon, since in E6-positive cells pRb only became hypophosphorylated. The presence of E2F under cell cycle arrest led to a classical "conflict situation" which finally induced apoptosis (Finzer et al, 2001; Finzer et al, 2002; Finzer et al, 2004). Hence, the knowledge how the transforming potential of HPV can be bypassed without switching off viral transcription could open new therapeutical perspectives for the treatment of cervical cancer (Acharya et al, 2006). The drug design on HPV are mainly tampering with the reactivity of E(early) protein.

2.3.1 Other labs approach

Rehmi and his group are mainly working on E2 proteins. The E2 protein from HPV 16 was selected as a molecular target and its known structures were exploited for broad scope of "hits" to be identified in the screening process. They compared both structure-based and ligand-based design approaches for virtual screening. Databases enriched in natural compounds were used for virtual screening based on molecular docking. In this study, they identified novel classes of HPV inhibitors by means of a structure-based drug-design protocol involving Pharmacophore based virtual screening with molecular docking simulation (Rehmi et al, 2009).

Baleja and his group have different approach, because they are using E6 protein as vaccine template. The E6 protein from the high-risk HPV types represents an attractive target for intervention because of its roles in viral propagation and cellular transformation. E6 functions in part by interaction with human cellular proteins, several of which possess a helical E6-binding motif. The role for each amino acid in this motif for binding E6 has been tested through structure determination and site-directed mutagenesis. These structural and molecular biological approaches defined the spatial geometry of functional groups necessary for binding to E6. This E6-binding information (the E6-binding pharmacophore) was transferred into a three-dimensional query format suitable for computational screening of large chemical databases. Compounds were identified and tested using in vitro and cell culture-based assays. Several compounds selectively inhibited E6 interaction with the E6-binding protein E6AP and interfered with the ability of E6 to promote p53 degradation. Such compounds provide leads for the development of new pharmacologic agents to treat papillomavirus infections and their associated cancers (Baleja et al, 2006).

2.3.2 Our approach

Our approach was done by Identification of a better *Homo sapiens* Class II HDAC inhibitor. The aim of this work is to analyze the interaction of *Homo sapiens* class II HDACs with SAHA and TSA that are already in the phase I/II clinical trials based on their binding affinity and pharmacological properties. Since, no theoretical works have been carried out in identifying the properties and specificity, we intend to identify the group that could act as potential binding inhibitors.

In this paper, we present homology models of six *Homo sapiens* Class II HDACs (HDAC4, HDAC5, HDAC6, HDAC7, HDAC9, and HDAC10) that are validated by comparison with the X-ray structure of HDAC4 and HDAC7, which became available during the course of our study. Two HDAC inhibitors (SAHA and TSA) are docked to the six homology models. The pharmacological properties of SAHA and TSA were identified using Molinspiration, Osiris Property, Tox- Boxes, and Toxmatch-v1.06. Therefore, the molecular binding interactions between the histone deacetylases with SAHA and TSA were analyzed to provide some insights into the molecular interactions and designing new HDAC inhibitors.

The certain types of HPV are involved in the development of cervical cancer. In attempts to find additional drugs in the treatment of cervical cancer, inhibitors of the histone deacetylases (HDAC) have received much attention due to their low cytotoxic profiles and the E6/E7 oncogene function of human papilomavirus can be completely by passed by HDAC inhibition. The histone deacetylase inhibitors can induce growth arrest, differentiation and apoptosis of cancer cells. HDAC class I and class II are considered the main targets for cancer. Therefore, the six HDACs class II was modelled and about two inhibitors (SAHA and TSA) were docked using AutoDock 4.2, to each of the inhibitor in order to identify the pharmacological properties. Based on the results of docking, SAHA and TSA were able to bind with zinc ion in HDACs models as a drug target. SAHA was satisfied almost all the properties i.e., binding affinity, the Drug-Likeness value and Drug Score with 70% oral bioavailability and the carbonyl group of these compound fits well into the active site of the target where the zinc is present. Hence, SAHA could be developed as potential inhibitors of class II HDACs and valuable cervical cancer drug candidate (Tambunan et al, 2010).

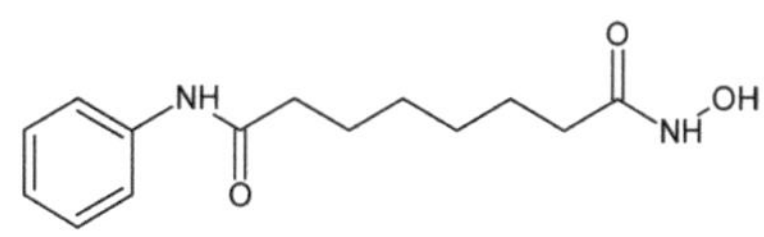

Suberoyl Anilide Hydroxamic Acid (SAHA)

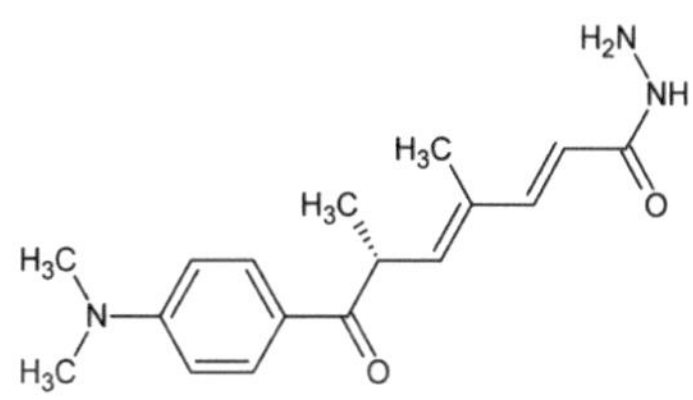

Trichostatin A (TSA)

Fig. 3. 2D Structure of SAHA and TSA. SAHA and TSA are hydroxamic acid derivatives that can be HDAV inhibitors.

Each ligand shows different affinity with class II HDAC, for example SAHA compound show best affinity with HDAC 5 based on Autodock calculation, and HDAC 10 based on APBS calculation. Whereas the same compound was found to be rank 2 with HDAC7 (-7.42 kcal/mol) based on AutoDock calculation and HDAC6 (-213.60 kJ/mol) based on APBS calculation, and rank 3 (-6.72 kcal/mol) with HDAC10 (AutoDock) and HDAC7 (-203.21 kJ/mol, APBS). Local free binding energy obtained from AutoDock of *Homo sapiens* class II HDACs complexed with an inhibitor showed that SAHA is a weaker inhibitor of HDACs than TSA. But, global binding energy of *Homo sapiens* class II HDACs and inhibitors obtained from APBS, showed that TSA to be a weaker inhibitor of HDACs than SAHA. There are differences in binding energy calculated with AutoDock
and APBS; this is because AutoDock does not calculate columbic contribution from all of atoms in protein like APBS.

The further descriptor analysis and the toxicity prediction helped in the identification of the better inhibitor. Drug Score and the Drug-Likeness are the two properties that are important for considering a compound to become a successful drug. TSA had a drug score of 0.37 and drug likeness property score of 1.24, which is higher than those for SAHA with respective scores of 0.35 and -8.87. The molecular weight of SAHA was 264.32 g/mol and that of TSA was 302.37 g/mol (Table 1), between the preferred range of molecular weight for drug

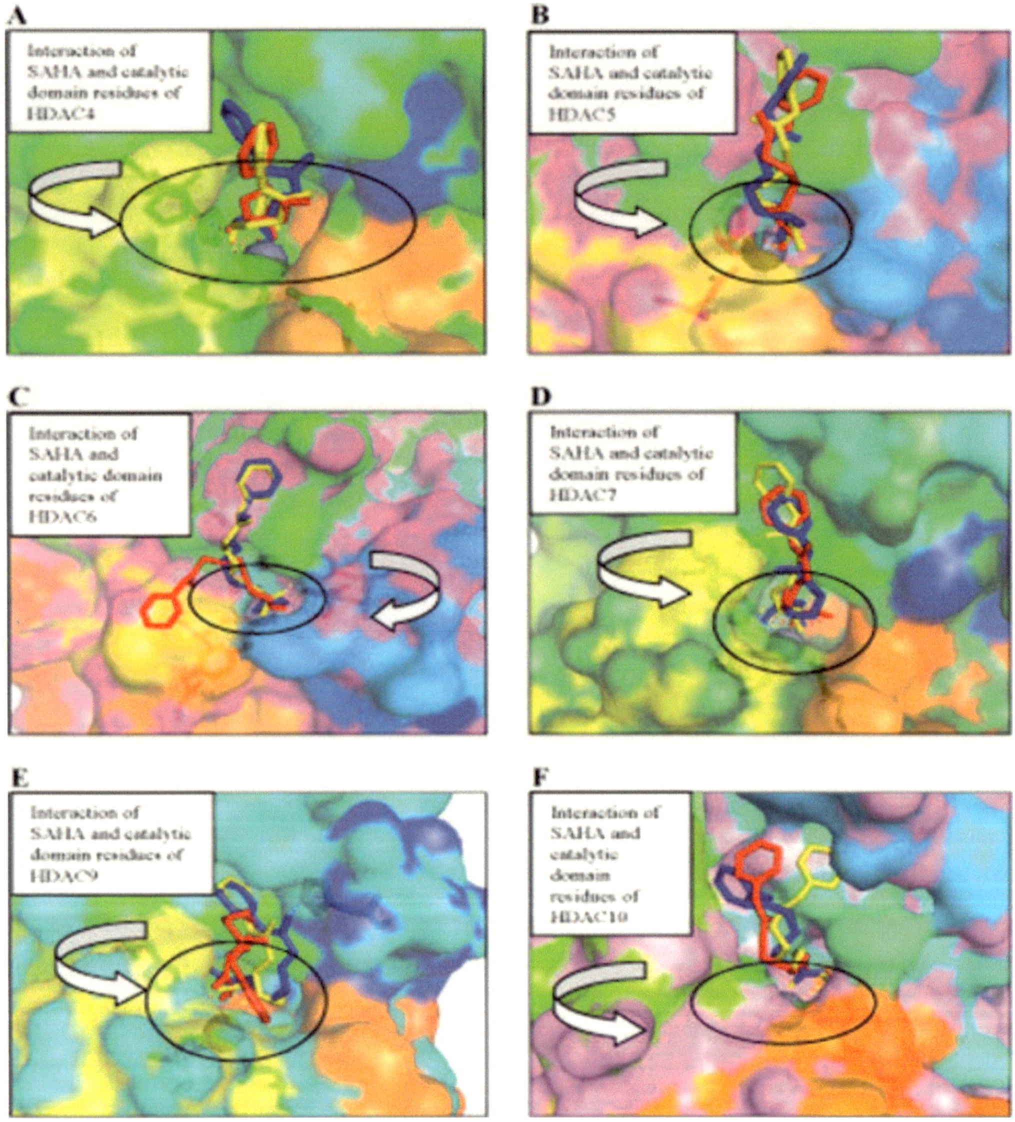

Fig. 4. Structures of docked SAHA with *Homo sapiens* Class II HDACs. Three Conformations of Structures of docked SAHA with (A)HDAC4, (B) HDAC5, (C) HDAC6, (D) HDAC7, (E) HDAC9 and (F) HDAC10. A surface representation of catalytic domain of Homo sapiens Class II HDACs bound to SAHA. The zinc ion is shown as gray sphere. SAHA are shown as stick models colored as per docked type: red, blue, and yellow. Amino acids coordinating the zinc and forming the trihedrally coordinates are shown as sticks. Some catalytic domain of Homo sapiens Class II HDACs residues interacting with the docked SAHA are shown as stick models. In HDAC4-SAHA, HDAC5-SAHA, HDAC6-SAHA and HDAC7-SAHA complexes, SAHA binds the catalytic zinc ion in a bidentate fashion, with its carbonyl and hydroxyl bound to catalytic zinc ion. Whereas, in HDAC9-SAHA and HDAC10-SAHA complexes bind the catalytic zinc ion in a monodentate fashion, with its carbonyl bound to catalytic zinc ion.

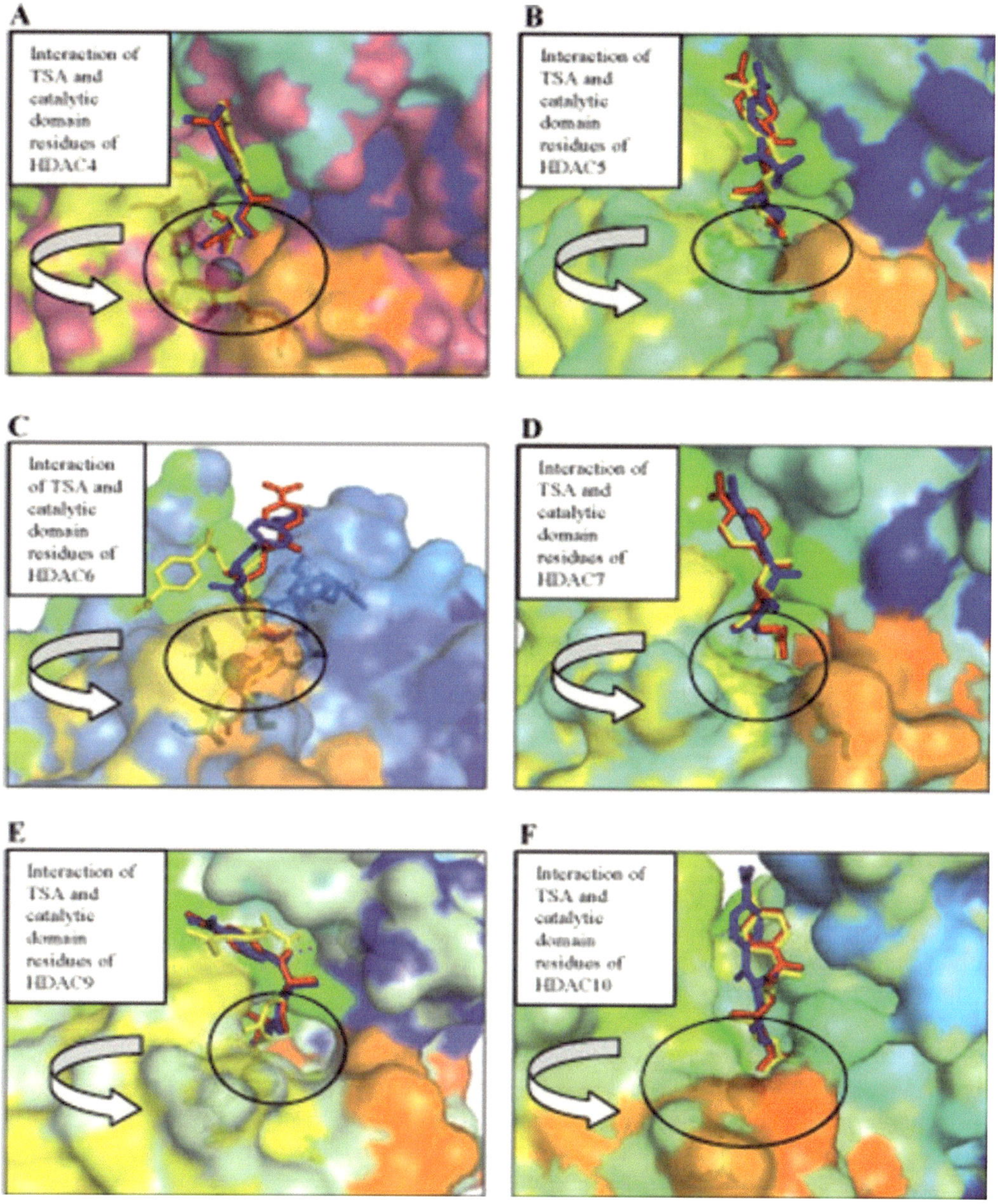

Fig. 5. Structures of docked TSA with HDAC Class II *Homo sapiens*. Three Conformations of Structures of docked TSA with (A) HDAC4, (B) HDAC5, (C) HDAC6, (D) HDAC7, (E) HDAC9 and (F) HDAC10. A surface representation of catalytic domain of *Homo sapiens* Class II HDACs bound to TSA. The zinc ion is shown as gray sphere. TSA are shown as stick models colored as per docked type: red, blue, and yellow. Amino acids coordinating the zinc and forming the trihedrally coordinates are shown as sticks. Some catalytic domain of *Homo sapiens* Class II HDACs residues interacting with the docked TSA are shown as stick models. Except HDAC5-TSA complex, all of *Homo sapiens* class II HDACs-TSA complexes bind the catalytic zinc ion in a monodentate fashion.

likeness property (160-480 g/mol). TSA was having tumorigenic property. SAHA was the compound that had the acceptable range for toxicity risk. These values were also taken into account to decide the best inhibitor. Thus, SAHA was the best drug candidate than TSA and also found to possess better global binding affinity score.
The ADME-TOX box results showed that the SAHA has an oral bioavailability of more than 70% i.e., good solubility and stability. It acts as a non-substrate and non-inhibitor of P-gp. SAHA does not undergo significant first-pass metabolism.

The three-dimensional models for six class II histone deacetylases (HDAC4, HDAC5, HDAC6, HDAC7, HDAC9, and HDAC10), which were built using homology modeling and validated by bioinformatics techniques and by comparison to an X-ray structures, were docked to SAHA and TSA. Our studies provide the structural view of the catalytic domain of a class II HDAC and reveal for this subclass specific features: (i) novel zinc binding motif that is likely to be involved in substrate binding and/or protein-protein interactions and may provide a site for modulation of activity, and (ii) a unique active site topology in catalytic activity. SAHA and TSA predicted to inhibit the class II HDACs are effective to all forms HDACs. SAHA was satisfied almost all the properties i.e., binding affinity scores of SAHA in the six class II HDAC enzymes was -156.94 kJ/mol, -171.77 kJ/mol, -213.60 kJ/mol, -203.21 kJ/mol, -179.29 kJ/mol & -263.15 kJ/mol respectively, the Drug Likeness value (1.24) and drug score (0.37) with 70% oral bioavailability and the carbonyl group of these com- pounds fits well into the active site of the target where the zinc is present. Hence, SAHA could be developed as potential inhibitors of class II HDACs and valuable anti cancer agents.

3. Conclusion

The IT industry has provided strong and robust computing power, with low cost expediture. Nowadays, a powerful low cost multiprocessor computers are available,which made the modeling of complicated proteins and sophisticated drug design possible. The major computer operating system, such as MacOSX, Linux, and Windows are already supporting open source bioinformatics software. They could do the functionalities of the commercial software, with the same robustness. Nowadays, the field of bioinformatics is growing. The In Silico (Bioinformatics) experiment will be considered as important as wet experiment by biologist and/or biotechnologist. The In silico approach did not designed to replace wet experiment, but it's in order to supplement it. Open source implementation will help bioinformaticians to solve viral threat in efficient and effective manner. There will be more robust bioinformatics tools available in the future for solving crucial virology related problems. Our laboratory has successfully designing primer and vaccine for therapeutics. However, the efficacy of the design must be proven in the wet labs experiment. Synthesizing them by using latest molecular biology instrument is crucial for progressing towards clinical trial. Conducting it will require us to form strong cooperation with faculty of medicine in our university. We already have cooperation with them, and will verify our design in the future.

HPV Bioinformatics is a growing and developing field. Our labs has sucessfully developed HPV Genome detection, Vaccine, and drugs design. We found 7 conserve region candidates for PCR design, HPV L1 cVLP for vaccine design, and SAHA/TSA drug design. In silico PCR Primer, Vaccine, and drugs design are possible with the newest development in algorithm and programming. Our labs and others has successfully developed them. The next challenges would be implementing them in the wet laboratory research.

4. Aknowledgement

This publication is supported by Universitas Indonesia. The authors are grateful to to Dr. Ridla Bakri, Chairman of Department of Chemistry, Faculty of Mathematics and Natural Science, University of Indonesia for his support.

5. References

Acharya, MR; Sparreboom, A; Sausville, EA; Conley, BA; Doroshow, JH; Venitz, J & Figg, WD. (2006). Interspecies differences in plasma protein binding of MS-275, a novel histone deacetylase inhibitor, *Cancer Chemotherapy and Pharmacology*, 57:275-81. ISSN: 1432-0843

Alfonso, M; Perla, F; Armando, G; Hueman, J; Emma, R; Arcadio, M; Mercedes, E; Rogelio, M & Loren, BK. (2006). In silico evaluation of a novel DNA chip based fingerprinting technology for viral identification, *Revista latinoamericana de microbiología*, 48 (2): 56-65

Baleja, JD; Cherry, JJ; Liu, Z; Gao, Hua; Nicklaus, MC; Voigt, JH; Chen, JJ & Androphy, EJ. (2006). Identification of inhibitors to papillomavirus type 16 E6 protein based on three-dimensional structures of interacting proteins, *Antiviral Research*, Volume 72, Issue 1, 2006, Pp 49-59, ISSN 0166-3542,

Clavel, C; Masure, M & Putaut, I. (1998). Hybrid Capture II, a new sensitive test for human *papillomavirus* detection. Comparison with hybrid capture I and PCR results in cervical lesions. *Journal of Clinical Pathology*, 51:737-740. ISSN: 1472-4146

Dahlgren, L. (2005). *Studies on the Presence and Influence of human papillomavirus (HPV) in Head and Neck Tumors*. ISBN: 91-7140-289-6. Karolinska University of Stockholms

De Groot, AS;, Sbai, H;, Aubin, CS; McMurry, J & Martin, W. (2002). Immuno-informatics: Mining genomes for vaccine components. *Immunology and Cell Biology. Nature Publishing Group*. Volume 80 issue 3. pp 255- 269. ISSN: 1440-1711

De Ruijter, AJ; van Gennip, AH; Caron, HN; Kemp, S & van Kuilenburg, AB. (2003). Histone deacetylases (HDACs): characterization of the classical HDAC family, *Journal of Biochem* , 370:737-49. ISSN: 1470-8728

Eom, J; Park, S & Zhang, B. (2004). Genetic Mining of DNA Sequence Structures for Effective Classification of the Risk Types of Human Papillomavirus (HPV). *Neural Information Processing: Lecture Notes in Computer Science*. Springer Berlin / Heidelberg. pp 1334-1343
Volume: 3316. ISSN: 0302-9743

Finzer, P; Krueger, A; Stöhr, M; Brenner, D; Soto, U; Kuntzen, C; Krammer, PH & Rösl, F. (2004). HDAC inhibitors trigger apoptosis in HPV-positive cells by inducing the E2F-p73 pathway. *Oncogene*, 23:4807-17.ISSN: 09509232

Finzer, P; Ventz, R; Kuntzen, C; Seibert, N; Soto, U & Rösl, F. (2002) Growth arrest of HPV-positive cells after histone deacetylase inhibition is independent of E6/E7 oncogene expression, *Journal of Virology*, 304:265-73. ISSN: 1096-0341

Finzer, P; Kuntzen, C; Soto, U; zur Hausen, H & Rösl, F. (2001). Inhibitors of histone deacetylase arrest cell cycle and induce apoptosis in cervical carcinoma cells circumventing human papillomavirus oncogene expression,*Oncogene* , 20:4768-76. ISSN: 09509232

Gupta, SK; Singh, A; Srivastava, M; Gupta, SK & Akhoon, BA. (2009) In silico DNA vaccine designing against human papillomavirus (HPV) causing cervical cancer, *Vaccine,* Volume 28, Issue 1, Pages 120-131, ISSN 0264-410X

Icenogle, J. (1995). *Analysis of the Sequences of the L1 and L2 Capsid Proteins of Papillomavirus.* Centers for Disease Control, Atlanta, Georgia.

Kaladhar, DSVGK; Devi, TU & Nageswara, RPV. (2010). An In Silico Genome Wide Identification, Characterization and Modeling of Human Papilloma Virus Strain 92. *International Journal of Engineering Science and Technology.*Vol. 2(9), 4288-4291. ISSN: 0975–5462.

Kolls, A & Sherris, J. (2000). *HPV Vaccines: Promoises and Challenges.* PATH Seattle.

Lee, I; Kim, S & Zhang, B. Multi-objective Evolutionary Probe Design Based on Thermodynamic Criteria for HPV Detection. PRICAI 2004: Trends in Artificial Intelligence. Lecture Notes in Computer Science. 2004. Springer Berlin / Heidelberg. pp: 742-750.Volume: 3157

Lorinez, A. & J. Anthony. (2001). Hybrid Capture method for detection of human papillomavirus DNA in clinical specimens: a tool for clinical management of equivocal Pap smears and for population screening, *Journal of obstetrics and gynaecology,* 12:145-154. ISSN: 1341-8076

Reshmi, G & Pillai, MR. (2009). In Silico Screening of Novel Inhibitors for HPV: A Rational Structure Based Approach (Docking Versus Pharmacophore Model Generation), *Letters in Drug Design & Discovery,* Volume 6 Issue 7.pp.494-501. ISSN: 1570-1808.

Subha, K & Kumar, GR. (2008). Assessment for the identification of better HDAC inhibitor class through binding energy calculations and descriptor analysis., *Bioinformation,* 3:218-222. ISSN: 0973-2063

Tambunan, USF; & Wulandari, EK. (2010).Identification of a better *Homo sapiens* Class II HDAC inhibitor through binding energy calculations and descriptor analysis, *BMC Bioinformatics* , 11(Suppl 7):S16. ISSN:1471-2105

Tambunan, USF & Parikesit, AA. (2010). Cracking The Genetic Code of Human Virus by using Open Source Bioinformatics tools, *Journal of Fundamental Science,* 6(1).ISSN: 1823-626X

Tambunan, USF; Parikesit, AA;, Tochary, TA & Sugiono, D. (2007). Computational Study of Post Translation Modification in Chimeric Virus Like Particles Vaccine of Human Papilloma Virus with Virion Capsid L1, *Makara Sains Journal,* 11(2): 56-62. ISSN: 1693-6671

Tambunan, USF; Butar-Butar ,HW; Umbas, R & Hidayah, Z. (2007). Conserved Region Analysis of Oncogenic Human Papillomavirus Genome., *Biotechnology,* (6)1: 93-96. ISSN: 16822978

Voet, D., Voet J.G. (1995). *Biochemistry,* John Willey and Sons Inc,. ISBN-13: 978-0471586517, New York

15

Therapeutic Exploitation of Targeting Programmed Cell Death for Cervical Cancer

Yang Sun and Jia-hua Liu
Department of Obstetrics and Gynecology, Fujian Provincial Hospital, Fujian Provincial Clinical Medical College, Fujian Medical University, Fuzhou, Fujian China

1. Introduction

Programmed cell death (PCD) is a basic biological phenomenon that plays an important role during development, preservation of tissue homeostasis, and elimination of damaged cells. Several nomenclature systems have been proposed to classify PCD. One widely accepted system describes three major morphologies of programmed cell death, and classifies PCD as type I, apoptosis; type II, autophagy; and type III, programmed necrosis[1,2].

Type I, apoptotic cell death, acts as part of a quality-control and repair mechanism by elimination of unwanted, genetically damaged, or senescent cells, and as such is critically important for the development of organisms. Highly conserved in both plants and animals, it is also the cell-death mechanism best characterized at both genetic and biochemical levels[3]. Type II, autophagic cell death, is a catabolic process conserved among all eukaryotes from yeast to mammals[4]; it is a mechanism by which organelles are removed. Autophagic cell death is the primary degradation mechanism for long-lived proteins, and thus maintains quality control for proteins and organelles to enhance survival under conditions of scarcity or starvation. Type III, programmed necrosis, is a passive process that usually affects large fields of cells; in contrast, apoptosis and autophagy are controlled and energy-dependent and can affect individual cells or clusters of cells. Perhaps the most remarkable characteristic of programmed necrosis is that this death outcome appears as a distinct entity, not by exclusive engagement of selected effectors, but rather, by combinatorial use of the effectors shared with other cell-death outcomes.

Although all three types of PCD can occur normally as a homeostatic mechanism to maintain the cell population in tissues, dysregulation of the delicate balance between cell life and PCD has tremendous pathological implications. The type of cell death that occurs depends on the stimulus and the cellular context, because every cell-death program is a net result of self-propagating signals and other signals that suppress the other cell-death programs[2]. Deficient cell death is frequently involved in early cancer development and tumour resistance to chemotherapy or radiotherapy[5]. Increasingly, evidence suggests that PCD is closely related to anti-cancer therapy. The cancer therapy is improved by targeting the PCD pathway.

Cervical cancer is the most prevalent malignancy of the female reproductive system. Several randomized controlled studies have shown survival benefits of platinum-based neoadjuvant chemotherapy followed by radical surgery in locally advanced cervical cancer. Survival benefit of neoadjuvant chemotherapy depends on high chemoresponsiveness. Considerable evidence indicates that platinum can kill cells through the induction of apoptosis; however, cancer cells, in their relentless drive to survive, hijack cell processes, resulting in resistance to apoptosis. This resistance underlies not only tumorigenesis, but also the inherent resistance of certain cancers to chemotherapy and radiotherapy. Fortunately, in addition to inducing apoptosis, a number of chemotherapeutic agents have been shown to induce nonapoptotic forms of cell death. The significance of nonapoptotic cell death in chemotherapy, and the mechanisms by which it is induced remain less well understood. Given the fact that most cancer cells have defects in the response to induction of apoptosis, it would be desirable if therapeutic agents could kill cancer cells resistant to apoptosis through alternative mechanisms.

In this chapter, we firstly review the main features and functions of all three types of programmed cell death, and further elucidate the intricate relationship between apoptosis, autophagy and necrosis. We discuss the dual roles of autophagy in cancer and highlighted their relationship to tumor suppression and tumor progression. We also review several key autophagic mediators that play pivotal roles in autophagic signaling networks in cancer. Understanding the signaling pathways involved in the regulation of autophagy as well as the autophagy process itself represents new directions in the development of cervical cancer therapies.

2. Basic features of PCD

Programmed cell death displays several cellular phenotypes affecting various intracellular organelles and membranes, and the cell nucleus. For example, the well-characterized processes of cytoplasmic and chromatin condensation, nuclear fragmentation, membrane blebbing, and formation of membrane-bound apoptotic bodies are part of apoptosis. Autophagy involves the formation of a double-membrane vesicle which encapsulates cytoplasm and organelles, and fuses with lysosomes, thus resulting in the degradation of the vesicle contents. Programmed necrosis is characterized by the presence of swelling organelles followed by the appearance of "empty" spaces in the cytoplasm that merge and make connections with the extracellular space. The plasma membrane is fragmented, but the nucleus is relatively preserved[6].

2.1 Apoptosis

The major biochemical features of apoptosis are activation of intracellular proteases especially caspases, and internucleosomal DNA fragmentation. Changes in several cell surface molecules also ensure that apoptotic cells are immediately recognized and phagocytized by neighboring cells in tissues, with the result that many cells can be deleted from tissues in relatively short time. Therefore, apoptosis results in the orderly elimination of cells without generating an inflammatory response[7].

The apoptosis cascade can be initiated via two major pathways, involving either activation of death receptors in response to ligand binding (extrinsic or death-receptor pathway), or the release of proapoptotic proteins, such as cytochrome c, from mitochondria to cytosol (intrinsic or mitochondrial pathway)[8]. Some evidence has indicated that the two pathways are linked and that molecules involved in one pathway can influence the other[9]. The death receptor pathway is activated through the tumour necrosis factor (TNF) family of cytokine receptors, and has a fundamental role in maintaining tissue homeostasis, particularly in immune recognition. The Bcl-2 family of proteins plays a central role in controlling the mitochondrial pathway. Different members of the Bcl-2 family localize to the cytoplasm or to different subcellular compartments in healthy cells. However, upon receiving a death stimulus, most of these proteins carry out their functions at various intracellular membranes, particularly the endoplasmic reticulum (ER) and mitochondrial membranes. More than 20 members of this family have been identified to date in humans, including suppressors (Bcl-2, Bcl-XL, Mcl-1, Bfl-1/A1, Bcl-W, Bcl-G) and promoters (Bax, Bak, Bok, Bad, Bid, Bik, Bim, Bcl-Xs, Krk, Mtd, Nip3, Nix, Nora, Bcl-B) of apoptosis[10].

The central players in both pathways are the caspases (the cysteine-dependent, aspartate-specific family of proteases), which also function as the executioner in apoptotic cell death[11]. Regulated at the post-translational level, caspases are synthesized as pro-caspases. Under stimulation of pro-apoptotic signals from different sources, pro-caspases are digested by protease to become active caspases. Mitochondrial dynamics contribute substantially to apoptotic pathways by stimulation of caspases, and by chromosomal fragmentation[12,13].

The extrinsic pathway is triggered at the cell surface through cytokine-induced death by receptor-mediated activation of caspase-8 or caspase-10, followed by activation of caspase-3 and -7[3]. The intrinsic pathway is characterized by mitochondrial dysfunction, resulting in cytochrome c release followed by formation of apoptosomes and subsequent activation of caspase-9 followed by caspases-3 and -7. Bid connects the extrinsic and intrinsic pathways. Cleavage of Bid by caspase-8 produces a truncated Bid fragment[14] that initiates mitochondrial outer membrane permeabilization (MOMP) through the multidomain pro-death molecules Bax or Bak[15]. In turn, Bax/Bak translocation to mitochondria induces the release of cytochrome c into the cytosol and subsequent activation of the executioner caspases.

An additional pathway involves T-cell-mediated cytotoxicity and perforin-granzyme-dependent cell death. The perforin/granzyme pathway can induce apoptosis via either granzyme A or granzyme B. The granzyme A pathway activates a parallel, caspase-independent cell-death pathway via single-stranded-DNA damage[16]. The extrinsic, intrinsic, and granzyme B pathways converge on the same terminal pathway.

2.2 Autophagy

Autophagy is a physiological process that plays an important role in the turnover of cellular proteins and other macromolecules. Moreover, it is the major catabolic route for eukaryotic cells to salvage essential molecules, and to maintain an adequate amino acid level to sustain protein synthesis during nutritional deprivation[17]. It is characterized by mitochondrial dilation, extensive intracellular membrane remodeling, and the generation of autophagosomes, large organelles that engulf various cellular constituents in double or multiple membranes. Autophagosomes subsequently fuse with lysosomes to become autolysosomes, where sequestered cellular components are digested[18]. Amino acids and fatty acids generated by this process can be used for protein synthesis, or can be oxidized by the mitochondrial electron transport chain to produce ATP for cell survival under starvation conditions[19]. In addition to promoting cell survival, autophagy can lead to cell death.

Based on the mechanisms used for the delivery of cargo to lysosomes, autophagy has been classified into three different types: macroautophagy, microautophagy, and chaperone-mediated autophagy (CMA)[20]. Unlike apoptosis, which relies on the activation of caspases that cleave hundreds of target proteins[21], autophagic cell death is caspase-independent[22]. Indeed, autophagic cell death has been demonstrated in cells with profound defects in the apoptosis machinery[23] and in cells grown in the presence of caspase inhibitors[24]. Cells undergoing autophagic cell death look different from cells undergoing apoptosis. The characteristic cellular morphology of apoptosis results from caspase cleavage of cytoskeletal and other structural proteins[21]; apoptotic cells show early degradation of the cytoskeleton, but preserve organelles until fairly late in the process. In contrast, autophagic cell death is associated with accumulation of large numbers of autophagic vesicles, which degrade organelles early in the process, while the cytoskeleton remains intact and functional until late in the process[25].

Morphologic changes, such as chromatin condensation or membrane blebbing, may also occur in autophagic cell death, but there is no DNA fragmentation or formation of apoptotic bodies[26]. Over 30 *ATG* genes have been identified in yeast and at least 11 (*ATG1, 3, 4, 5, 6, 7, 8, 9, 10, 12* and *16*) have orthologs in mammals, *ATG6* is also known as *BECN1* (Beclin 1) and *ATG8* is commonly called *LC3* in mammals.

2.3 Programmed necrosis

Accumulating evidence supports a 'sequence' of events that characterize necrotic cell death at both the phenomenological and the biochemical level, thereby reflecting a programmed course of events in the dying necrotic cell, and contributing to a definition of necrotic cell death. In addition, in some circumstances the 'occurrence' of necrotic cell death is also programmed. Type III PCD, programmed necrosis, is not due to one well-described signalling cascade, but is the result of interplay between several signalling pathways.

The lack of caspase and lysosomal involvement distinguishes programmed necrosis from other types PCD. Programmed necrosis is characterized by early swelling of intracellular organelles such as mitochondria, ER, and Golgi apparatus, followed by loss of plasma membrane integrity. After signalling- or damage-induced lesions, necrosis can include signs of controlled processes such as mitochondrial dysfunction, enhanced generation of reactive oxygen species, ATP depletion, or proteolysis by calpains and cathepsins[27]. In addition, programmed necrosis is also typically associated with nuclear degradation that is accompanied by the release of nuclear factors such as high mobility group box 1 (HMGB1) that triggers a potent inflammatory response[28,29]. Recent reports describe that this programmed necrosis is firmly regulated and, depending on the cell-death system and/or PCD insult, implicates different proteins, such as TRAIL, TRADD, TRAF2, JNK1, RIP1, XRCC1, AIF, calpains, Bax, or Drp1[6,30-32].

3. PCD-based therapeutic strategies against cancer

Deregulation of the cellular pathways leading to PCD in mammals can cause a number of disease states, including neurodegenerative diseases, autoimmunity, and most prominently, various cancers[33].

3.1 Apoptosis based therapeutic strategies

Apoptosis is a major defense mechanism against malignant transformation. In fact, failures in normal apoptotic pathways contribute to carcinogenesis by creating a permissive environment for genetic instability and the accumulation of gene mutations. Tumour cells use a variety of molecular mechanisms to suppress apoptosis.

Cancer cells can acquire resistance to apoptosis by the expression of anti-apoptotic proteins such as Bcl-2 or by the down-regulation or mutation of pro-apoptotic proteins such as Bax. The expression of both Bcl-2 and Bax are regulated by the product of the *P53* tumour suppressor gene, a transcription factor that regulates the cell cycle, and which mutation occurs in over half of all human tumors. Among the remaining tumors, although they may process a wild-type *P53*, the pathways of *P53*-induced cell-cycle arrest and apoptosis are deficient. Therefore, *P53* serves as a unique molecular target for cancer therapy. PRIMA-1 (*P53* reactivation and induction of massive apoptosis) is the second class of compounds reported to have the capability of restoring tumor-suppressor function to mutant *P53*, and it does not appear to have an effect on wild-type *P53*. This makes PRIMA-1 unique among all the chemotherapeutics currently used in the clinic[34]. In addition, p73 belongs to a small but important family of p53-related proteins (p53, p63, p73). The *Trp73* gene contains two promoters that drive the expression of two major groups of p73 isoforms with opposing cellular actions: The TAp73 isoforms contain the p73 transactivation domain (TA) and exhibit proapoptotic activities, whereas the ΔNp73 isoforms lacking the N-terminal TA domain are anti-apoptotic. It has been proposed that a loss of p73 function might lead to tumorigenesis[35], and that TAp73 down-regulation may be coupled with ΔNp73 up-regulation in some tumors[36]. Therefore, ΔNp73 is a marker of poor prognosis in many cancers, and pharmacological attempts are being made to inhibit ΔNp73 expression. Another mechanism of apoptosis-suppression in cancer involves evasion of immune surveillance[37].

An agent that can selectively induce cell death in transformed cells without affecting normal cells would be an ideal anti-cancer chemotherapeutic agent. In fact, the molecular mechanisms that control and execute apoptotic cell death in cancer growth and resistance have been coming into focus and are enabling a new era of drug development for cancer treatment[38].

A variety of experimental approaches have been explored in the development of anti-cancer compounds that block Bcl-2 function. These include the use of antisense oligonucleotides to Bcl-2 that target gene expression at the mRNA level, peptides that mimic BH3 domains and bind to the pocket of Bcl-2 where pro-apoptotic BH3-only proteins would normally bind, and small molecule inhibitors of Bcl-2 function. The first attempt to introduce an agent that specifically targets Bcl-2 was made by Genta with their antisense DNA agent, oblimersen. On the basis of preclinical studies that found that antisense inhibition of Bcl2 levels could induce death in cancer cell lines, they designed a phosphorothioate DNA molecule complementary to Bcl2. More recently, in a study of chronic lymphocytic leukaemia (CLL), an improvement in response rate was observed in relapsed CLL patients when oblimersen was added to fludarabine and cyclophosphamide[39]. Albeit limited and not as diverse, some studies have also designed gene therapy approaches to enhance the activities of pro-death Bcl-2 proteins. Adenoviral vectors expressing these genes have recently been constructed with the goal of delivering them into cancer cells. Adenovirus-mediated overexpression of Bax, Bcl-Xs, Bik and others has been a successful strategy for killing various cancer cell lines[40,41]. In addition, Cancer cells produce higher levels of ROS (reactive oxygen species) than normal cells due to increased metabolic stress and proliferative rate.[42-44] Excessive ROS production may increase the permeability of lysosomal membranes, leading to release of lysosomal proteases, which further contribute to mitochondrial membrane impairment[11] and cancer progression[43-45]. It has been reported[42] that increasing ROS generation selectively sensitizes oncogenically transformed cells to β-phenylethyl-isothiocyanate-induced cell death, suggesting that increasing ROS generation in cancer cells could be a strategy for cancer therapy.

The selective activation of caspases might be a valuable strategy for combating cancer where pathogensis is related to insufficient cell death. Several strategies that trigger caspase activation have been developed, and several drugs that act in this way are currently being tested in preclinical trials. Therapeutic strategies have included adenovirus-mediated expression of caspases-3, -6, -8 and -9, which has resulted in both *in vivo* and *in vitro* anti-tumourogenic activities[46]. In addition, adenoviral gene therapy approaches have also been used in the delivery of caspase constructs that can be activated on demand by the addition of a compound readily able to penetrate the cell membrane. The strategy relies on the fusion of caspases to one or chimeric "death switches", which can be activated by chemical inducers of dimerization specific for a given construct[47]. There is considerable evidence that cysteine cathepsins play an important role in executing the apoptotic program in several tumour cell lines induced by death ligands such as TNF-α[48,49] or TNF-related apoptosis inducing ligand (TRAIL)[50]. In the last few years, an apoptosis inducing agent, TRAIL, that was shown to target cancer cells specifically without damaging normal cells and tissues has received special interest in cancer therapy. Several groups recently discovered a cathepsin-mediated proteolytic event in the apoptotic pathway triggered by TRAIL. First, the inhibition of TRAIL-induced apoptosis was observed upon treatment of oral squamous carcinoma cells with cathepsin inhibitors[51]. Subsequently, the pathway for apoptosis induction through Bid activation was confirmed in several other tumour cell lines[50,52,53].

3.2 Autophagy based therapeutic strategies

In tumour cells in which the quality control mechanisms of both apoptosis and autophagy are disabled, failure to maintain energy homeostasis accelerates the generation of damaged cells[54]. This failure of protein/organelle quality control to curtail the accumulation of damaged proteins and organelles through autophagy may have a broad impact on cellular functions, leading either directly or indirectly to genome damage that promotes tumourigenesis. This may mean that autophagy is one of the mechanisms that contribute to the breakdown of cell growth control in cancer [55].

In contrast to the potential cancer-promoting effect of autophagy, numerous observations have demonstrated that loss-of-function mutations in the autophagy pathway are associated with tumour progression[56,57]. Furthermore, constitutive activation of the PI3K pathway is one of the most common events in human cancer[58], and the downstream kinase mTOR restricts autophagy induction in response to starvation[59]. Although many human cancers exhibit mutations in pro-autophagy genes, and several tumour suppressor genes (*e.g.*, *DAPK*, *PTEN*, and *TP53*) can stimulate autophagy[60], the molecular mechanism through which autophagy inhibits oncogenesis is currently unclear.

Therapeutically induced autophagic cell death is another method for tumour-cell killing. Especially in apoptosis-defective cells, autophagy is often induced by cytotoxic drugs; the excessive cellular damage and attempt to remediate that damage through progressive autophagy can promote autophagic cell death[23]. Inhibition of autophagy is important in cancer therapy. The process of cancer metastasis necessarily requires that tumour cells survive in isolation from the primary tumour, without its nutrient support system. Thus, early metastases may be particularly susceptible to inhibition of autophagy.

Potential synergy with proteasome inhibitors is another reason for the use of autophagy inhibitors. The ubiquitin-mediated proteasome protein degradation pathway is functionally compensatory with protein turnover by lysosomal degradation through the autophagy pathway[61,62]. Therefore, protein degradation that is mediated by autophagy and proteasomes may be lethally exclusive to tumour cells with a high metabolic rate, or with increased susceptibility to the production of unfolded proteins. The ubiquitin-proteasome pathway is an intracellular proteolytic system which regulates the degradation of a broad spectrum of intracellular proteins, including diverse regulators of cell proliferation or apoptosis. Both bortezomid- and lenalidomide-based therapies are especially active, with bortezomib in particular being shown to provide a platform for combination, which is able to overcome resistance in this setting. Bortezomib, a first-in-class proteasome inhibitor, represents the prototypic member of a class of peptide boronate proteasome inhibitors of 26S proteasome activity, and has been approved by the US Food and Drug Administration, shows efficacy in treating multiple myeloma[63].

3.3 Programmed necrosis based therapeutic strategies

Type III PCD, programmed necrosis, is usually defined in a negative fashion, as a type of cell demise that involves rupture of the plasma membrane without the hallmarks of apoptosis and without massive autophagic vacuolization. Necrosis lacks specific biochemical markers apart from the presence of plasma membrane permeabilization, and can be detected only by electron microscopy. Necrosis is considered to be harmful because it is often associated with pathological cell loss and because of the ability of necrotic cells to promote local inflammation that may support tumour growth[64]. However, necrotic cell death is induced in cancer cells by the therapeutic administration of alkylating DNA damaging agents[65] and photosensitizing molecules that preferentially accumulate in tumour cells and generate ROS following excitation with light from various spectra[66,67].

4. The relationship of PCD to cervical cancer therapy

The ultimate goal of anticancer therapy is to kill cancer cells quickly and effectively. Over the past two decades, it has become clear that cell death, in both malignant and non-malignant cells, can be an active, regulated program. Thus, elucidation of the programmed cell-death pathways will provide new insight into tumour biology, revealing novel strategies for combating cancer. Tumour cells can only persist if they ignore the requirement for senescence that is imposed on all cells of organisms. Failure to execute PCD is usually a reflection of defective or absent molecular components of the cell-death machinery. Cervical cancer is second only to breast cancer in women as the most common of gynecologic malignancies, and it remains one of the most important causes of mortality in women worldwide. In recent years, cervical cancer has been affecting younger women. Because radiation therapy will negatively affect ovarian function in women of reproductive age, chemotherapy for cervical cancer has been receiving increased attention from clinicians. Although platinum-based neoadjuvant chemotherapy is an attractive option for chemotherapy given prior to surgery, and can reduce tumor size and lead to improvement in overall survival, cancer cells often harbor mutations that confer resistance to apoptosis, suggesting the need for other therapeutic approaches that would exploit non-apoptotic cell modes of death or enhance cell apoptosis for cervical cancer therapy.

4.1 Apoptosis autophagy and cervical cancer therapy

The mechanism of tumour cell killing by an anti-cancer agent determines the way that the agent selects for resistance to the therapy. A drug that induces apoptosis might provide quite different selective pressures on the tumour cell compared with a drug that induces autophagic cell death. Thus, drugs with different mechanisms of action would be expected to have different levels of efficacy against a particular tumour[68]. On the other hand, the close connections between the apoptosis machinery and other PCD machinery under investigation would be expected to result in simultaneous activation of these PCD processes.

When treating cancer, we often use drugs that cause severe damage to the cell. Regulation of PCD using caspase activators/inhibitors can constitute a treatment for cancer or for other PCD defective/excessive diseases[69]. Blockage of caspase activation causes degradation of catalase; the resultant increase in ROS generation leads to cell death. Degradation of catalase is also mediated by autophagy, thus suggesting a role for autophagy in caspase-independent cell death[70]. So, when cancer cells are treated, the induction of autophagy, and the interactions between autophagy and apoptosis could have profound effects on the outcome for the tumour cell.

Some connections occur upstream of the apoptotic and autophagic machinery where signalling pathways regulate both processes. For example, the autophagy gene beclin1 is part of a Type III PI3 kinase complex that is required for the formation of the autophagic vesicle, and that interacts with Bcl-2. A study found that the protein level of Beclin1 is lower in cervical cancer tissues than in normal tissues, and is closely related to pelvic lymph node metastases and histologic tumor grade[71]. Overexpression of Beclin1 in human cervical cancer SiHa and HeLa cell lines may induce the massive cells from to autophagy and inhibit tumor cell growth[72,73]. Another experiment indicates that beclin1 may be the critical molecular switch that plays an important role in fine tuning the autophagy and apoptosis through caspase-9 in cervical cancer cells[72]. Beclin1 also interacts with the other major anti-apoptotic Bcl family protein (Bcl-xL). It has been shown that autophagy can be regulated by this interaction. In addition to inhibiting apoptosis by binding to and interfering with the action of the pro-apoptotic proteins Bax and Bak, Bcl-2/Bcl-xL also inhibits autophagy by binding with beclin1. This latter interaction is particularly important in the regulation of starvation-induced autophagy[74]. Bcl-2 can inhibit autophagy not only by interacting with beclin1, but also by blocking calcium release from the ER[75]. Conversely, DRAM (damage-regulated autophagy modulator), a well known component of the autophagic machinery, is essential also for p53-mediated apoptosis[76]. Similarly, activation of the PI3 kinase/Akt pathway, a well-known way to inhibit apoptosis, also inhibits autophagy[77]. Thus important signalling pathways apparently simultaneously increase and decrease both autophagy and apoptosis. In our laboratory, we achieved stable transfectants expressing Beclin1 in cervical cancer CaSki cells, and observed that Beclin1 induced cell arrest in the G0/G1 phase. We then selected several drugs that can induce apoptosis to cancer cells by various mechanisms, including a anti-microtubule agent (paclitaxel), a platinum agent (cisplatin), an anti-metabolite (5-fluorouracil), and an anthracycline (epirubicin), to detect the role of Beclin1 in chemosensitivity. We found that Beclin1 overexpression in CaSki cells reduced cell survival following exposure to all four anti-cancer drugs. However, down-regulation of endogenous Beclin1 by siRNA in the CaSki cells did not lead to obvious resistance to the anti-cancer drugs. Taken together, these data provide evidence that Beclin1 is associated with chemosensitivity and the level of expression causes changes in response to chemotherapeutic drugs in cervical cancer, at least *in vitro,* despite the distinct damage mechanisms to cancer cells of these drugs[78, 79].

It has been suggested the mitochondrion may be the central organelle that integrates apoptosis and autophagy[80]. A positive feedback mechanism can be elicited by the activation and maturation of pre-apoptotic factors from autophagic processes in mitochondria, and lead to cell destruction through apoptotic and autophagic mechanisms. Autophagy can stop cells from undergoing apoptosis by sequestration of damaged mitochondria[81]. Moreover, some of the signals that are involved in apoptosis may also be involved in autophagy. For example, in both apoptosis and autophagy, there is the coordinated regulation of Akt and p70S6 kinase. Other proteins that may be part of the network connecting the two types of cell death include DAPK, Beclin1, BNIP3, HSpin1, or protymosin-α[82]. In our previous study[73], we found that both autophagy and apoptosis were activated during carboplatin-induced death of cervical cancer cells. Beclin1 may act as an orchestrator, integrating apoptotic and autophagic activities. Another study demonstrated that autophagy and apoptosis contribute to etoposide-induced CaSki cervical cancer cell death, and autophagy may be the predominant mechanism of etoposide-induced cell death[83]. In addition, multiple death stimuli converge on mitochondria to provoke MOMP and release of apoptogenic factors such as cytochrome c, Smac/Diablo, Omi/HtrA2, Endonuclease G (Endo G), or AIF. Once released into the cytosol, these proteins initiate apoptosis, autophagy, or programmed necrosis[30,31,84].

4.2 Programmed necrosis and cervical cancer therapy

Increasing evidence indicates that programmed necrosis can occur as a result of the activation of specific signal transduction cascades, and subsequently can be actualized only on inhibition of apoptosis and/or autophagy. Thus, it might be therapeutically desirable to trigger necrotic cell death in tumour cells that might have been selected to resist apoptotic or autophagic cell death.

Studies suggest that cell death that usually manifests with an apoptotic morphology can be shifted to a more necrotic morphology when caspase activation is prevented by pharmacological inhibitors, or by the elimination of essential caspase activators such as Apaf-1[85]. In some situations, caspase inhibition can even sensitize cells to the induction of necrosis, thereby reducing the dose of TNFa required to kill some cell lines[86]. A study found that heat treatment can induce cervical cancer CaSki cell apoptosis and necrosis[87]. Of the thermal conditions, 45°C exhibited the best induction of apoptosis, while 47°C induced direct fierce necrosis. This was further demonstrated by examining the expression level of several key apoptosis-related genes: caspase-3, Smac and Survivin. During apoptosis, caspase-3 and Smac levels were up-regulated, whereas anti-apoptotic Survivin was down-regulated, enhancing programmed cell death. Similarly, inhibition of autophagy by transfection with constitutively active Akt protein kinase, or knockout of one of the alleles encoding the Beclin1 protein also determines a shift from type II (autophagy) to type III (programmed necrosis) cell death[56]. Another study[88] also suggests that necrotic cell death induces an immune response against the dying cell through the release of pro-inflammatory cytokines, which help to initiate the repair of damaged tissue. In this way, programmed necrosis differs fundamentally from apoptosis. Death by programmed necrosis is passive, causes cellular contents to be released into the extracellular space, and often causes inflammation. In addition, oxidative-stress-induced cell death is not completely blocked by inhibiting either apoptosis or autophagy. Indeed, in the hypoxic region of a tumour, where both apoptosis and autophagy are inhibited, increased necrosis with infiltration of macrophages and production of cytokines and chemokines has been observed in mouse models[56]. What specifically triggers necrosis is unknown, but ATP production insufficient to maintain plasma-membrane integrity results in metabolic catastrophe, making cell lysis highly probable[89]. Thus, it is also reasonable to assume that cells under oxidative stress could undergo cell death through multiple pathways including necrosis.

5. Summary

PCD is a genetically regulated process that allows for the maintenance of tissue homeostasis and cell numbers, and provides protection against damaged or infected cells that threaten this balance. It is becoming increasingly clear that PCD is involved in cancer formation and survival; the process of PCD responds to several forms of cancer treatments. Elimination of cancer cells might occur not only via apoptosis, but could also be mediated by other forms of cell death such as autophagy and programmed necrosis. In recent years, the PCD-based pharmacological therapies were mainly focused on apoptosis and the main regulators of this PCD pathway, the caspase family of cysteine proteases. Drug resistance limits the effectiveness of existing medical treatments, and is still a major challenge in the current research on PCD. To better understand the pathology and the potential therapeutic strategies for human cancer that are characterized by enhanced cell death, it is crucial to elucidate the death mechanism(s) directly involved in each cancer. Treatment should depend on the actual mechanism of cell death that plays a role in disease onset. Modulation of the autophagic pathway may be a novel way of sensitizing cervical cancer cells to anti-cancer drug therapy[90], and further studies of autophagy, apoptosis and necrosis may provide new insights into the mechanisms accommodating or contributing to PCD, thereby unveiling new strategies for cervical cancer therapy.

6. Acknowledgements

This project was supported by the Natural Science Foundation of Fujian Province of China (No 2011J01132 and No 2009J01113).

7. References

[1] Gozuacik D, Kimchi A. Autophagy and cell death. Curr Top Dev Biol 2007;78:217–45.
[2] Clarke PGH. Apoptosis: from morphological types of cell death to interacting pathways. Trends Pharmacol Sci 2002;23:308–9 (author reply 310)
[3] Hengartner MO. The biochemistry of apoptosis. Nature 2000;407:770-6.
[4] Klionsky DJ. The molecular machinery of autophagy: Unanswered questions. J Cell Sci 2005;118:7–18.
[5] Mashima T, Tsuruo T. Defects of the apoptotic pathway as therapeutic target against cancer. Drug Resist Updat 2005;8:339–43.

[6] Boujrad H, Gubkina O, Robert N, Krantic S, Susin SA. AIF mediated programmed necrosis: A highly regulated way to die. Cell Cycle 2007;6:2611-8.
[7] Edinger AL, Thompson CB. Death by design: apoptosis, necrosis and autophagy. Curr Opin Cell Biol 2004;16:663-9.
[8] Green DR, Reed JC. Mitochondria and apoptosis. Science 1998;281:1309-12.
[9] Igney FH, Krammer PH. Death and anti-death: tumour resistance to apoptosis. Nat Rev Cancer 2002;2:277-88.
[10] Iannolo G, Conticello C, Memeo L, De Maria R. Apoptosis in normal and cancer stem cells. Crit Rev Oncol Hemet 2008;66:42-51.
[11] Danial NN, Korsmeyer SJ. Cell death: critical control points. Cell 2004;116:205-19.
[12] Heath-Engel HM, Shore GC. Mitochondrial membrane dynamic, cristae remodeling and apoptosis. Biochim Biophys Acta 2006;1763:549-60.
[13] Kim R, Emi M, Tanabe K, Murakami S, Uchida Y, Arihiro K. Regulation and interplay of apoptotic and non-apoptotic cell death. J Pathol 2006;208:319-26.
[14] Li HL, Zhu H, Xu CJ, Yuan JY. Cleavage of BID by caspase 8 mediates the mitochondrial damage in the Fas pathway of apoptosis. Cell 1998;94:491-501.
[15] Desagher S, Osen-Sand A, Nichols A, Eskes R, Montessuit S, Lauper S, et al. Bid-induced conformational change of Bax is responsible for mitochondrial cytochrome c release during apoptosis, J Cell Biol 1999;144:891-901.
[16] Martinvalet D, Zhu P, Lieberman J. Granzyme A induces caspase- independent mitochondrial damage, a required first step for apoptosis. Immunity 2005;22:355-70.
[17] Maiuri MC, Zalckvar E, Kimchi A, Kroemer G. Self-eating and self-killing: crosstalk between autophagy and apoptosis. Nat Rev Mol Cell Biol 2007;8:741-52.
[18] Reggiori F, Klionsky DJ. Autophagosomes: biogenesis from scratch? Curr Opin Cell Biol 2005;17:415-22.
[19] Levine B, Yuan J. Autophagy in cell death: an innocent convict? J Clin Invest 2005;115: 2679-88.
[20] Sun Y, Peng ZL. Autophagy, beclin1, and their relation with oncogenesis. Labmedicine. 2008;39:287-90.
[21] Luthi AU, Martin SJ. The CASBAH: a searchable database of caspase substrates. Cell Death Differ 2007;14:641-50.
[22] Tsujimoto Y, Shimizu S. Another way to die: autophagic programmed cell death. Cell Death Differ 2005;12(Suppl 2):1528-34.
[23] Shimizu S, Kanaseki T, Mizushima N, Mizuta T, Arakawa-Kobayashi S, Thompson CB, et al. Role of Bcl-2 family proteins in a non-apoptotic programmed cell death dependent on autophagy genes. Nat Cell Biol 2004;6:1221-8.
[24] Yu L, Alva A, Su H, Dutt P, Freundt E, Welsh S, et al. Regulation of an ATG7-beclin1 program of autophagic cell death by caspase-8. Science 2004;304:1500-2.
[25] Cuervo AM. Autophagy: in sickness and in health. Trends Cell Biol 2004;14:70-7.
[26] Codogno P, Meijer AJ. Autophagy and signaling: their role in cell survival and cell death. Cell Death Differ 2005;12 (Suppl. 2):1509-18.
[27] Golstein P, Kroemer G. Cell death by necrosis: towards a molecular definition. Trends Biochem Sci 2007;32:37-43.
[28] Lotze MT, Tracey KJ. High-mobility group box 1 protein (HMGB): Nuclear weapon in the immune arsenal. Nat Rev Immunol 2005;5:331-42.
[29] Zeh HJ, Lotze MT. Addicted to death - Invasive cancer and the immune response to unscheduled cell death. J Immunother 2005;28:1-9.

[30] Bras M, Yuste VJ, Roue G, Barbier S, Sancho P, Virely C, et al. Drp1 mediates caspase-independent type III cell death in normal and leukemic cells. Mol Cell Biol 2007;27:7073–88.

[31] Moubarak RS, Yuste VJ, Artus C, Bouharrour A, Greer PA, Menissier-de Murcia J, et al. Sequential activation of poly(ADP-ribose) polymerase 1, calpains, and Bax is essential in apoptosis-inducing factor-mediated programmed necrosis. Mol Cell Biol 2007;27:4844–62.

[32] Vanden Berghe T, Van Loo G, Saelens X, Van Gurp M, Brouckaert G, Kalai M, et al. Differential signaling to apoptotic and necrotic cell death by Fas-associated death domain protein FADD. J Biol Chem 2004;279:7925–33.

[33] Okada H, Mak TW. Pathways of apoptotic and non-apoptotic death in tumour cells. Nat Rev Cancer 2004;4:592-603.

[34] Bykov VJ, Issaeva N, Selivanova G, Wiman KG. Mutant p53-dependent growth suppression distinguishes PRIMA-1 from known anticancer drugs: a statistical analysis of information in the National Cancer Institute database. Carcinogenesis 2002; 23:2011–18.

[35] Flores ER, Sengupta S, Miller JB, Newman JJ, Bronson R, Crowley D, et al. Tumorpredisposition in mice mutant for p63 and p73: Evidence for broader tumor suppressor functions for the p53 family. Cancer Cell 2005；7：363–73.

[36] Zaika AI, Slade N, Erster SH, Sansome C, Joseph TW, Pearl M, et al. ΔNp73, a dominant-negative inhibitor of wild-type p53 and TAp73, is upregulated in human tumors. J. Exp. Med.2002; 196: 765–80.

[37] Smyth MJ, Godfrey DI, Trapani JA. A fresh look at tumor immunosurveillance and immunotherapy. Nat Immunol 2001;2:293–9.

[38] Reed JC. Apoptosis-targeted therapies for cancer. Cancer Cell 2003; 3:17-22.

[39] O'Brien S, Moore JO, Boyd TE, Larratt LM, Skotnicki A, Koziner B, et al. Randomized phase III trial of fludarabine plus cyclophosphamide with or without oblimersen sodium (Bcl-2 antisense) in patients with relapsed or refractory chronic lymphocytic leukemia. J Clin Oncol 2007;25:1114–20.

[40] Naumann U, Schmidt F, Wick W, Frank B, Weit S, Gillissen B, et al. Adenoviral natural born killer gene therapy for malignant glioma. Hum Gene Ther 2003;14:1235-46.

[41] Roy S, Bayly CI, Gareau Y, Houtzager VM, Kargman S, Keen SL, et al. Maintenance of caspase-3 proenzyme dormancy by an intrinsic "safety catch" regulatory tripeptide. Proc Natl Acad Sci U S A 2001;98:6132-7.

[42] Trachootham D, Zhou Y, Zhang H, Demizu Y, Chen Z, Pelicano H, et al. Selective killing of oncogenically transformed cells through a ROS-mediated mechanism by beta-phenylethyl isothiocyanate. Cancer Cell 2006;10:241–52.

[43] Schumacker PT. Reactive oxygen species in cancer cells: live by the sword, die by the sword. Cancer Cell 2006;10:175–6.

[44] Waris G, Ahsan H. Reactive oxygen species: role in the development of cancer and various chronic conditions. J Carcinog 2006; 5:14.

[45] Pelicano H, Carney D, Huang P. ROS stress in cancer cells and therapeutic implications. Drug Resist Update 2004;7:97–110.

[46] Philchenkov A. Caspases: potential targets for regulating cell death. J Cell Mol Med 2004;8:432-44.

[47] Shariat SF, Desai S, Song W, Khan T, Zhao J, Nguyen C, et al. Adenovirus-mediated transfer of inducible caspases: A novel "death switch" gene therapeutic approach to prostate cancer. Cancer Res 2001;61:2562-71.

[48] Foghsgaard L, Wissing D, Mauch D, Lademann U, Bastholm L, Boes M, et al. Cathepsin B acts as a dominant execution protease in tumor cell apoptosis induced by tumor necrosis factor. J Cell Biol 2001;153:999-1010.
[49] Liu J, Guo Q, Chen B, Yu Y, Lu H, Li YY. Cathepsin B and its interacting proteins, bikunin and TSRC1, correlate with TNF-induced apoptosis of ovarian cancer cells OV-90. FEBS Lett 2006;580:245-50.
[50] Nagaraj NS, Vigneswaran N, Zacharias W. Cathepsin B mediates TRAIL-induced apoptosis in oral cancer cells. J Cancer Res Clin Oncol 2006;132:171-83.
[51] Vigneswaran N, Wu J, Nagaraj N, Adler-Storthz K, Zacharias W. Differential susceptibility of metastatic and primary oral cancer cells to TRAIL-induced apoptosis. Int J Oncol 2005;26:103-12.
[52] Garnett TO, Filippova M, Duerksen-Hughes PJ. Bid is cleaved upstream of caspase-8 activation during TRAIL-mediated apoptosis in human osteosarcoma cells. Apoptosis 2007;12:1299-315.
[53] Guicciardi ME, Bronk SF, Werneburg NW, Gores GJ. cFLIPL prevents TRAIL-induced apoptosis of hepatocellular carcinoma cells by inhibiting the lysosomal pathway of apoptosis. Am J Physiol Gastrointest Liver Physiol 2007;292:G1337-46.
[54] Jin S, White E. Role of autophagy in cancer. Autophagy 2007;3:28–31.
[55] Levine B. Cell biology: autophagy and cancer. Nature 2007;446:745–7.
[56] Degenhardt K, Mathew R, Beaudoin B, Bray K, Anderson D, Chen GH, et al. Autophagy promotes tumor cell survival and restricts necrosis, inflammation, and tumorigenesis. Cancer Cell 2006;10:51–64.
[57] Karantza-Wadsworth V, Patel S, Kravchuk O, Chen GH, Mathew R, Jin S, et al. Autophagy mitigates metabolic stress and genome damage in mammary tumorigenesis. Genes Dev 2007;21:1621–35.
[58] Manning BD, Cantley LC. AKT/PKB signaling: navigating downstream. Cell 2007;129:1261–74.
[59] Guertin DA, Sabatini DM. Defining the role of mTOR in cancer. Cancer Cell 2007;12:9–22.
[60] Kondo Y, Kondo S. Autophagy and cancer therapy. Autophagy 2006;2:85–90.
[61] Ding WX, Ni HM, Gao WT, Yoshimori T, Stolz DB, Ron D, et al. Linking of autophagy to ubiquitinproteasome system is important for the regulation of endoplasmic reticulum stress and cell viability. Am J Pathol 2007;171:513–24.
[62] Pandey UB, Nie ZP, Batlevi Y, McCray BA, Ritson GP, Nedelsky NB, et al. HDAC6 rescues neurodegeneration and provides an essential link between autophagy and the UPS. Nature 2007;447:859–63.
[63] Roccaro AM, Hideshima T, Richardson PG, Russo D, Ribatti D, Vacca A, et al. Bortezomib as an antitumor agent. Curr Pharm Biotechnol 2006;7:441–8.
[64] Vakkila J, Lotze MT. Opinion - Inflammation and necrosis promote tumour growth. Nat Rev Immunol 2004;4:641–8.
[65] Zong WX, Ditsworth D, Bauer DE, Wang ZQ, Thompson CB. Alkylating DNA damage stimulates a regulated form of necrotic cell death. Genes Dev 2004;18:1272–82.
[66] Agostinis P, Buytaert E, Breyssens H, Hendrickx N. Regulatory pathways in photodynamic therapy induced apoptosis. Photochem Photobiol Sci 2004;3:721–9.
[67] Almeida RD, Manadas BJ, Carvalho AP, Duarte CB. Intracellular signaling mechanisms in photodynamic therapy. Biochim Biophys Acta 2004;1704:59–86.
[68] Hippert MM, O'Toole PS, Thorburn A. Autophagy and cancer: good bad or both? Cancer Res 2006;66:9349–51.
[69] Blagosklonny MV. Prospective strategies to enforce selectively cell death in cancer cells. Oncogene 2004;23:2967–75.

[70] Yu L, Wan F, Dutta S, Welsh S, Liu Z, Freundt E, et al. Autophagic programmed cell death by selective catalase degradation. Proc Natl Acad Sci USA 2006;103:4952–7.
[71] Wang ZH, Peng ZL, Duan ZL, Liu H. Expression and clinical significance of autophagy gene Beclin1 in cervical squamous cell carcinoma. Sichuan Da Xue Xue Bao Yi Xue Ban 2006;37: 860–3.
[72] Wang ZH, Xu L, Duan ZL, Zeng LQ, Yan NH, Peng ZL. Beclin 1-mediated macroautophagy involves regulation of caspase-9 expression in cervical cancer HeLa cells. Gynecol Oncol 2007;107:107–13.
[73] Sun Y, Zhang J, Peng ZL. Beclin1 induces autophagy and its potential contributions to sensitizes SiHa cells to carboplatin therapy. Int J Gynecol Cancer 2009;19:772-6.
[74] Pattingre S, Tassa A, Qu X, Garuti R, Liang XH, Mizushima N, et al. Bcl-2 antiapoptotic proteins inhibit beclin 1-dependent autophagy. Cell 2005;122:927–39.
[75] Hoyer-Hansen M, Bastholm L, Szyniarowski P, Campanella M, Szabadkai G, Farkas T, et al. Control of macroautophagy by calcium, calmodulin-dependent kinase kinase-beta, and Bcl-2. Mol Cell 2007;25:193–205.
[76] Crighton D, Wilkinson S, O'Prey J, Syed N, Smith P, Harrison PR, et al. DRAM, a p53-induced modulator of autophagy, is critical for apoptosis. Cell 2006;126:121–34.
[77] Mathew R, Karantza-Wadsworth V, White E. Role of autophagy in cancer. Nat Rev Cancer 2007;7:961-7.
[78] Sun Y, Liu JH, Jin L, Lin SM, Yang Y, Sui YX, Shi H. Over-expression of the Beclin1 gene upregulates chemosensitivity to anti-cancer drugs by enhancing therapy induced apoptosis in cervix squamous carcinoma CaSki cells. Cancer Lett 2010;294:204-10
[79] Sun Y, Jin L, Liu J, Lin S, Yang Y, Sui Y, Shi H. Effect of autophagy on paclitaxel-induced CaSki cell death. Zhong Nan Da Xue Xue Bao Yi Xue Ban 2010;35:557-65.
[80] Jin SK. Autophagy, mitochondrial quality control, and oncogenesis.Autophagy 2006;2:80-4.
[81] Ravikumar B, Berger Z, Vacher C, O'Kane CJ, Rubinsztein DC. Rapamycin pre-treatment protects against apoptosis. Hum Mol Genet 2006;15:1209–16.
[82] Klionsky DJ, Emr SD. Autophagy as a regulated pathway of cellular degradation. Science 2000;290:1717–21.
[83] Lee SB, Tong SY, Kim JJ, Um SJ, Park JS. Caspase-independent autophagic cytotoxicity in etoposide-treated CaSki cervical carcinoma cells. DNA Cell Biol 2007;26:713-20.
[84] Boya P, Gonzalez-Polo RA, Casares N, Perfettini JL, Dessen P, Larochette N, et al. Inhibition of macroautophagy triggers apoptosis. Mol Cell Biol 2005;25:1025–40.
[85] Golstein P, Kroemer G. Redundant cell death mechanisms as relics and backups. Cell Death Differ 2005;12 (Suppl 2): 1490–6.
[86] Degterev A, Yuan J. Expansion and evolution of cell death programmes. Nat Rev Mol Cell Bio 2008;9:378-90.
[87] Zhou J, Wang X, Du L, Zhao L, Lei F, Ouyang W, Zhang Y, Liao Y, Tang J. Effect of hyperthermia on the apoptosis and proliferation of CaSki cells. Mol Med Report 2011;4:187-91
[88] Zong WX, Ditsworth D, Bauer DE, Wang ZQ, Thompson CB. Alkylating DNA damage stimulates a regulated form of necrotic cell death. Genes Dev 2004;18:1272–82.
[89] Jin S, Dipaola RS, Mathew R, White E. Metabolic catastrophe as a means to cancer cell death. J Cell Sci 2007;120:379–83.
[90] Sun Y, Liu JH, Sui YX, Jin L, Yang Y, Lin SM, Shi H. Beclin1 Over-expression Inhibitis Proliferation, Invasion and Migration of CaSki Cervical Cancer Cells. Asian Pacific J Cancer Prev 2011;12:1269-73

16

Antiproliferative Effect and Induction of Apoptosis by *Inula viscosa* L. and *Retama monosperma* L. Extracts in Human Cervical Cancer Cells

L. Benbacer[1], N. Merghoub[1,2,3], H. El Btaouri[3], S. Gmouh[4], M. Attaleb[1], H. Morjani[3], S. Amzazi[2] and M. El Mzibri[1,*]

[1]*Unité de Biologie et Recherche Médicale, Centre National de l'Energie, des Sciences et Techniques Nucléaires (CNESTEN), Rabat*

[2]*Laboratoire de Biochimie-Immuniologie, Faculté des Sciences, Rabat*

[3]*MEDyC CNRS UMR 6237, UFR Sciences et UFR Pharmacie, Reims*

[4]*Unités d'Appui Technique à la Recherche Scientifique, Centre National pour la Recherche Scientifique et Technique, Rabat*

[1,2,4]*Morroco*

[3]*France*

1. Introduction

Worldwide cervical cancer is the second most common malignancy in women with nearly a half million new cases diagnosed and 250,000 deaths each year Almost 80% of cases occur in low-income countries, where cervical cancer is the most common cancer in women (WHO, 2009). In spite of recent advances in the development of new anticancer agents, cancer continues to be one of the major causes of death worldwide. Resistance to chemotherapeutic agents remains a principal obstacle in the successful treatment of cancer. Therefore, development and search of novel and effective anticancer agents to overcome resistance have become very important issues.

As other cancers, radiotherapy and chemotherapy are the conventional cancer treatment used nowadays and remain the routine method for the treatment of cervical cancer. These approaches present sole limits related to the cost, problems of unstable efficiency and severe side effects whose reduce the quality of life and discourage patients to observe medication protocols which then lead to the progression of cancer and associated complications. In addition, many of these treatments present limited anti-cancer activities

[*] Corresponding Author

(Mans, 2000). Therefore, development and search of novel and effective anticancer agents to overcome resistance and without severe side effects have become very important issues.

During last decades, natural products have been an important source of chemotherapeutics, more than half of effective cancer drugs can be traced to natural origins (Ma, 2009). Approximately 60% of drugs currently used for cancer treatment have been isolated from natural products (Gordaliza, 2007; Newman, 2007). Currently, medicinal plants constitute a common alternative for cancer treatment in many countries around the world (Gerson-Cwilich, 2006; Tascilar, 2006).

Many candidate compounds that are able to arrest proliferation and induce apoptosis in neoplastic cells have been discovered. These include *Vinca* Alkaloids; *Taxus* diterpenes; *Camptotheca* Alkaloids; and *Podophyllum* lignans. Currently, there are 16 new plant-derived compounds being tested in clinical trials and of these 13 are being tested in phase I or II, and 3 are in phase III. Among these compounds, flavopiridol, isolated from the Indian tree *Dysoxylum binectariferum* and mesoindigo, isolated from the Chinese plant *Indigofera tinctoria,* have been shown to exhibit anti-cancer effects with lesser toxicity than conventional drugs (Saklani A, 2008).

In Morocco, medicinal plants have always been associated with cultural behaviour and traditional knowledge. Herbal remedies are frequently used to treat a large variety of ailments and symptoms, like a fever, inflammation, and pain (Gonzalez-Tejero, 2008). However, there is little information about their anti-cancer properties.

Drug discovery from natural sources involves a multidisciplinary approach combining ethnobotanical, phytochemical and biological techniques to provide new chemical compounds for the development of new drugs against various pharmacological targets, including cancer and related complications. Cytotoxic screening models provide important preliminary data to select plant extracts with potential antineoplastic properties. The initial screenings are cell-based assays using established cell lines, in which the toxic effects of plant extracts or isolated compounds can be measured. Most of the clinically used antitumor agents possess significant cytotoxic activity in cell culture systems (Cardellina, 1999).

In the course to contribute to development of new anticancer drugs against cervical cancer, the human cervical carcinoma SiHa and HeLa cell lines, has been used as a model system in this study for screening promising plant materials from folk Moroccan medicine possessing anticancer effect. Thus, seven medicinal plants: *Inula viscosa* L. (Ait.), *Retama monosperma* L. (Boiss.), *Ormenis mixta* L. (Dumont.), *Ormenis eriolepis* Coss., *Rhamnus lycioides* L., *Berberis hispanica* Bois. and *Urginea maritima* L. (Baker.) were collected and evaluated for the *in vitro* cytotoxic effect against SiHa and HeLa cell lines. The selection was made on the basis of their reputation as folk medicines and ethnobotanic informations to treat different illnesses and diseases. The selected plants have been described to exhibit several biological activities. However, the antiproliferative and apoptotic effects of these plants against cervical cancer cells have not yet been explored. The second part of this study, the most active plants were then selected and were evaluated for their potential antiproliferative effects against SiHa and HeLa cells. Furthers assays were used to elucidate its cytotoxic mechanism.

2. Materials and methods

2.1 Plant species

Seven plant species were collected from different regions of Morocco and were identified by Dr. M. Fennane from the Scientific Institute of Rabat. Voucher specimens are kept in the herbarium of institute. Table 1 shows the ethnobotanical data of the investigated plant species, including botanical names, local names, ethnomedical uses, as well as the plant parts employed in this study.

Plants species (Family)	Place of collection	Part plant collected	Traditional use	pharmacological activities
Inula viscosa L. Ait (Asteraceae)	Ain atik Temara	Leaves	Skin diseases, treats cutaneous abcesses, wound healing, Tuberculosis, bronchial infections (Bellakhdar, 1997)	Anti-inflammatory effects (Hernandez, 2007; Máñez, 2007) Antimicrobial activity (Maoz., 1998) Antifungal activity (Cafarchia, 2002)
Retama monosperma L. Bois (Fabaceae)	Sidi-Boughaba Mahdia	Leaves	Purgative, vermifuge, antihelmintic, abortive and disinfectant (Benrahmoune, 2003)	No information available
Berberis hispanica Bois and Reut. (Berberidaceae)	Tamahdit	Bark roots	Blood pressure, digestive, disorders, anorexia, urinary system, nephritic, liver and astrointestinal disorders, ocular affections, febrifuge, antileishmania, antitumoral (Bellakhdar, 1997)	Antimicrobial activity (Ai-Rong, 2007) Antitumor activities (Fukuda, 1999; Meenakshi, 2007)
Ormenis eriolepis Coss. (Asteraceae)	Ouarzazat	Aerial part	Stomachic, anthelmintic and antidiabetic (Bellakhdar, 1997)	Antibactrial activities (El Hanbali, 2004) Antileishmania activities (El Hanbali, 2005) Antifungic activity (Amani, 2008)
Ormenis mixta (Asteraceae)	Sidi-Boughaba Mahdia	Aerial part	Drain the buttons, healing wounds (Haddad, 2003)	Antimicrobial activity (Satrani, 2007)
Rhamnus lycioides ssp. *Oleoides* (Rhamnaceae)	Sidi-Boughaba Mahdia	Leaves	Laxative, diuretic and hepatic affections (Hmamouchi, 2001)	Hypotensive activity (Terencio, 1990)
Urginea maritima L. *Baker* (Lemnaceae)	Sidi-Boughaba Mahdia	Bulbs	Cardiac failures, whooping-cough, pneumonia, abortive, vipers bites, aphrodisiac, cough, bronchitis and the jaundice, diuretic and internal tumours (Bellakhdar, 1997)	Cytotoxic and antimalarial activities (Sathiyamoorthy, 1999)

Table 1. Ethnobotanical data and some reported pharmacological activities of plants species used in this study.

2.2 Plant extracts preparation

The seven Plants were dried and ground finely. 20g of each powdered plant were extracted by absolute methanol (100 ml, three times) for 72 h at room temperature. The extracts were evaporated to dryness under reduced pressure at 40°C. A total of 40 mg of obtained extract were dissolved in dimethyl sulfoxide (DMSO) to give a solution stock to 40 mg/ml and conserved at -20°C until use.

In second part of the study, the most actives plants were submitted to extraction with solvents with different polarities. *Inula viscosa* L. and *Retama monosperma* L. were extracted successively in a Soxhlet with *n*-hexane and methanol. The resulting extracts were then evaporated by Rotavapor to give dried extracts. The methanol concentrated extract was dissolved in distilled water and was successively extracted with dichloromethane and ethyl acetate. The solvent was evaporated to obtain the crudes extracts, and kept in the dark at +4 °C until tested.

2.3 Cell lines

Human cervical cancer SiHa and HeLa cell lines were used in this study. Cells were grown as monolayers in Minimum Essential Medium (MEM) supplemented with 10% heat-inactivated fetal calf serum and 1% Penicillin-Spreptomycin mixture. Cultures were maintained at 37°C in 5% CO2. SiHa and HeLa cell lines were kindly provided by Dr. P. Coursaget, INSERM U618, University François Rabelais, Tours, France.

2.4 Cytotoxicity assay

Cytotoxicity of the plant extracts was determined using the MTT Assay as described previously (Mosmann, 1983). Cells were seeded in 96-well microplates. After 24 h of culture, the cells were treated with different concentrations ranging from 15.6 to 500 µg/ml, in quadruplicate for 48h or 72h incubation. 10µL MTT (5mg/mL) was added to each well. After 4 hours incubation, 150µL DMSO were added to dissolve purple formazan crystals, and absorbance was then determined using a spectrophotometer at 590nm. Mitomycin C and vinblastin (~ 95 % HPLC, sigma-Aldrich) were used as a positive control.

2.5 Detection of the morphological changes associated with apoptosis

SiHa and HeLa cells were cultured on glass chamber slides in 2 well plates and were treated with the IV-HE, IV-DF and Rm-DF for 24h , 48h and 72h at a concentration of 20µg/ml. After incubation, cells were washed with PBS twice and fixed with (4% paraformaldehyde and 0.1% Triton X-100) for 5 min. The cells were then washed with PBS and incubated with Hoecsht 33342 (10µg/ml) (Sigma) at 37 °C for 30min. The cells were visualized through fluorescence inverted microscope (Axiovert 200M Zeiss, Germany) equipped with an LD achroplan 40X objective. The images were collected with a CCD cooled camera (Coolsnap HQ, Ropper Scientific).

2.6 Mitochondrial membrane potential ($\Delta\Psi_m$) measurement

Analysis of mitochondrial membrane potential was carried out using the lipophilic cationic probe, JC-1 (Molecular Probes, Eugene, OR) whose monomer emits at 530 nm (green) after excitation at 500 nm. Depending on the mitochondrial membrane potential, JC-1 is able to form J-aggregates respectively from green to yellow-orange fluorescence emission (590 nm) as mitochondrial membrane becomes more polarized. Therefore, the I_{590}nm/I_{530}nm emission ratio value allows observation of mitochondrial dysfunction. SiHa and HeLa cells were treated with the extract for 24 h or 48h. JC-1 reagent (10µM) was added for 20 min at 37 °C in the dark. Cells were then washed with PBS and centrifuged at 1500 rpm, 4°C for 5 min. The pellet was resuspended in 1 ml ice-cold PBS and the measurements were performed using the Spectrofluorometer (RF-5301PC, Shimadzu, Tokyo, Japan). Residual mitochondrial potential as percentage of control was expressed as follows: (R treated/R control) x 100; R = I_{590} nm/I_{530} nm.

2.7 Reactive oxygene species (ROS) production

Production of ROS (reactive oxygen species) was monitored via oxidation of the carboxydichlorofluorescein analog probe, C2938. SiHa and HeLa cells (2 x10^5) were seeded into a 6-well plate and treated with the appropriate concentration of the extract for 24 h. Control and treated cells were washed and stained with 10 µM C2938 (30 min, 37°C). Fluorescence emission from the oxidized probe was quantified with a Spectrofluorophotometer (RF-5301PC, Shimadzu) (excitation: 488±1 nm; emission: 518±1 nm).

2.8 Western blot analysis

Cells were treated with 20 µg/ml of extracts for (24h, 48h and 72h), scrapped, washed with PBS and lysed in ice-cold lysis buffer (10 mM Tris pH 7.4, 150 mM NaCl, 5 mM EDTA, 1 mM Na_3VO_4, 1mM dithiothreitol, 10µg/ml Leupeptin , 10µg/ml aprotinin, 10% glycerol, 1%Brij (v/v)) , placed on ice for 20 and centrifuged at 14,000g for 15 min at 4 °C. The amount of protein was determined using the Bio-Rad protein quantification kit. Equal amounts of proteins (25-30µg/ml) was subjected to electrophorese on SDS-polyacrylamide gels and, transferred to a Nitrocellulose membrane by electroblotting. After blocking non-specific sites, the membrane was incubated overnight with appropriate primary antibodies: Monoclonal anti- pro-Caspase 3 (1/700), Monoclonal anti-β actin (dilution 1/5000), Monoclonal anti-BCl_2 (1/700) and polyclonal anti- PARP (1/1000). Horseradish peroxidase-conjugated goat anti-rabbit or anti-mouse IgG were used as secondary antibodies and proteins were detected using an enhanced chemiluminescence (ECL) kit.

2.9 Gas chromatography/mass spectrometry (GC/MS) analysis

The identification of the compounds from *I. viscosa* hexanic fraction (IV-HE) and *R. monosperma* dichloromethane fraction (Rm-DF) was performed by (GC/MS) analysis using a Hewlett Packard 5890 II Gaz Chromatograph, equipped with a HP 5972 Mass selective detector and a VB5 (5% phenyl ; 95% methylpolisyloxane) capillary column (30 m, 0.25 mm, film thickness 0.25 µm). Injection volume was 1 µl with a splitless; the injector and detector temperatures was held constant at 250. For GC/MS detection an electron ionization system with ionization energy of 70 eV was used. Helium was used as the carrier gas with an inlet pressure of 10.48 psi, corresponding to a flow rate of 1.0 ml/min. The analytical conditions worked the following programme: oven temperature from 60 to 280°C at rate of 16°C min^{-1}, the final temperature of 300°C was held for 10 min. Tentative identification of the compounds was based on the comparison of their relative retention time and spectral mass with those of Nist and Wiley7 library data of the GC/MS system.

2.10 Statistical analysis

Data are presented as means ± SD of at least triplicate or quadruplicate determinations of three different assays. The statistical analysis was performed by student's-test with Microsoft excel software. Significant differences are indicated by $*p < 0.05$; $**p < 0.01$; $***p < 0.001$.

3. Results and discussion

3.1 Cytotoxic effect of the medicinal plants extracts from Morocco

Crude extracts of selected plants were made by exhaustive methanol extraction. These plants extracts were tested for their potential cytotoxic effects, SiHa and HeLa cells were treated with plants extracts at different concentrations ranging from 15 to 500 µg/ml for 48h. The cells viability were determined by MTT assay. Among the 7 medicinal plant extracts, methanolic extract from *Inula viscosa* L. and *Retama monosperma* L. have been found to exhibit marked cytotoxic effect on both SiHa and HeLa cell lines. Their IC_{50} values were 54±12 and 99±1 µg/ml in SiHa cells and 60±8 and 112±4 µg/ml in HeLa cells, respectively. The methanolic extract of *Ormenis eriolepis* Coss., *Ormenis mixta* L. and *Berberis hispanica* Boiss. have lower cytotoxic effect on the cancer cell lines tested (Table 2). However, *Urginea maritime* L. and *Rhamnus lycioides* L. had insignificant or no cytotoxic effects at tested concentration with IC_{50} >500µ/ml.

Methanolic extracts	IC_{50} ± SD (µg/ml)	
	SiHa	*HeLa*
Inula viscosa L.	54 ± 12	60 ± 8
Ormenis eriolepis Coss.	94 ± 4	112 ± 4
Ormenis mixta L.	383 ± 26	311± 14
Berberis hispanica Boiss.	178 ± 5	224 ± 10
Retama Monosperma L.	99 ± 1	96 ± 4
Urginea maritime L.	› 500	› 500
Rhamnus lycioides L.	› 500	› 500
Mitomycin C	6 ± 1	1 ± 0.30

Table 2. Cytotoxic activity of methanolic extracts of some medicinal plants from Morocco on SiHa and HeLa cervical cancer cell lines.

Inula viscosa L. (Ait.) and *Retama monosperma* L. methanolic extracts showed the highest cytotoxic activity with lowest IC_{50} values. Previous studies have reported interesting biological activities with potential therapeutic applications of these plants. *Inula viscosa* L. is used in Moroccan folk medicine as antihelmintic, diuretic, anemia and as cataplasm for rheumatic pain (Hmamouchi, 2001), tuberculosis, expectorant and treatment of bronchitis

(Bellakhdar, 1997). The aerial part of this plant is used as decoction in the treatment of diabetes, hypertension and renal diseases (Eddouks, 2002). This plant has been described to exhibit several biological activities such as anti-inflammatory (Hernández, 2007), antimicrobial (Maoz, 1998) and antifungal effects (Cafarchia, 2002). *Retama monosperma* L. is used in the traditional medicine of many countries, as a purgative, vermifuge, antihelmintic and abortive (Bellakhdar, 1997). Moreover, it has been reported that R*etama Genus* for a various pharmacological effects, including an hypoglycemic and diuretic (Maghrani, 2005a; Maghrani, 2005b), cytotoxic (Conforti, 2004; Hayet, 2007; López-Lázaro, 2000), antioxidant and antiviral (Edziri, 2010) and antihypertensive (Eddouks, 2007).

Cells were exposed to different concentrations of extracts for 48h. Data are expressed as IC_{50} values (µg/ml) and are means ± SD of three experiments. Mitomycine was used as positive control.

The cytotoxic effect of extracts from *Inula viscosa* L. and *Retama monosperma* L.

As evidenced by MTT assays, we found that hexanic (IV-HE) and dichloromethane (IV-DF) extracts from *Inula viscosa* were able to inhibit cell growth in dose-dependent manner after 72h of treatment, in both cell lines. The IC_{50} values for IV-HE on SiHa and HeLa were 9.56±1.68 and 13.17±0.79 µg/ml, respectively. However, for IV-DF, the IC_{50} values on SiHa and HeLa were respectively 6.54±1.46 and 22.04±3.31 µg/ml. *Retama monosperma* dichloromethane fraction (Rm-DF) was the most active extract, exhibiting also cytotoxic activity against both cells lines in dose-dependent manner. Values of IC_{50} obtained were 14± and 21±µg/ml, in SiHa and HeLa cell lines respectively (Table 3). The American National Cancer Institute assigns a significant cytotoxic effect of promising anticancer product for future bio-guided studies if it exerts an IC_{50} value <30 µg/ml (Suffnes, 1990). The obtained results indicate that IV-HE and IV-DF and Rm-DF were shown to induce significant and dose-dependent inhibitory activities against human cervical cancer cell lines SiHa and HeLa.

Extracts	IC_{50} (µg/ml)	
	SiHa	HeLa
Retama monosperma L. extracts		
Hexane extract (Rm-HE)	› 80	› 80
Methanol extract (Rm-ME)	› 80	› 80
Dichloromethane fraction (Rm-DF)	14.57±4.15	21.33±7.88
Acetate ethyle fraction (Rm-AF)	27.54±5.64	77.47±2.25
Inula viscosa L. extracts		
Hexane extract (IV-HE)	9.56 ± 1.68	13.17±0.79
Methanol extract (IV-ME)	52.83±3.28	› 80
Dichloromethane fraction (IV-DF)	6.54±1.46	22.04±3.31
Ethyl acetate fraction (IV-AF)	63.62±10.55	› 80
Vinblastin	10.88±0.78	6.28±0,35

Table 3. Cytotoxic effect of extracts and fractions of *Retama monosperma* L. and *Inula viscosa* L. extracts against SiHa and HeLa cervical cancer cells.

Cells were exposed to different concentrations of extracts for 72h. As determined by MTT assay. Data are expressed as IC_{50} values (µg/ml) and are means ± SD of three experiments. Vinblastin was used as a positive control.

3.2 Chemical identification of plants extracts

Analyses of the most active extracts by gas chromatography (GC) coupled with and GC-mass spectrometry (MS) revealed the presence of a sesquiterpene acid: isocostic acid (46.05%) and two sesquiterpenes lactones: tomentosin (33.27%) and inuviscolide (13.04%), as major compounds in IV-HE extract (Table 4). In the fact, *Inula viscosa* L. is source of a number of bioactives compounds as well as flavonoids (Hernandez, 2007) and sesquiterpene derivatives (Fontana, 2007).

Extracts	Compounds	RT	Area (%)
IV-HE	1-Amino-1-ortho-chlorophenyl-2-(2-quinoxalinyl)ethene	12.79	0.21
	3-(4'-Methoxyphenyl)-1-acetyl-2-phenylindolizine	24.99	1.68
	Isocostic acid	40.56	46.05
	Isoaromadendrene epoxide	41.38	1.44
	Phenanthrene, 7-ethenyl-1,2,3,4,4α,4β,5,6,7,8,10,10α-dodecahydro-4α,7-dimethyl-1-methylene-, [4αS-(4αα',4βα',7α',10αα')]-	42.74	0.69
	Iso-velleral	46.26	1.87
	6,9,12,15-Docosatetraenoic acid, methyl ester	46.82	0.37
	Quercetin 7,3',4'-trimethoxy	46.93	0.22
	Tomentosin	47.27	33.27
	Inuviscolide	47.39	13.04
	Tetracosane	54.32	0.77
	6-Imino-8-(3',5'-dichlorolphenyl)-3,4-dihydro-2H, 6H-pyrimido[2,1-β][1,3]thiazine-7-carbonitrile	57.78	0.39
IV-DF	Benzeneacetic acid, α',4-bis[(trimethylsilyl)oxy]-, trimethylsilyl ester	18 .91	10.44
	9H-pyrrolo[3',4':3,4]pyrrolo[2,1-a]phthalazine-9,11(10H)-dione,10-ethyl-8-phenyl	24.99	47.85
	Isocostic acid	40.56	2.29
	1 ,2-longidione	44.54	5.03
	10 hydroxy-1 ,4,5,8-Tetramethyl anthrone	44.84	2.54
	Chiapin B	46.27	1.55
	2,4,7 Trimethyl-5 ,6-diphenyl-1H-isoindol-1 ,3(2H)-dione	47.01	9.12
	Tomentosin	47.26	13.93
	Methyl 2,3-Dideoxy-4-O-propargyl-6-O-(tert-butyldimethylsilyl)-α-D-erythro-hex-2-enopyranoside	55.92	7.24

Area (%):(%): area percentage (peak area relative to the total peak area percentage).
RT : Retention time (min).

Table 4. Compounds present within *Inula viscosa* L. extracts identified by CG/MS.

However, CG/MS analysis of Rm-DF (Table 5) revealed the presence of five known quinolizidine alkaloids as well as, sparteine (10.97%), L- methyl cytisine (9.11%), 17-oxosparteine (3.49%), lupanine (0.93%) and anagyrine (39.63%). The Retama species have been reported to contain alkaloids (Abdel Halim, 1997) and flavonoids (Kassem, 2000). Fifteen quinolizidine and 3 dipiperidine alkaloids were isolated from the leaves of flowering plants of *R. monosperma* collected from Morocco (Touati, 1996).

Extracts	Compounds	RT	Area(%)
Rm-DF	α-Pinene	9,89	2.73
	1,8-Cineole	13,79	8.03
	Benzeneacetic acid, α,4-bis[(trimethylsilyl)oxy]-,	18.91	4.71
	trimethylsilyl ester		
	9H-pyrrolo[3',4':3,4]pyrrolo[2,1-a]phthalazine-9,	24.99	19.05
	11(10H)-dione,10-ethyl-8-phenyl		
	Sparteine	38,98	10.97
	Hexadecanoic acid	42,71	0.86
	L methyl cytisine	44,23	9.11
	17- oxosparteine	46,67	3.49
	4-(N-(3-trifluoromethylphenyl)-amino)-5,6-dimethyl-7H-pyrro[2.3-d]pyrimidine	47.78	0.50
	Lupanine	48,78	0.93
	Anagyrine	53 ,73	39.63

Area (%):(%): area percentage (peak area relative to the total peak area percentage).
RT : Retention time (min).

Table 5. Compounds present within *R. monosperma* L. extracts identified by CG/MS.

3.3 Molecular mechanisms of apoptosis signalling pathways

Induction of apoptosis constitute an important mechanism for anticancer effects of many naturally occurring and synthetic agents. Activation of apoptotic pathways seems to be an effective strategy against tumor progression (Brown, 2005). The caspase pathway plays a pivotal role in the induction, transduction and amplification of intracellular apoptotic signals. Among the caspase family proteins, capase-3 is responsible for the proteolytic cleavage of many key proteins such as PARP, which is considered as a marker of apoptosis (Kothakota, 1997; Wang, 2005).

3.4 IV-HE, IV-DF and Rm-DF induced apoptosis in SiHa and HeLa cells

In order to determine whether plant extracts induced cell death was due to apoptosis, we analyzed chromatin condensation and nuclear fragmentation by Hoechst 33342 staining and fluorescence microscopy (Kerr, 1994). SiHa and HeLa cells were treated with IV-HE, IV-DF and Rm-DF for 24h, 48h and 72h. As shown in Figure 1, the rate of apoptotic cells was increased significantly in a time-dependant manner after treatment with IV-HE, IV-DF and Rm-DF (Figure.1).

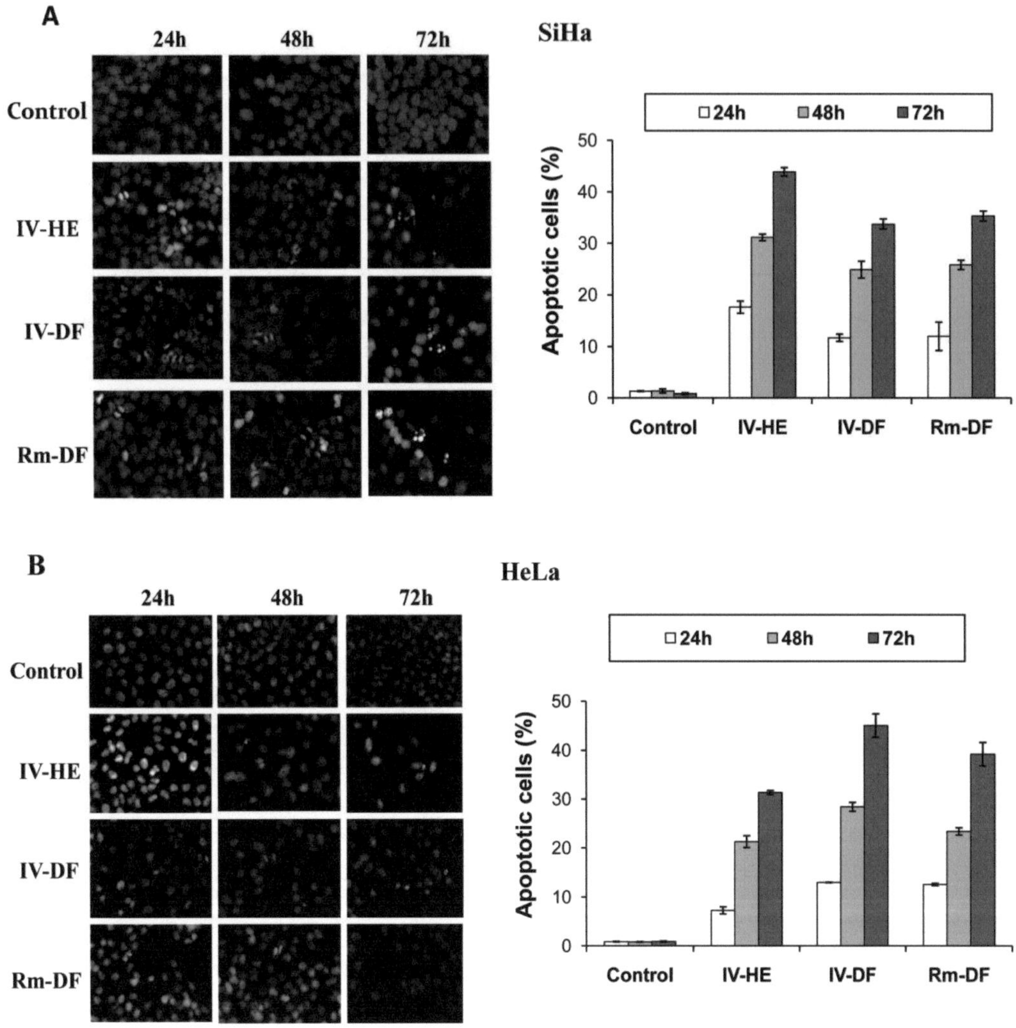

Fig. 1. IV-HE, IV-DF and Rm-DF induce apoptosis of cervical cancer cells. SiHa (A) and HeLa (B) cells were treated IV-HE, IV-DF and Rm-DF and stained with Hoechst 33342. Condensed, fragmented nuclei and apoptotic bodies were seen in the treated cells. The stained nuclei were visualized and photographed with an inverted fluorescence microscope (Axiovert 200M Zeiss). Data represent at least two experiments (Magnification: x 400).

3.5 Expression of Pro-caspase, Bcl2 and PARP cleavage

Inula viscosa and *Retama monosperma* extracts were able to induce apoptosis in HeLa and SiHa cells as evidenced by western blot analysis. Activation of caspase-3 causes the cleavage of poly-(ADP-ribose)-polymerase (PARP), a hallmark of apoptosis, to produce an 85 kDa fragment during apoptosis (Tewari, 1995). After treatment of cells, a procaspase-3 cleavage and cleavage of poly (ADP-ribose) polymerase (PARP) were observed in time- and dose-dependent manner. IV-HE, IV-DF and Rm-DF caused the proteolytic cleavage of PARP with accumulation of the 85 kDa fragment in SiHa and HeLa cells (Figure 2.A; 2.B). This

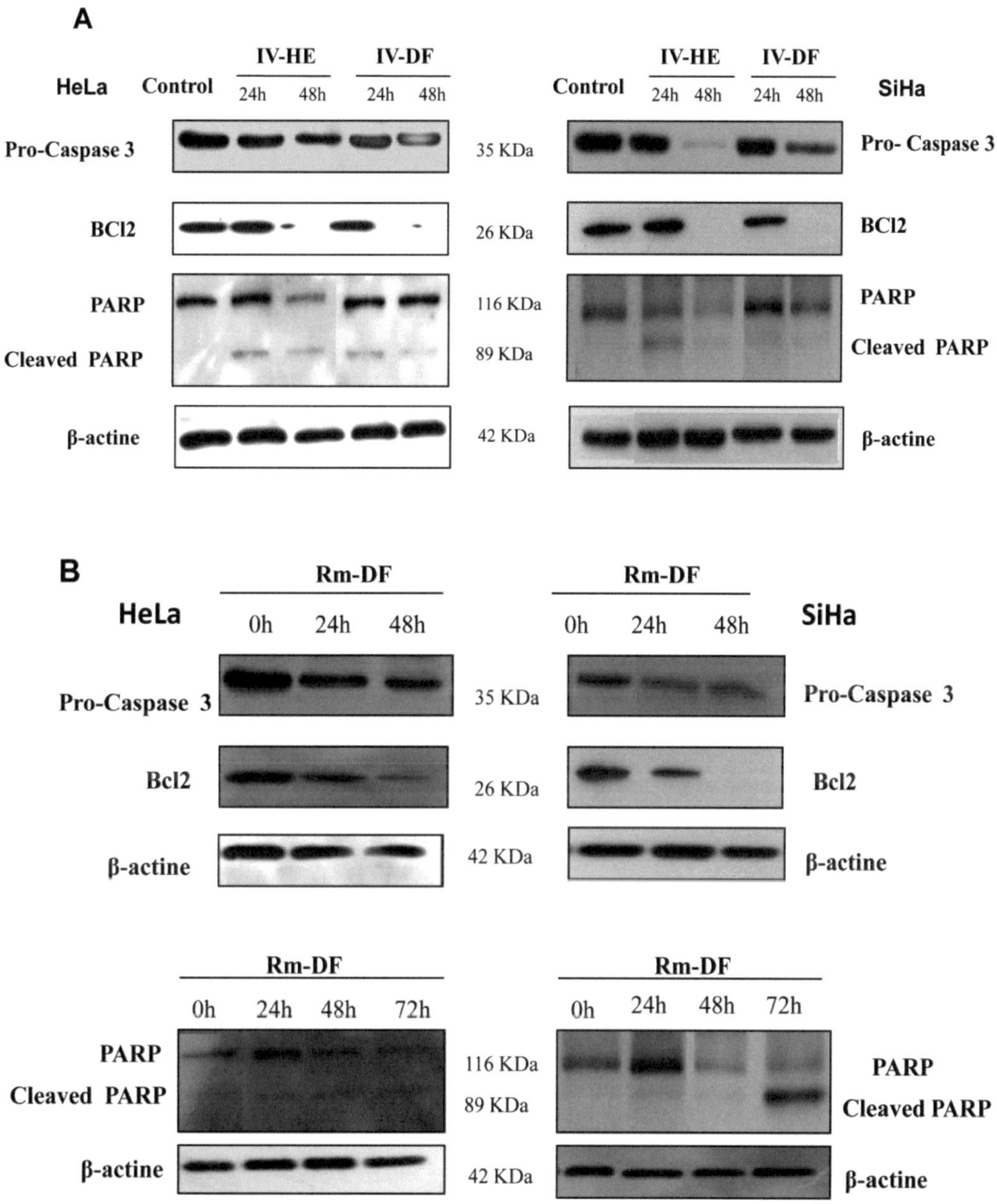

Fig. 2. Expression of Pro-caspase 3 , Bcl-2 and PARP proteins in HeLa and SiHa treated-cells analysed by Western blot. After treatment with 20μg/ml of IV-HE, IV-DF (A) and Rm-DF (B) during 24h and 48 h or 72h, cell lysates were prepared and the proteins were separated on SDS-polyacrylamide gel and transferred into nitrocellulose membranes. The membranes were probed with the indicated antibodies. β-actin was used as a control for protein loading. The results shown here were from two or three representative experiments.

suggests that apoptosis induced by IV-HE, IV-DF and Rm-DF could be associated with a caspase-dependent pathway.

The activation and function of caspases are regulated by various key of molecules, such as inhibitors of apoptosis protein, Bcl-2 protein family. Increased expression of the anti-apoptotic protein Bcl-2 causes resistance to chemotherapeutic drugs, while decreasing Bcl-2 expression may promote apoptotic responses to anticancer drugs (Reed J.C., 1994). Our investigations showed a significant decrease in Bcl-2 expression after 24h treatment with IV-HE, IV-DF and Rm-DF (Figure 2A, 2B).

3.6 Statut of mitochondrial membrane potential

Mitochondrial dysfunction has been shown to participate in the induction of apoptosis. Indeed, opening of the mitochondrial permeability transition pore has been demonstrated to induce depolarization of the transmembrane potential ($\Delta\Psi m$), release of apoptogenic factors and loss of oxidative phosphorylation (Zimmermann, 2001). To characterize the effect of IV-HE, IV-DF and Rm-DF on the mitochondrial apoptotic pathway, we measured the mitochondrial membrane potential ($\Delta\Psi_m$) in SiHa and HeLa cells after treatment for 24h. As shown in (Figure.3), IV-HE, IV-DF and Rm-DF, induced a significant decrease in mitochondrial membrane potential ($\Delta\Psi m$), in both SiHa and HeLa cells.

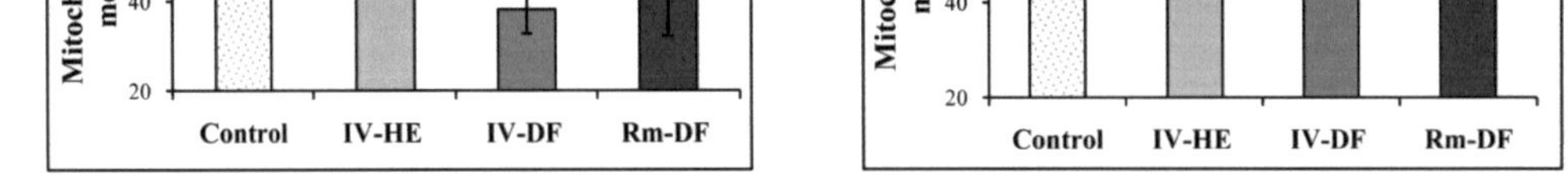

Fig. 3. Mitochondrial membrane potential state in treated cells with IV-HE, IV-DF and Rm-DF, measured by spectrofluorometry and JC-1 probe in SiHa (A) and HeLa (B). Cells are treated with 20µg/ml of extracts for 24h as described in Materials and Methods. The results are presented as the mean ± SD of three independent experiments.

3.7 Measurement of ROS production

Mitochondria are a source of ROS during apoptosis and reduced mitochondria membrane potential leads to increased generation of ROS and apoptosis (Zamzami, 1995). We investigate whether the intracellular ROS are involved in the signal transduction pathways of apoptosis. ROS generation was measured after cells treatment with IV-HE, IV-DF and Rm-DF (20µg/ml) for 24h, using a ROS-sensitive fluorescent C2938 probe.

Tested extracts showed a dose-dependent increase in the intracellular ROS production when compared to the control (Figure.4). This indicate that ROS generation induced by IV-HE, IV-DF and Rm-DF in SiHa and HeLa cells can contribute to apoptosis via the mitochondrial pathway.

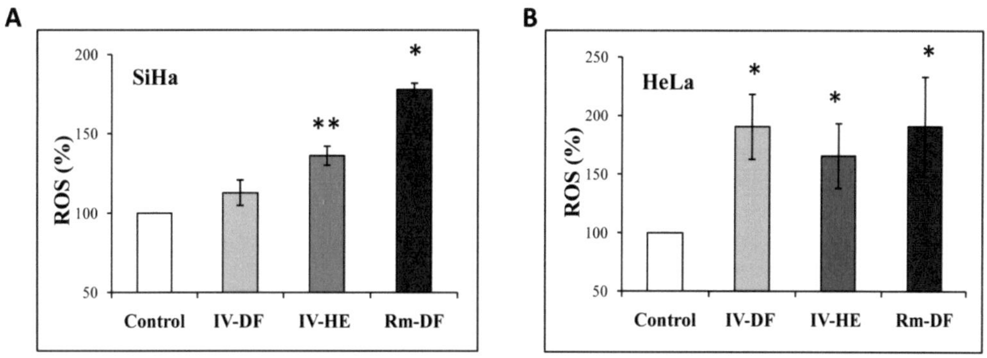

Fig. 4. ROS production in treated cells with IV-HE, IV-DF and Rm-DF, using an oxydation-sensitive fluorescent C2938 probe in SiHa (A) and HeLa (B). Cells are treated with 20µg/ml of extracts for 24h as described in Materials and Methods. The results are presented as the mean ± SD of three independent experiments.

Taken together, these results show clearly that the hexanic extract of *Inula viscosa* and dichloromethane fractions of both *Inula viscosa* and *Retama monosperma* have cytotoxic effects against cervical cancer cell lines SiHa and Hela by inducing apoptotic process. Previous studies have showed that some plant extracts with pronounced cytotoxic in vitro had marked effects in vivo and showed promising potential to be used as an anticancer drugs. Indeed, sesquiterpene lactones, isolated from *Carpesium rosulatum*, have recently been largely studied for their pharmacological proprieties as anti-neoplastic agents (Ma G, 2009; Moon, 2011; Robinson, 2008; Taylor, 2008). Sesquiterpenes lactones, artemisinin, thapsigargin and parthenolide and many of their synthetic derivatives, are in advanced stage for clinical trials (Ghantous, 2010).

Phytochemicals contained in *Inula viscosa* L. extracts including like tomentosin and inuviscolide, as evidenced by CG/MS analysis, have been shown recently to possess an antiproliferative and apoptotic effects on human melanoma cell lines (Rozenblat, 2008).

Quinolizidine alkaloids are known to present in *Retama monosperma* as main active constituents. Quinolizidine alkaloids contained in the dichloromethane fraction of *Retama monosperma* L. extract, may act as potential *in vitro* cytotoxic agents against human cervical cancer cells through the induction of apoptosis. In fact, previous reports have shown that quinolizidine alkaloids have been found to elicit a range of biological activities, including antiviral (Ding, 2006), antihypoglycemic (Brukwicki, 2009) and anti-tumoral (Zhang, 2010) activities.

4. Conclusion

The hexanic extract of *Inula viscosa* and dichloromethane fractions of both *Inula viscosa* and *Retama monosperma* showed pronounced cytotoxic effects against cervical cancer cell lines through the inhibition of proliferation and induction of apoptosis caspase-dependent and involving a mitochondria-mediated signaling pathway. Our findings suggest that these extracts might provide compounds which could be potential sources of anticancer drug leads. Further investigation into the isolation, characterization and mechanism of cytotoxic compounds from the selected plants extracts and in vivo are necessary. Moreover it will be interesting to use some *in vivo* models to evaluate the anti-tumor activity of these plant extracts.

5. References

Abdel Halim O.B., Abdel Fattah H., Halim A.F., Murakoshi I. (1997). Comparative chemical and biological studies of the alkaloidal content of Lygos species and varieties growing in Egypt. *Acta Pharm Hung* 67: 241-247.

Ai-Rong L., Zhu Y., Li X.N., Tian X.J. (2007). Antimicrobial activity of four species of Berberidaceae. *Fitoterapia* 78: 379–381.

Amani H., Rouhi R., Idrissi Hassani L.M. (2008). Étude anatomique et screening phytochimique de trois espèces du sud marocain: Chamaecytisus mollis, Retama monosperma et Hesperolaburnum platycarpum. Détermination du potentiel antifongique des extraits aqueux. Agadir, Maroc. *The 3rd International Symposium on Aromatic and Medicinal Plants (SIPAM3).The first International symposium on Bioactive Molecules (CIMB1) Oujda –Morocco 29th and 30th of May;.*

Bellakhdar, J (1997). La pharmacopée marocaine traditionnelle. Médecine arabe ancienne et savoirs populaires. *Ed. Ibis press.*

Benrahmoune I.Z. (2003). Invitation à l'Amour des plantes - Réserve biologique de Sidi-Boughaba. *Ed. Scriptra.* 114: 228-227.

Brown J.M., Attardi L.D. (2005). Opinion: the role of apoptosis in cancer development and treatment response *Nat. Rev. Cancer* 5: 231–237.

Brukwicki T., Włodarczak J., W., W (2009). The spatial structure of 13a-hydroxy-2-thionosparteine - a potential hypoglycemic agent - and some related compounds. *Journal of Molecular Structure* 928: 189-194.

Cafarchia C., De Laurentis N., Milillo M.A., Losacco V., Puccini V., (2002), Antifungal activity of essential oils from leaves and flowers of Inula viscosa (Asteraceae) by Apulian region. *Parassitologia* 44: 153-156

Cardellina J.H., Fuller R.W., Gamble W.R., Westergaard C., Boswell J., Munro M.H.G., Currens M., Boyd M.P. (1999). Evolving strategies for the selection dereplication and prioritization of antitumor and HIV- inhibitory natural products extracts. In: Bohlin, L., Bruhn, J.G. (Eds), Bioassay Methods in natural product Research and Development. *Kluwer Academic Publishers, Dordrecht,* 25- 36.

Conforti F., Statti,G., Tundis R., Loizzo M.R., Bonesi M., Menichini F., Houghton P.J. (2004). Antioxidant and cytotoxic activities of Retama raetam subsp. Gussonei. *Phytother Res* 18: 585-587.

Ding P.L., Huang H., Zhou P., D.F., C (2006) Quinolizidine alkaloids with anti-HBV activity from Sophora tonkinensis. *Planta Med* 72: 854-856.

Eddouks M., Maghrani M., Lemhadri A., Ouahidi M.L., Jouad H. (2002). Ethnopharmacological survey of medicinal plants used for the treatment of diabetes mellitus, hypertension and cardiac diseases in the south-east region of Morocco (Tafilalet). *J Ethnopharmacol* 82: 97-103.

Eddouks, M, Maghrani, M, Louedec, L, Haloui, M, Michel, JB (2007). Antihypertensive activity of the aqueous extract of Retama raetam Forssk. leaves in spontaneously hypertensive rats. *J Herb Pharmacother* 7: 65-77.

Edziri, H, Mastouri, M, Cheraif, I, Aouni, M (2010). Chemical composition and antibacterial, antifungal and antioxidant activities of the flower oil of Retama raetam (Forssk.) Webb from Tunisia. *Nat Prod Res* 24: 789-796.

Fontana, G, La Rocca, S, Passannanti, S, Paternostro, MP (2007). Sesquiterpene compounds from Inula viscosa. *Nat Prod Res* 21: 824-827.

Fukuda K., Hibiya Y., Mutoh M., Koshiji M., Akao S., Fujiwara H. (1999). Inhibition by berberine of cyclooxygenase-2 transcriptional activity in human colon cancer cells. *J Ethnopharmacol.* 66: 227-233.

Gerson-Cwilich R., Serrano - Olvera A., Villalobos - Prieto A (2006). Complementary and alternative medicine (CAM) in Mexican patients with cancer. *Clinical and Transitional Oncology* 8: 200 - 207.

Ghantous A., Gali-Muhtasib H., Vuorela H., Saliba N.A., Darwiche N. (2010). What made sesquiterpene lactones reach cancer clinical trials? *Drug Discov Today* 15: 668-678.

Gonzalez-Tejero M.R., Casares-Porcel M., Sanchez-Rojas C.P., Ramiro-Gutierrez J.M., Molero-Mesa J., Pieroni A., Giusti M.E., Censorii E., de Pasquale C., Della A., Paraskeva-Hadijchambi D., Hadjichambis A., Houmani Z., El-Demerdash M., El-Zayat M., Hmamouchi M., Eljohrig S. (2008). Medicinal plants in the Mediterranean area: synthesis of the results of the project Rubia. *J Ethnopharmacol* 116: 341-357.

Gordaliza M. (2007). Natural products as leads to anticancer drugs. *Clin Transl Oncol* 9: 767-776.

El Hanbali F., Mellouki F., Akssira M., Balasquez A. (2004). Etude Comparative des Compositions Chimiques et de l'Activité Antibactérienne des Huiles Essentielles de Chamaemelum eriolepis Maire et Chamaemelum Africana J.&Four. *1er Congrès Maroco-Espagnol sur la Chimie Organique et 4ème Rencontre Andalou-Marocaine sur la Chimie des Produits Naturels* 16-18 sept.

El Hanbali F., Oulmoukhtar A.S., Lemrani M., Akssira M., Mellouki F. (2005). Activité anti-leishmanienne des huiles essentielles de deux camomilles : Ormenis eriolepis et Ormenis africana. *International Congress On Medicinal Plants, Errachidia* March 16-19, Morocco.

Haddad P.S., Depot M., Settaf A., Chabli A., Cherrah Y. (2003). Comparative study on the medicinal plants most recommended by traditional practitioners in Morocco and Canada. *J. Herbs Spices Med. Plants* 10: 25-45.

Hayet E., Samia A., Patrick G., Ali M.M., Maha M., Laurent G., Mighri Z., Mahjoub L. (2007). Antimicrobial and cytotoxic activity of Marrubium alysson and Retama raetam grown in Tunisia. *Pak J Biol Sci* 10: 1759-1762.

Hernández V., Recio M.C., Manez S., Giner R.M., Rios J.L. (2007). Effects of naturally occurring dihydroflavonols from Inula viscosa on inflammation and enzymes involved in the arachidonic acid metabolism. *Life Sci* 80: 480-488.

Hmamouchi M. (2001). Les plantes Médicinales et aromatiques Marocaines. *2ème édition Impri Fédala (Mohammadia)*: 108-109.

Kassem, M, Mosharrafa, SA, Saleh, NA, Abdel-Wahab, SM (2000). Two new flavonoids from Retama raetam. *Fitoterapia* 71: 649-654.

Kerr J.F., Winterford C.M., Harmon B.V., (1994). Apoptosis. Its significance in cancer and cancer therapy. Cancer 73: 2013-2026.

Kothakota S., Azuma T., Reinhard C., Klippel A., Tang J., Chu K., McGarry T.J., Kirschner M.W., Koths K., Kwiatkowski D.J., Williams L.T., (1997). Caspase-3-generated fragment of gelsolin: effector of morphological change in apoptosis. *Science* 278: 294-298.

López-Lázaro M., Martin-Cordero C., Cortes F., Pinero J., Ayuso M.J. (2000). Cytotoxic activity of flavonoids and extracts from Retama sphaerocarpa Boissier. *Z Naturforsch C* 55: 40-43.

Ma G., Chong L., Li Z., Cheung A.H., M.H., T (2009). Anticancer activities of sesquiterpene lactones from Cyathocline purpurea in vitro. *Cancer Chemother Pharmacol* 64: 143-152

Ma X. , Wang Z. (2009). Anticancer drug discovery in the future: an evolutionary perspective. *Drug Discovery Today* 14: 1137-1142.

Maghrani M., Michel J.B., Eddouks M., (2005). Hypoglycaemic activity of Retama raetam in rats. *Phytother Res* 19: 125-128.

Maghrani M., Zeggwagh N.A., Haloui M., Eddouks M. (2005). Acute diuretic effect of aqueous extract of Retama raetam in normal rats. *J Ethnopharmacol* 99: 31-35.

Máñez S., Hernández V., Giner R.M., Ríos J.L., Recio M.C. (2007). Inhibition of pro-inflammatory enzymes by inuviscolide, a sesquiterpene lactone from Inula viscosa. *Fitoterapia* 78: 329–331.

Mans D.R., da Rocha A.B., Schwartsmann G., (2000). anticancer drug discovery and development in Brazil: targeted plant collection as a rational strategy to acquire candidate anticancer compounds. *Oncologist* 5: 185- 198.

Maoz M., Neeman I. (1998). Antimicrobial effects of aqueous plant extracts on the fungi Microsporum canis and Trichophyton rubum and on three bacterial species. *Lett. Appl. Microbiol* 26: 61-63.

Meenakshi S., Srivastava S. (2007). Antimicrobial activities of Indian Berberis species. *Fitoterapia* 78: 574-576.

Moon H.I., Zee O. (2011). Anticancer activity of sesquiterpene lactone from plant food (Carpesium rosulatum) in human cancer cell lines. *Int J Food Sci Nutr* 62: 102-105.

Newman D.J., Cragg G.M. (2007). Natural products as sources of new drugs over the last 25 years. *Journal of Natural Products* 70: 461-477.

Reed J.C. (1994). Bcl-2 and the regulation of programmed cell death. *J Cell Biol* 124: 1-6.

Robinson A., Kumar T.V., Sreedhar E., Naidu V.G., Krishna S.R., Babu K.S., Srinivas P.V., Rao J.M. (2008). A new sesquiterpene lactone from the roots of Saussurea lappa: structure-anticancer activity study. *Bioorg Med Chem Lett.* 18: 4015-4017.

Rozenblat S., Grossman S., Bergman M., Gottlieb H., Cohen Y., Dovrat S. (2008). Induction of G2/M arrest and apoptosis by sesquiterpene lactones in human melanoma cell lines. *Biochem Pharmacol* 75: 369-382.

Saklani A., Kutty S.K. (2008). Plant-derived compounds in clinical trials. *Drug Discov Today* 13: 161-171.

Satrani B., Ghanm M., Farah A., Aafi A., Fougrach H., Bourkhiss B., Boust D., Talbi M. (2007) Composition chimique et activité antimicrobienne de l'huile essentielle de Cladanthus mixtus. . *Bull. Soc. Pharm.* 146: 85-96.

Sathiyamoorthy P., Lugasi-Evgi H., Schlesinger P., Kedar I., Gopas J., Pollack Y., Golan-Goldhirsh A. (1999). Screening for Cytotoxic and Antimalarial Activities in Desert Plants of the Negev and Bedouin Market Plant Products. *Pharmaceutical Biology (Formerly International Journal of Pharmacognosy)* 37: 188-195.

Suffness M., Pezzuto J.M. (1990). Assays related to cancer drug discovery. In: Hostettmann, K. (Ed). Methods in Plant Biochemistry: Assays for Bioactivity. *Academic Press, London* 6: 71-133.

Tascilar M., de Jong F. A., Veinweij J., Mathijssen R.H., (2006). Complementary and alternative medicine during cancer treatment: beyond innocence. *Oncologist* 11: 732-741.

Taylor P.G., Dupuy Loo O.A., Bonilla J.A., Murillo R. (2008) Anticancer activities of two sesquiterpene lactones, millerenolide and thieleanin isolated from Viguiera sylvatica and Decachaeta thieleana. *Fitoterapia* 79: 428-432.

Terencio M.C., Sanz M.J., Paya M. (1990). A hypotensive procyanidin-glycoside from Rhamnus lycioides ssp. Lycioides. *J Ethnopharmacol.* 30: 205-214.

Tewari M., Quan L.T., O'Rourke K., Desnoyers S., Zeng Z., Beidler D.R., Poirier G.G., Salvesen G.S., Dixit V.M. (1995). Yama/CPP32 beta, a mammalian homolog of CED-3, is a CrmA-inhibitable protease that cleaves the death substrate poly(ADP-ribose) polymerase. *Cell* 81: 801-809.

Touati D., Allain P., Pellecuer J., Fkih-Tetouani S.A., (1996). Alkaloids from Retama monosperma ssp. Eumonosperma. *Fitoterapia* 67: 49-52.

Wang Z.B., Liu Y.Q., Cui.Y.F., (2005). Pathways to caspase activation. *Cell Biol Int* 29: 489-496.

WHO (2009). Strengthening cervical cancer prevention and control. *Report of the GAVI-UNFPA-WHO meeting* /RHR/10.13 (www.who.int).

Zamzami N., Marchetti P., Castedo M., Decaudin D., Macho A., Hirsch T., Susin S.A., Petit PX.., Mignotte B., Kroemer G., (1995). Sequential reduction of mitochondrial transmembrane potential and generation of reactive oxygen species in early programmed cell death. *J Exp Med* 182: 367-377.

Zhang Y., Liu H., Jin J., Zhu X., Lu L., Jiang H., (2010). The role of endogenous reactive oxygen species in oxymatrine-induced caspase-3-dependant apoptosis in human melanoma A375 cells. *Anticancer Drugs* 21: 494-501.

Zimmermann K.C., Green D.R. (2001). How cells die: apoptosis pathways. *Journal of Allergy and Clinical Immunology* 108: 99-103.